THERAPEUTIC INEQUALITIES

ANTHROPOLOGIES OF AMERICAN MEDICINE: CULTURE, POWER, AND PRACTICE

General Editors: Paul Brodwin, Michele Rivkin-Fish, and Susan Shaw

Therapeutic Inequalities

Mood Disorder Self-Management in Chicago

Talia Rose Weiner

NEW YORK UNIVERSITY PRESS

New York

NEW YORK UNIVERSITY PRESS
New York
www.nyupress.org

© 2025 by New York University
All rights reserved

Please contact the Library of Congress for Cataloging-in-Publication data.

ISBN: 9781479817627 (hardback)
ISBN: 9781479817634 (paperback)
ISBN: 9781479817641 (library ebook)
ISBN: 9781479817658 (consumer ebook)

This book is printed on acid-free paper, and its binding materials are chosen for strength and durability. We strive to use environmentally responsible suppliers and materials to the greatest extent possible in publishing our books.

The manufacturer's authorized representative in the EU for product safety is Mare Nostrum Group B.V., Mauritskade 21D, 1091 GC Amsterdam, The Netherlands. Email: gpsr@mare-nostrum.co.uk.

Manufactured in the United States of America

10 9 8 7 6 5 4 3 2 1

Also available as an ebook

CONTENTS

FIGURES

It is hard to suppress an awkward giggle as a string quartet begins its solemn rendition of "Pomp and Circumstance" and my cohort-mate Miranda and I march, in our slippery black robes and tasseled caps, across a long classroom to receive our diplomas. The musical cliché, though the proximate cause of the moment's absurdity, is in fact but a small contributor to my overall sense of bemused alienation: There is also the fact that the Chicago School for Psychoanalytic Psychotherapy (CSPP),[1] from which I am graduating, is the third program I have attended in as many years in my quest to earn a clinical credential; that my new credential as of today—a Master's in Clinical Counseling—is a significant departure from the doctorate in clinical psychology that I had initially set out to acquire; that said departure, and the general circuitousness of my educational trajectory, has resulted in my possession of *three* master's degrees but (to the endless dismay of my parents) no gainful employment; and that because of a series of institutional and interpersonal dramas—most of which took place before I arrived on the scene at CSPP—my graduating class consists only of Miranda and myself.

In spite of the intimacy that Miranda and I have developed by virtue of our shared—and emotionally intense—psychodynamic training experience, our approaches to the morning's rite of passage highlight the divide between our respective relationships to the field that we are formally entering. Beneath her robe, Miranda wears an embroidered evening gown, impressive heels, and a strand of pearls. Several members of her immediate and extended family are seated in the audience, including Miranda's until-recently-estranged mother. Many more family members and friends will toast Miranda's achievements later in the afternoon at a catered party—complete with a "shrink"-themed cake featuring a fondant *DSM-5* reclining atop an analytic couch—that she and her spouse will host in honor of the occasion. For Miranda, this morning's ceremony marks the end of her graduate studies and the beginning of her membership within a professional community to which she is already devoted: A longtime recipient of psychotherapy herself, Miranda is unequivocal in her belief in the talking cure and her intention to become a practitioner of it. As I stand beside her, my less meticulously coordinated sartorial selections and lack of invited guests at the graduation betray a greater ambivalence about the field of counseling and my place within it. Although I am relieved to have completed the master's program, I have always treated my clinical training as one small component of my doctoral studies—the end of which still seems woefully remote. Added to that is the fact that I have read too much social theory *not* to maintain a hearty skepticism of clinical encounters—particularly psychotherapeutic ones. Moreover, I actively work to retain this skepticism and the discomfiting experience of not-quite-fitting-in that goes with it; hanging on to that degree of critical distance, I tell myself, is what enables me to survive as an ethnographer of my own professional milieu.

If I am truly honest with myself, though, I must admit that there is a more profound awkwardness to my experience of the graduation than that which stems from my carefully cultivated position of clinician/critic/outside observer. That awkwardness is the product of an uncanny recognition of my sociological *belonging* among the quirky community of therapists at CSPP. As I glance around the classroom at the small crowd of fifty or so clinicians who have come to take part in the event, I note the presence of several of my neighbors, who provide private psychotherapy to my peers and hold faculty, administrative, and board of trustee positions at CSPP. I see my own former therapist, a clinician-anthropologist whose academic interests overlap with mine, and who has served on my colleagues' dissertation committees. I see individuals whose faces are familiar because they participated in the memorial conference of a late professor from my doctoral department—an esteemed psychoanalyst with whom I once collaborated on a publication. I see, in short, the sociologically overdetermined contributors to my arrival at this particular professional juncture refracted back at me in the guise of a group of (predominantly) white, Jewish, middle-class, educated, politically left-leaning therapists.

The keynote speaker for the graduation ceremony—Dr. Miriam Levine—is introduced, and I suddenly feel as though I am watching a parody about the incestuousness of the psychoanalytic community. The person giving the introduction is a former dean of CSPP and a graduate of the school's doctoral program. Miranda—who is always more up-to-date on the institutional gossip than I am—whispers to me that she is also the spouse of the analyst of one of our former classmates. The former dean rattles off the long list of affiliations and accomplishments of Dr. Levine, who happens to be her aunt, and jokes that their family connection is not the reason why the speaker was chosen to address us today.

The topic of Dr. Levine's warm and personal keynote lecture is the narrative of her own life journey to become an analyst and clinical educator. She begins by declaring that this moment, in the company of her niece and in the special space that is CSPP, is an appropriate one in which to reflect on her own experience; to think about "how it's evolved, and what in the end I've come to accept as being of most help to patients theoretically and clinically."

I find myself interpellated as Dr. Levine begins to describe her lifelong fascination with stories—both literary ones and the lived stories shared with her by other people. I am reminded of my own excess of academic credentials when she recounts how, over the course of earning two doctorates and then undergoing classical Freudian psychoanalytic training, she eventually discovered that she was "on a mission to learn more about the inner emotional lives of people, especially what makes them strong and vital, what in their development might interfere with that process, and how they might need help to gain or to regain a consolidated self-experience." For Dr. Levine, this learning process turned on her exposure to contemporary psychoanalytic theory—the same approach taken by most of the faculty at CSPP—and her experience of the contemporary relational orientation as resonating with her "literature-based understanding of what it means to be human." Whereas Dr. Levine's classical—and deeply patriarchal—psychodynamic training had insisted that the truth of the patient's experience was to be determined by the analyst, in the contemporary psychoanalytic theories of Heinz Kohut, Stephen Mitchell, Melanie Klein, Robert Stolorow (all names whose mention elicits satisfied nods of recognition among the roomful of listeners), and others, she had found a paradigm that privileged the *patient's* phenomenological truth. With this comparison, we arrive at the heart of the keynote address—a characterization of the clinical and intellectual community into which we are being initiated, along with a piece of advice to carry forward with us. Contemporary psychoanalytic theory, Dr. Levine concludes,

> acknowledges that meaning is always indeterminate, co-constructed, and contextual, displacing the therapist as the only one who knows. . . . We've come a long way from the imposition of the therapist's theoretical truth to be accepted by the patient, to a process of co-creating a subjective, narrative truth that is anchored in the patient's experience. . . . So that's my story. I imagine—in fact, I *hope*—that yours is different. What is important is for each of us to arrive at our own, comfortable ways of thinking and being with patients. . . . With all of your learning, and with all of your experience, it's time for you to throw away the book and be yourselves!

Listening to the keynote speaker's words, I am struck—not for the first time—by the ways in which contemporary psychoanalysis overlaps with those aspects of ethnography to which I am existentially and epistemologically drawn:[2] Both paradigms gravitate toward complexity and particularity; both subordinate an interest in describing objective reality to a process of understanding local meaning; both recognize that one's own incomplete, situated, historically contingent subjectivity is a vital tool—not a hindrance—for gathering and interpreting data; and both acknowledge that certain sorts of truths can only be found within the intersubjective space that comes into being over the course of a sustained social relationship (Briggs 2008; Hollan 2008; Kirmayer 2008). For a brief moment, reflecting on these similarities, I abandon my efforts to peer in at my graduation experience from the safety of the disciplinary margins and indulge in the fantasy of having actually arrived at the ideal conjuncture of cultural anthropology and clinical practice. Perhaps, I muse, I will come to feel at home in my newly bestowed professional identity.

Only six weeks later, during my first interview for a clinical counseling position, I begin to appreciate how far removed my graduation day concerns are from the quotidian experience of providing community mental health services as an entry-level therapist in Chicago. I had applied for several jobs posted on a massive, undifferentiable-to-me list of openings at RecoveryNet—a not-for-profit social services and community mental health organization. RecoveryNet, whose many programs and facilities cover most regions of Chicago and sprawl out as far as 100 miles south and west of the city, was undergoing a period of rapid growth at the time, in part because it had recently contracted with the Chicago Department of Public Health (CDPH) to become one of the city's private "community partners." As hundreds of clients who had previously been receiving psychiatric and psychotherapeutic services directly from the CDPH were "transitioned" (as the CDPH termed it) to these partnering providers, agencies such as RecoveryNet had been scrambling to keep up with intakes and new staffing needs, setting up makeshift workspaces or holding therapy sessions entirely in the field. As it happened, the position for which I had applied and was now interviewing was one in which I would serve as part of a Community Support Team (CST)—a designation derived from an Illinois Department of Human Services, Division of Mental Health (DHS/DMH) Rule 132 Medicaid billing category.[3] The team, which had only recently been created but already needed to look for new clinicians due to staff turnover, was operating for the time being out of a trailer in an industrial area on the West Side of Chicago. It had the distinction—though unbeknownst to me when I applied for the job—of being one of the few programs at RecoveryNet and within community mental health more broadly that was not beholden to a fee-for-service reimbursement model:[4] Whereas, in general, all Illinois state-contracted providers since the first decade of the twenty-first century were subject to a strictly audited system of payment advance and reconciliation that purportedly enforced standards of efficiency and accountability (Spitzmueller 2016), this team was part of a pilot program in which Medicaid managed care paid RecoveryNet a flat rate, and did not track specific services provided.

My job interview consists of shadowing the clinical team leader, Maya, for four hours as she goes about her day's work driving around the South Side of Chicago to meet with clients at their homes.[5] CST, I learn, means that the team acts collectively as one therapist, sharing a caseload of clients among the group. Maya explains that these are higher-needs clients—though they are not the lowest functioning individuals served by RecoveryNet—who may require more-than-weekly visits with a community support worker. I cannot help but think about my senior colleagues at CSPP, many of whom still offer traditional, three-days-a-week, on-the-couch psychoanalysis, as I am told that the reasoning behind Community Support Team services is to have multiple workers assigned to cases that are too time-consuming or demanding for any one therapist to handle on their own.

As we make our way to the first client of the day, Maya attempts to divide her attention between following the navigation orders from the GPS, watching the road, maintaining conversation with me, and fielding a steady stream of phone calls and text messages from the team members that she supervises. She asks me how I heard about RecoveryNet, but before I can answer, the phone chirps again. Maya quickly taps out a reply at a red light, simultaneously explaining to me that she gets a lot of questions right now because all of the team members are fairly new to the job. *Turn left onto West 93rd Street*, commands Maya's phone. *Arrived.*

We park, and then enter the stale-smelling callbox area of a multi-unit brick building. Maya types in the client's apartment number and waits for several minutes as the callbox rings and rings. After a second attempt, she concludes: "I guess he's not home. Let's go back to the car and we'll write a note saying we stopped by." "Is there a backyard or someplace that we should look?" I ask. "Or can we call his cell?" Maya says she'll swing back later in the day if there is time; otherwise, another team member will try again tomorrow. It dawns on me that we had not made an appointment to meet with the client or even let him know that we were on our way over, and Maya confirms that this is usually the case with CST visits. As she enters our next client's home address into her phone's GPS, Maya comments that in this sort of situation, it is a relief that her program operates on a flat rate of insurance reimbursement. "I could imagine that if this job were fee-for-service, it would be a nightmare! Like, if we don't see somebody—like, if they're not home—you would have to be working to try to find somebody else to see." On the other hand, Maya notes, her program's unusual payment structure means that Maya and her team are ineligible for the biannual billing performance-based bonuses that RecoveryNet offers the rest of the organization's clinicians. "That part sucks," Maya admits. "The bonus kind of reeled me in [to RecoveryNet]. I wish we could get it anyway, because we work *really* hard in this program. We should at least get something, like, maybe from the insurance companies. Like, you guys saved all this money because of us! Just throw us a thousand or so bonus or *something!*"

Maya starts the engine, but then turns her car back off as the phone rings with yet another call from a team member. "Hey!" she answers. "Uh huh. . . . The seventy dollars, is that for the week? . . . So it's like 270 per week? . . . Also could you explore with her, like, where her money's at? . . . Yeah, find out where her SSI check is, and what's going on with that. You know, how she's gonna pay the 500 before she moves into her place. . . . Alright. Alright." Maya hangs up and sighs, offering by way of explanation only that this client had recently returned from living out of state, and that she wishes the team had not taken the client back.

As we begin our drive toward the next visit, Maya and I chat about my long-term career plans and research interests, and about politics on the South Side of Chicago. We talk about our hopes for the upcoming mayoral election, and about which of the candidates that are running against the incumbent mayor Rahm Emanuel will do the most to address the city's many mental health-related inequalities within schools, prisons, and the police force. Maya mentions that her intention is to remain in the team leader position at RecoveryNet just long enough to sit for her clinical licensing examination, and then to open a not-for-profit mental health consultation firm for the South Side community. I am vaguely surprised to learn that Maya is only a marginally more experienced clinician than I am, and that she does not already hold a license in clinical social work or counseling.

Our next stop brings us into the house of a client who is in the midst of a crisis. The living room and the client are both in disarray. When Maya introduces me as the shadowing prospective employee, the client compliments my shoes and apologizes for the mess and the cigarette smoke. "Don't be sorry, this is your home," I stammer guiltily.

The client appears to live with an older man. I cannot discern whether he is her boyfriend or father, or neither. Together, they explain to Maya and me that the client has been in "real bad shape" for the past several days—drinking and sleeping all day, crying constantly, and unable to keep down any food. Maya asks for details about when each symptom began, inquires as to whether the client is in pain, and asks if she is feeling like she wants to hurt herself. The client insists that her main problem is that she needs a prescription for daytime depression and anxiety medications. She had recently taken Ativan with good results while in prison for several months, but since her release, had been unable to find a psychiatrist who accepts Medicaid to renew the prescription. "I *thought* a psychiatrist was supposed to be here today," the client says pointedly. Maya takes a bulky laptop out of her bag and tells the client that although the psychiatrist cannot come to her home, one of the benefits of our program is that she can speak to a psychiatrist face-to-face through a video call that is "kind of like Skype."[6]

Maya continues to interview the client about her appetite and treatment history as she logs in to the video conferencing software, fails to connect with the psychiatrist, calls the RecoveryNet office, and eventually reaches the psychiatrist by text message. "Ok, she will be on in a bit," Maya tells all of us. Eventually, there is a crackling sound, and a face appears on the screen. Maya hands the laptop over to the client, who repeats her request to "get my Ativan prescription re-upped by a psychiatrist." They talk for a few minutes, and the psychiatrist asks the client when she last consumed alcohol. "Ten minutes ago?" the client guesses. The psychiatrist explains that you can't take benzodiazepine drugs like Ativan while you are drinking, and suggests that the client go to a detox program instead. When the video call ends, the client protests to Maya: "I just don't feel like it will be a lot of help. I've been through so many detoxes I could do their class *for* them, you know what I mean? I know everything the counselors know!" Besides, the client continues, she needs help *now*, and the detox centers will not let her come in until the next morning. Moreover, when she leaves detox she still will not have an ongoing psychiatrist or prescriptions for daytime psychotropic medications. Maya nods empathically while she uses her phone to locate a detox center that has an opening for the next morning. She convinces the client to try going through the full program one more time, assuring her that the RecoveryNet team will call to see how things are going and come back to visit afterward. "I heard [the detox center] is not the *best* place around, but they do their job," Maya promises. Strangely, the client appears to relax upon hearing this less-than-ringing endorsement, and makes small talk with us as we pack up and head back to Maya's car.

The purpose of my juxtaposing the scenes above is not simply to foreground the differences—though they are profound—between the concerns and practices of private psychoanalytic therapists and those of community mental healthcare workers. Nor is it to suggest that the client I visited with Maya received inappropriate or inadequate care, or that she would necessarily have been better served by a CSPP-style therapeutic intervention. Rather, my aim is to present a set of questions that frame and guide this book: How does one give an account of a profession that can produce both a Dr. Levine and a Maya, sometimes even (as in my own case) within a single person? What are the conditions of possibility for the emergence of distinct forms of therapeutic disposition, orientation, and relationships with clients—and how do these intersect with the processes and trajectories of professional socialization? What sorts of therapeutic interventions become thinkable and enactable across different class milieux, and on what grounds are those interventions understood to be clinically appropriate? How do clinical interactions and goals articulate with the political economy and public policies of a particular place and historic moment, absorbing and expanding upon that moment's ideological commitments?

In this book, I address these and related questions through a multi-sited, clinical ethnographic exploration of the mental healthcare landscape in contemporary Chicago, Illinois. More specifically, this ethnography traces some of the institutional, political, professional, and discursive pathways by which mental health treatment differences—or what some might even term treatment *disparities*—are brought into being, naturalized, and reproduced. I begin with the observation that what might appear to be a fundamental or universal aim of mental healthcare—say, to paraphrase Dr. Levine, the facilitation of a patient's experience of strength and vitality—in practice gets translated across geographic and sociopolitical space into an array of incommensurable projects. These projects, I argue, produce and foreclose distinct possibilities for patient subjectivity and moral agency (Myers 2015; Blacksher 2002)—some perhaps more livable or empowering than others. The book then moves outward to examine the various interlocking systems and structures that come together to render the disparities across mental health treatment settings intractable and mutually reinforcing.

A particular focus of this book's project is the role of a mode of thinking and embodied practice that I gloss as *self-management*.[7] It argues that although self-management was originally developed to enable patients with physical ailments such as arthritis to gain self-confidence in their ability to control their own symptoms, it drew on the powerful ideology of American individualism to assert that a disease is "something that you have, but not who you are." In doing so, this idea of self-management promoted the notion that patients have both the ability and responsibility to manage their own diseases.

But while self-management might be attainable in the context of physiological diseases like arthritis, it seems less realistic in the case of, for instance, mood disorders, where the patient faces challenges relating to their mental status. In this book, I argue that when the expert discourses of public health officials and clinicians portray self-management as a technology that any patient can learn and practice on their own to take charge of their mood disorder or related psychiatric illness, they fail to acknowledge the role of sociopolitical context. Self-management can, indeed, potentially be helpful for those who have resources to draw on to support them as they manage their condition. But given that depressive and similar disorders disproportionally affect adults who are unemployed, less educated, or of a lower socioeconomic status, the self-management paradigm sets up an approach that raises the likelihood of harming the very individuals who are at greatest risk for these mental illnesses. Moreover, this book illuminates the circumstances through which therapists themselves come to embrace self-management approaches as a means to sustain their own sense of self-worth as they confront the structural bounds of their work.

As you read this book, you will encounter various kinds of self-managers—mood disorder support group members, community mental health workers, psychoanalysts, psychiatric consumer activists, and neighborhood coalitions—engaging in diverse forms of self-management. You will see how the impetus for self-management, and the practices that self-management entails, shift with the actor and their circumstances—and that there is a vast range in the extent to which self-management is volitional or even conscious. Self-management, you will find, is the connective tissue holding together a broken system of mental healthcare; but it may be the case that by pointing a critical spotlight on self-management—by naming the work that self-management does for us, the unlivable boundaries that it erects, and the power relations that it obfuscates—we can begin to imagine an outside to that system.

Introduction

Crossing the Midway: The Inequitable Landscape of Self-Management

Hyde Park, Chicago, 2012–2013. To the right of my apartment building was the posh home of the psychoanalyst next door. She was a faculty member at the Chicago School for Psychoanalytic Psychotherapy, where I had recently matriculated in a master's degree program. If you turned left, you would come to an upscale Italian restaurant and pastry shop, where you could sip an espresso and read social theory while looking out at the north façade of the Museum of Science and Industry—an architectural landmark housed in the Palace of Fine Arts that was built for the 1893 Chicago World's Fair. A few blocks to the east was Promontory Point—my neighborhood's beloved peninsular park that jutted into Lake Michigan and that, for a reported $125,000, Mayor Rahm Emanuel rented out for ten days in the summer of 2013 as the private venue for George Lucas's star-studded wedding reception (Perlstein 2015a).

Several blocks to the west of my apartment were the Gothic-style buildings and manicured quadrangles of the University of Chicago, where I had been working toward my doctoral degree for the past five years. It was in that direction that I was headed this evening, to attend a lecture by Alex Lickerman—a physician and the vice president for Student Health and Counseling Services at the University of Chicago—on the topic of "Constructing an Indestructible Self." I entered a beautiful campus building gifted to the university by John D. Rockefeller, Jr. in 1932, and was seated in an oak-paneled hall with cathedral windows and a Steinway grand piano. For the next hour, I listened as Dr. Lickerman outlined his approach to the "things every person can do on a daily basis that will put you at the top of your range of resilience"—a capacity that he defined as "not just surviving but *thriving* in the face of adversity, in the face of heartbreaking loss; finding a way not just to get through it, but to actually become even happier as a result." Among Dr. Lickerman's recommendations were to cultivate "explanatory flexibility," strategically choosing to account for your misfortunes with "causes that empower you to help you feel as though you can overcome what has challenged you"; and, moreover, to shift from a "sense-making" to a "benefit-finding" orientation toward your own experiences of suffering and loss.

In the Q&A session that followed, I summoned the nerve to ask Dr. Lickerman about something that had been bothering me throughout his presentation—namely, that none of the styles of explanation for which he advocated seemed to include a consideration of any structural, political, or institutional causes of adversity. In the face of real social injustices in the world, I inquired, was the best path to happiness or empowerment truly just to adjust your attitude, look for the positive side of the situation, and work on becoming an "indestructible self"?

"So," Dr. Lickerman replied,

you're bringing it out to a larger context of: when there's a social injustice, for example, what was the cause? And I was thinking about the use of self-explanatory style on more of a personal level . . . because certain things happen to us that seem to be outside of our control, and a person with more explanatory flexibility will recognize that and ask themselves "what cause is related to this that I *do* have control over?" I think we in society . . . presume we understand the causes of events far more often than we actually do. So I hadn't really put much thought into—in the context of resilience—applying the idea of understanding causes of large social events, because really what it comes down to is "how do I as an individual react to this event?" And how I react to it depends on what I understand its cause to be. . . . My perspective is that to the degree that we can't always know the cause, we can *pick* the cause that empowers us the most . . . So I think more on the individual level is how I was thinking about this. The other way is interesting, but I don't know, off the top of my head, how that would necessarily empower the individual.

Dr. Lickerman's response—his equation of empowerment with individual choice and self-control, and his rejection of the potential merit of locating an understanding of a person's struggles within their broader social context—is a manifestation of the logic of self-management that I trace and problematize throughout this book. It is tied to a vision of humanity that valorizes autonomy and self-mastery over interconnection and social support. And it subscribes to the premise that each of us, on our own, can triumph over internal and external adversity essentially through sheer willpower—a premise that I, following Bateson (1972) and others, believe to be not only erroneous but dangerous as well.

But self-management does not always look the same way, or mean the same thing. Ironically, for a logic that hinges on the erasure of the significance of social context, self-managerial ideologies, practices, and outcomes vary rather dramatically depending on the sort of setting in which they occur. As troubling as it was for me to listen to Dr. Lickerman's exhortation to construct an indestructible self in an opulent room full of academics and clinicians, I needed only to cross the Midway Plaisance—a well-maintained, mile-long public green space that functions as the dividing line between affluent Hyde Park and the poor, predominantly African American neighborhood of Woodlawn to its south—to witness firsthand how dire the logic of self-management could become.

I first became acquainted with the Mental Health Coalition (MHC) in the spring of 2012. At that time, the MHC was in the midst of protesting Mayor Emanuel's slated closure of the city-run mental health clinic in Woodlawn where, for decades, many of its members had found community and received vital psychiatric services. Members of the MHC initially attempted to "occupy" the Woodlawn clinic ahead of its scheduled closing date (which was only two weeks away) by barricading themselves inside of the building. A police SWAT team raid, twenty-three arrests, and a night in jail rapidly ensued. After that, the MHC relocated its occupation to a vacant lot across from the Woodlawn clinic. There, for over two months, MHC members pitched tents (which, before long, were forcibly removed by the Chicago Police Department), set up a long table for donated food, and used a makeshift grill to keep warm. I would periodically stop by the encampment between classes to chat with consumer activists and hear updates about their fight for the right to a public mental healthcare safety net for Chicago's poor and uninsured. Eventually, I joined the MHC and participated in many of its meetings and actions.

During the second week of the occupation, the MHC held a day-long health fair, where members of the Woodlawn community were offered free blood pressure readings, depression screenings, and educational sessions about mental health (Lydersen 2013). Several days later, the Woodlawn city clinic—the facility where MHC members had once been able to receive the very services that they now had to provide for themselves in a vacant lot—was permanently shuttered by the Chicago Department of Public Health. Five weeks after that, a Mental Health Coalition member with severe bipolar disorder, who had frequently declared to Chicago city officials that she would not survive the closure of her public clinic, was found dead in her apartment. The official cause of death was a heart attack, but if you asked any of her friends in the MHC, they would tell you that she died of a broken heart. In my view, she died of self-management.

What Is Self-Management?

Self-management can take an economic, political, narrative, organizational, or clinical form. It is a mode that is at times actively claimed by, at times forced upon, and often subtly diffused into its subjects. Highly resonant with neoliberal ideals of individual sovereignty (Brijnath and Antoniades 2016; Clarke 2005; Teghtsoonian 2009; Lemke 2001), self-management in each of its forms retains the quality of bestowing (wanted or unwanted) moral agency upon the individual by means of a kind of political economic mystification that eclipses the social networks and structural constraints in which the individual is embedded. Moreover, the duty to exercise sovereign self-management in the contemporary United States—to triumph over various forms of structural vulnerability through autonomous acts of agency, entrepreneurship, and rational choice—is disproportionally placed on the shoulders of individuals or communities who, by virtue of their sociopolitical positioning, are far from truly sovereign.

This book's engagement with self-management toggles between two interrelated senses of the term: In the narrow sense, self-management refers to a clinical modality for the treatment of (mental) illness that envisions the patient as both capable of and responsible for objectifying and controlling their own (psychiatric) disorder. Because the modality focuses on the self's managerial relationship with *itself*—or, more accurately in the parlance of the clinical literature, the self's relationship with a separable pathology that is within but not identical to itself—it takes the appearance of a technology that is politically neutral and context-free. I argue, however, that even in this narrow clinical sense, self-management contains and transmits to patients a set of disparate, historically contingent, sociopolitically laden beliefs and expectations about selfhood, responsibility, and agency. So disparate, in fact, are these sets of beliefs that the discourses and practices comprising clinical self-management can be diametrically opposed to each other in one class setting versus another.

Thus, this book contends that the very structures and ideologies to which clinical self-management appears indifferent are in fact inextricably woven into the fabric of the therapeutic technology; whether practiced by an individual alone with their self-help handbook, a team of community support workers with their client, a psychoanalyst and their longtime patient, or a marginalized coalition of mental health consumer activists, self-management interventions absorb and reproduce the structural contradictions and class-differentiated neoliberal logics that pervade the broader mental healthcare apparatus in the contemporary United States. By asking what is meant by the very notion of mental illness self-management across diverse clinical contexts—and under what conditions an act or process of self-management is deemed appropriate or successful—this book begins to unravel the ways in which self-management as a therapeutic mode takes up and promotes class inequalities and health disparities. Conversely, one might argue, self-management in the narrow sense constantly exceeds the confines of the therapeutic scene, reverberating across—and instantiating itself within—various nodes of the wider healthcare landscape. I address self-management in a second, more metaphorical sense in this book to characterize these reverberations and their effects—and to show how, collectively, they work to simultaneously disavow and sustain a political economic order.

The ethnographic portion of this book loosely mirrors these migrations and flows of self-management as ideology and clinical practice. We begin in a depression and bipolar disorder support group, where we discover that the act of expertly enacting autonomous self-management becomes an exercise in demonstrating the futility of the task at hand. We then follow self-management to the heart of the book—a pair of chapters that describe how mental healthcare workers in disparate class settings engage in their own forms of self-management in order to reconcile, within their professional narratives and practices, the structural constraints in which they are bound. Echoing Paul Brodwin (2008, 2013) and others who observe that the everyday work of front-line clinicians entails an attempt to preserve ethical integrity within a compromised system of care, these chapters zero in on the clinician as unwitting "translator" between self-management as political/theoretical apparatus and self-management as practice. In particular, the chapters offer an explanation of how it is that therapists—many of whom are drawn to their professions out of a desire to intervene in the plights of the structurally vulnerable—end up with no alternative but to discursively erase structural conditions and socioeconomic inequalities if they are to maintain a sense of themselves as moral agents. In effect, clinicians imbibe a set of self-managerial logics and contradictions that arise out of a neoliberal healthcare system and are conveyed to them via professional socialization processes. Faced with an impossible-to-fulfill social mission, irreconcilable professional norms, everyday workplace frustrations, disappointed therapeutic ideals, and low status, they then attempt to lay claim to some degree of moral agency through acts of what I term "narrative self-management" that refigure structurally produced compromises as acts of choice grounded in principles of therapeutically appropriate care. This refiguration ultimately supports the constitution and naturalization of disparate clinical spaces, with correspondingly disparate notions of what it means for patients to responsibly manage their mental illnesses. In later chapters, we investigate how the logic of self-management insinuates itself among and between communities of disenfranchised consumers faced with community mental health privatization and state abandonment, bringing into being certain forms of political solidarity while simultaneously reproducing structural inequalities and free market competitions. Finally, we consider the clinical management of physical, affective, and ideological boundaries around selfhood as a matter of epistemic justice (Chapman and Carel 2022) and explore the conditions of possibility for access to cybernetic modes of being that are transformative and liberatory.

This book is a clinical ethnography of *the political economy of self-management*. That is to say, a central aim of the volume is to destabilize the notion of self-management as a unitary or apolitical technology and instead trace the many "uneven" or "variegated" forms (Brenner et al. 2010) that self-management (like neoliberalization) takes as it is distributed and enacted across a political economic field.[1] This book thus seeks to address questions such as: What forms of self-management are demanded of what sorts of people in what settings—and with what consequences? At the same time, the book is also a study of *the self-management of political economy*—meaning the ways in which, though self-management, structural and systemic problems are converted into individualized projects that fail to interrogate and thereby perpetuate the very forces sustaining their existence. This symmetrical duality in the book's attentions reflects the fact that self-management can be viewed as both vehicle and mechanism, at once conveying sociopolitically stratified neoliberal ideologies regarding responsibility and (in)dependence, and enabling the misrecognition of such ideologies through a transfer of focus to the individual.

Mood Disorders and Self-Management

The research project on which this ethnography is based was conceived as an examination of the relationship between the socioeconomic context of psychotherapeutic treatments for depression and the discourses, clinical practices, experiences, and outcomes associated with these treatments. The analysis was to center on the treatment modality known as "mood disorder self-management," tracking how its use—and, ultimately, its very meaning—differed according to class setting. Over the course of the two years that I spent undergoing my own clinical training, collecting ethnographic data, and analyzing these data, the project's focus shifted and expanded in significant ways: I rapidly discovered in the field, for instance, that it is generally not possible to study depression in isolation from other psychiatric and psychosocial problems. I also began to see "self-management" as a useful metaphor for thinking about the components of a broader mental healthcare apparatus that produced and sustained the class-based treatment differences that I had set out to document (Weiner 2025). By virtue of my own social positioning as clinical trainee and worker, the study came to focus more on therapists' own structural dilemmas and professional self-management strategies than I had initially envisioned. And as in any ethnographic research process, there were unexpected phenomena and events that caught my attention and steered the thematic turns of the eventual book.

But even given these detours and outgrowths, self-management—as a type of clinical treatment and beyond—remains a central analytic. Moreover, mood disorders, inasmuch as they represent a class of mental illness especially likely to invite usage of the self-management paradigm, still occupy a significant place in the research. Thus, it is instructive to begin with a review of the entwined histories of mood disorders and clinical self-management in the United States.

A Public Health Epidemic and an Enticing Remedy

Mood disorder self-management rose to prominence in relation to the conjuncture of neoliberal austerity measures (Crawshaw 2012; Clarke 2005; Brijnath and Antoniades 2016) and a perceived "epidemic" of depression in the United States. In recent years, mood disorders such as unipolar and bipolar depression have reportedly constituted the leading cause of disability in this country. Every year, we are told, they strike 9.5% of the adult population, cost $23 billion in workplace losses, and are responsible for 90% of the nation's suicides (World Health Organization 2008; DBSA 2017a; Greenberg et al. 2003).

In response to these alarming statistics, US public health officials have expressed a commitment to understanding and treating mood disorders as diseases of the brain. This biomedical framing is believed to decrease the stigma associated with diagnosis and to legitimize these mental illnesses as "real," physiological diseases—rather than signs of frailty—that warrant state attention (Dumit 2003). Indeed, an influential *JAMA* commentary by Thomas Insel, then-director of the National Institute of Mental Health (NIMH), argued in 2005 that

> *psychiatry's impact on public health will require that mental disorders be understood and treated as brain disorders.* In the past, mental disorders were defined by the absence of a so-called organic lesion. Mental disorders became neurological disorders at the moment a lesion was found.

With the advent of functional neuroimaging, patterns of regional brain activity associated with normal and pathological mental experience can be visualized, including detection of abnormal activity in brain circuits in the absence of an identifiable structural lesion. (Insel and Quirion 2005, 2221, emphasis added)

Insel reaffirmed this position in 2013 when, just weeks before the American Psychiatric Association's much-anticipated release of the fifth edition of its authoritative *Diagnostic and Statistical Manual of Mental Disorders*, he announced that the NIMH would be withdrawing its support for the *DSM-V* and reorienting its research agenda around a new taxonomic scheme, the Research Domain Criteria (Insel 2013; Belluck and Carey 2013). Citing a lack of validity in the *DSM*, Insel wrote that in order to receive funding from the NIMH, proposed studies would need to conceptualize psychiatric diseases in terms of underlying "brain circuits that implicate specific domains of cognition, emotion, or behavior" (Insel 2013).[2] At around the same time as the NIMH made its announcement, President Barack Obama launched the $100 million "Brain Research through Advancing Innovative Neurotechnologies" (BRAIN) Initiative, which proclaimed that a comprehensive mapping of the human brain is a necessary first step "if we are ever to develop effective ways of helping people suffering from [depression and other psychiatric disorders]" (NIH 2017).

However, this national will to biomedicalize mood disorders has not necessarily led to an increase in state resources being directed toward the provision of mental health services to help those currently suffering from depression. On the contrary, it has helped justify and popularize the use of the therapeutic modality of *self-management* as a cost-effective way to treat mood disorders. As noted earlier, self-management was originally developed to enable patients with chronic arthritis to "gain self-confidence in their ability to control their [own] symptoms" (Stanford Medicine 2017a). Calling forth a powerful ideology of American individualism, self-management discourses relentlessly assert that a disease is "something that you have, but not who you are" (Miklowitz 2002, 63). In drawing this distinction, such discourses promote the idea that patients have both the ability and the responsibility to manage their own diseases. That is, in the same move in which self-management recuperates the patient as a full person whose identity is not compromised or defined by their chronic disease, it seeks to recruit the patient into the role of sovereign, self-responsible citizen—a figure that has long been valorized in the United States (Myers 2010). Many laud the self-management approach, claiming that it "empowers" patients to objectify and independently control their conditions (Depp et al. 2009). And as policymakers continue to stress the equivalence of psychiatric disorders to physiological diseases, the rationale of empowering the patient with the duty to self-manage has increasingly been extended to mental illnesses—especially mood disorders, which are often described in contrast to psychotic disorders as severe and chronic, but eminently "manageable."

If this ideal of rational self-management by a fully autonomous individual is perhaps attainable in the context of physiological diseases like arthritis and diabetes,[3] it appears *particularly* unrealizable in the case of mood disorders such as bipolar depression, where the rationality of the patient is always in question (Martin 2007), and the boundary between self and disease is often elusive. Indeed, as we will see, the experience of attempting to self-manage a mood disorder on one's own often produces heightened distress and uncertainty rather than empowerment: To enact expertise as self-managers, individuals diagnosed with mood disorders must—paradoxically—express constant suspicion toward their thoughts and emotions as potential signs of illness. They also must articulate distrust of their imagined future selves, as they anticipate scenarios where their judgment is compromised and construct contingency plans for regaining control. At best, the process of trying to autonomously self-manage a mood disorder leads diagnosed individuals to model a form of discontinuous selfhood and of partial, distributed agency (Weiner 2011). Moreover, in those instances when mood disorder self-management is successful, it succeeds precisely *because* the diagnosed individual has access to the resources necessary to distribute responsibility for the management of their disease beyond the boundaries of the autonomous "self" (see Ungar 2019). In other words, as noted earlier, when the expert discourses of public health officials and clinicians portray mood disorder self-management as a technology that any patient can learn and practice on their own, they fail to acknowledge the deterministic role of self-management's sociopolitical context—specifically, of the human and nonhuman actors, institutions, and other social and material re-sources that shape self-management's processes and outcomes. Given that depressive disorders are known to disproportionally affect adults who are unemployed, less educated, or of lower socioeconomic status (Fryers et al. 2004; Zimmerman and Katon 2005; Blacksher 2002), there is reason for concern that the self-management paradigm may be caus-ing inadvertent harm to the very individuals who are at greatest risk for these mental illnesses.

It seems no accident that mood disorder self-management programs are proliferating in the United States in a historic moment defined by neoliberal anxieties regarding budget scarcity, entitlement services, and citizen dependence; that amidst austerity measures, in a "culture of man-aged care" (Cohen et al. 2006, 255), the moment that mood disorders be-come articulable as a public health crisis is the moment they begin to fall under the purview of a paradigm whose therapeutic mechanism entails shifting the burden of management from the public to the individual. If self-management is to be held up as a viable alternative to a rapidly disappearing infrastructure of public mental health services, I contend, then it is critical that we interrogate whether its forms and consequences are in fact inextricably tied to the very socioeconomic context that the paradigm seems to obscure.

Self-Management: The History of an Unstable and Overdetermined Signifier

The earliest public discourse about psychiatric patient empowerment and self-determination in the United States came from a political "anti-psychiatry" emancipatory movement that fought for change in the early 1970s. The spokespersons for this movement were well-educated "ex-patients" from wealthy families. Many had experienced forced, prolonged hospitalization and, consequently, had come to oppose psychiatric institutions, the use of psychotropic medications, and the acceptance of any form of financial support from the government. The goal of the movement's members at this founding moment was to free themselves from dependency on a mental health system that they found more debilitating and oppressive than helpful (McLean 2000; Chamberlin 1984).

During the same time period, physician Thomas Creer and his colleagues at the Children's Asthma Research Institute and Hospital in Denver were researching behavioral contributions to the rehabilitation of chronically ill children. They coined the term *self-management* in their book *Rehabilitation Literature* (Creer and Christian 1976) to describe what they believed to be the health benefits of a patient's active participation in treatment. In developing the self-management concept, Creer drew on the early writing of Canadian psychologist Albert Bandura, who proposed the construct of *self-efficacy*—the belief in one's "capacity to exercise control over one's own thought processes, motivation, and action"—as central to human agency (Bandura 1989, 1175; Lorig and Holman 2003).

Creer's notion of self-management was elaborated, operationalized, and eventually developed into a full educational protocol by Kate Lorig, a graduate student research associate (and, later, Professor of Medicine and Patient Education Director) at Stanford Medical School in the late 1970s. Lorig's protocol became a program called "The Arthritis Self-Help Course," which is now offered to thousands of patients with arthritis worldwide, and has served as a prototype for HIV/AIDS, back pain, and many other chronic disease self-management programs (Stanford Medicine 2017b). According to Lorig's model, two essential elements define self-management education: First, patients must learn problem-solving skills so that they may identify problems from their own (i.e., rather than the physician's) point of view and devise "action plans" for solving these problems. The successful design and achievement of an action plan is considered more important than the plan itself, since it enhances patients' self-efficacy or "confidence in managing their disease, confidence that fuels internal motivation" (Bodenheimer et al. 2002, 2472). Lorig and her colleagues include a role for physicians in this aspect of self-management, but they describe a paradigm shift wherein patients and physicians become "collaborators," and patients are credited with "an expertise similar in importance to the expertise of professionals" (Bodenheimer et al. 2002, 2470). This patient-physician partnership, in which patients "are encouraged to solve their own problems with information, but not orders, from professionals," is viewed as motivating and empowering patients to "accept responsibility to manage their own conditions" (2470). The second element of self-management education according to the Stanford model is that these problem-solving skills are applied to three aspects of chronic illness: medical or behavioral management, social/role management, and emotional management. Thus, in contrast with the psychiatric ex-patients' approach, this formulation sees patient empowerment as deriving from actively managing rather than eschewing medical treatment, as well as from accepting individual responsibility for "creating new meaningful behaviors or life roles" and "deal[ing] with the emotional sequeli [*sic*] of having a chronic condition" (Lorig and Holman 2003, 1).

As Lorig's model grew increasingly prevalent for the treatment of patients with chronic physiological diseases, changes in the demographic composition of the psychiatric ex-patient movement, in connection with broader mental healthcare policy shifts and the ascendancy of biomedical psychiatry in the United States, led to a gradual convergence of the ex-patient movement's prevailing concerns with many of Lorig's principles of self-management.[4] In the wake of federally mandated psychiatric deinstitutionalization, many ex-patients turned their attention to the problem of homelessness and the dire social and economic conditions to which patients were subject when discharged into the community (McLean 2000). Arguing that the ex-patient movement was too disorganized and weak to effectively address these kinds of issues, they began to advocate for change through lobbying, litigation, and dialogue with mental health professionals. This reformist turn led to a profound split within the ex-patient movement when members interested in these new social concerns agreed to collaborate with the Community Support Program (CSP) of the National Institute of Mental Health (NIMH) in order to establish a national consumer organization, while the more radical contingent of the ex-patient movement remained wary of any such collaborations. The CSP, for its part, had been initiated by the NIMH in 1977 as a corrective to problems resulting from deinstitutionalization. Recognizing the inadequacies of the medical model's focus on the individual, its original aim had been to produce a comprehensive model of community care that would be sensitive to clients' multiple and diverse needs. However, in order to gain congressional support for the CSP, the NIMH partnered with and helped fund an incipient family movement called the National Alliance for the Mentally Ill (NAMI).[5] NAMI members, indignant over their history of being wrongfully blamed for family members' mental illnesses, were committed to promoting the biomedical model of psychiatry. NAMI also advocated for a partnership ethos that would foster consumer choice and participation in the treatment marketplace (McLean 2000). By the time the psychiatric ex-patient movement began collaborating with the CSP, NAMI's influence over the NIMH had succeeded in moving the CSP in a direction that aligned closely with many of the concepts undergirding Lorig's self-management model.

By 1985, following the first annual Alternatives Conference for consumers and ex-patients funded by the CSP, two national psychiatric consumer organizations—the more conservative National Mental Health Consumers' Association, and the anti-medical model National Association of Psychiatric Survivors[6]—were founded. In spite of some remaining ideological differences between these two organizations, their creation signaled the end of the anarchist element of the ex-patient movement, which thereafter became a more organized, if more heterogeneous, body of consumers, ex-patients, and survivors willing to work with the mental health system and government agencies (McLean 2000). Together with other groups including health administrators, mental health providers, state associations, and civil rights organizations, the reformed ex-patient movement began to mobilize around the issue of the right to treatment—and the right to participate as a consumer in *choices* about treatment—rather than fighting for the right to *refuse* treatment as the movement's more radical founding contingent had once done.

Thus, over the course of just two decades, shaped by competing interests and alliances, discourses relating to psychiatric self-determination or management shifted from connoting a wholesale rejection of medicalized categories to (often) indicating a deep consonance with them—one that facilitates a seemingly unproblematic translation of physiological disease self-management concepts to the domain of mental illnesses (see Carr 2021). Furthermore, these shifts enabled the primary referent of such discourses to transform from a refusal to receive psychiatric treatment to a desire to actively participate in, and take responsibility for, the treatment of one's own psychiatric disease.

It can be said that, in addition to these dramatic shifts, another transformation in the meaning of psychiatric self-management has also been underway since the rapid expansion of managed care in the United States in the mid-1990s,[7] and perhaps especially under the conditions of "late liberalism" following the global financial credit crisis of 2008 (Povinelli 2011). Designed to reduce unnecessary healthcare costs through various mechanisms, managed care growth was spurred by the Health Maintenance Organization Act of 1973, which offered economic benefits to federally qualified HMOs. Beginning in 1993 under the Clinton administration, the federal government indicated a new willingness to provide waivers for states to enroll their eligible Medicaid beneficiaries in managed care programs, leading many states to embrace managed care as their principal cost-control strategy (Hackey 1998). Currently, managed care (comprising both for-profit and not-for-profit programs) is the most common type of Medicaid healthcare delivery system, and is nearly ubiquitous among Americans with private health insurance (Cohen et al. 2006). Its ethos of efficiency and cost containment has ushered in what many scholars critique as a distinctly corporatized "culture of managed care" that privileges budgetary concerns and profit-making over the quality of patient services, and imposes changes on the everyday practices of clinicians (Cohen et al. 2006; see also Lester 2009, 2017; Angell 1993; Donald 2001; Kirschner and Lachicotte 2001; Brodwin 2010; Spitzmueller 2016; Hopper 2001; Gostin 2000; Lammers and Geist 1997). Viewed within the context of this managed care culture and its priorities, self-management arguably begins to represent not only or primarily the interests of psychiatric consumers, but also those of the state.

Moreover, since the 2008 financial collapse, debates over the status of entitlement services in the United States have intensified, and consequently the notion of patient self-management has become morally fraught: While the figure of the independent, self-responsible citizen that underlies the self-management paradigm has long been valorized in the United States through the tropes of "enlightened self-interest" (Myers 2010, 2015) and "rugged individualism," it seems to carry *particular* rhetorical force in a contemporary moment in which purported budget scarcity has required a shift in the responsibility for health from the state to the individual (Clarke and Bennett 2013; Greco 1993). Whereas psychiatric ex-patients once sought independence from state and institutional apparatuses, self-managers today must contend with state abandonment (Povinelli 2011), and it is the state that now fears citizen dependency (e.g., Eberstadt 2012). The rhetoric of poor and disabled people's pathological "dependence" on government assistance had begun to crystallize in the late 1990s, when President Clinton signed the Personal Responsibility and Work Opportunity Reconciliation Act of 1996, "ending welfare as we know it" (Carr 2011, 24). One need only recall a controversy from 2012—when US presidential candidate Mitt Romney stated during a campaign fundraiser that it was not his job to worry about the 47% of American voters "who are dependent upon government" and who, he claimed, could never be convinced to "take personal responsibility and care for their lives" (MacAskill 2012)—to recognize how readily questions surrounding an individual's ability or obligation to self-manage now invoke strong, morally laden ideologies of legitimate personhood and political belonging. More recently, US leadership has adopted this sort of anti-dependency ideology as a cornerstone of its political platform and policy initiatives: At a GOP retreat in Philadelphia in early 2017, President Trump told Republican congressional leaders: "We want to get our people off of welfare and back to work. So important. It's out of control. It's out of control" (McDonnell 2017). A similar logic pitting the state's obligation to offer open-ended entitlement services to its low-income citizens against American ideals such as "flexibility" and "choice" was evident in Trump's proposed "World's Greatest Healthcare Plan of 2017" (Congress.gov 2017), an amendment to Obama's Affordable Care Act that included a rolling back of the expansions to Medicaid that were made under Obamacare (Lane 2017).[8] In an era such as the current one, an adequate analysis of psychiatric self-management cannot presume that the patient's best interests are always being served by this treatment approach; instead, it must attend to the politics that compel certain kinds of individuals to fulfill a moral "duty to be well" (Greco 1993) and that may produce "unwilling selves" (Clarke et al. 2007) or perpetuate social isolation and suffering. Also, crucially, the analysis must interrogate how those politics scale (Carr and Lempert 2016) from national governance to therapeutic governance.

Clinicians studying the outcomes of psychiatric self-management have noted in passing that self-management is a difficult research object to define because "it can range from formalised patient education programmes that aim to provide information and condition management skills . . . to the daily activities in which an individual must engage in order to control the impact of their condition on their health" (Jones et al. 2011, 584). The same term is used to refer both to professionally guided techniques and to interventions that are undertaken independent of professional contact (584). In light of the historically and politically shifting interests that continue to shape how different clinician and patient populations make (or disavow) claims to self-management, this book takes the multiplicity of self-management meanings as central, rather than incidental, to an understanding of the phenomenon. Thus, the aim of this book is not to distill a unitary definition of mood disorder self-management and its consequences in the contemporary United States, but rather to trace the range of practices and subjectivities that are produced under its rubric—and to better understand how these multiple practices and subjectivities relate to political economy at a historic moment marked by an unprecedented degree of anxiety over citizens' obligations to manage their own lives and bodies.

Global Reverberations

While this book's central concerns are with the politics of self-management in the United States, it is important to recognize the ways in which neoliberal ideals of self-care and biomedical models of mental illness intersect and circulate globally. Recent social scientific research has documented the ubiquity of self-management "in government policies and strategies, health promotion campaigns and patient intervention programs across most of the Western world, including Australia, UK, Canada and the US" (Brijnath and Antoniades 2016). Crawshaw (2012) describes, for example, how "a range of 'soft' or 'libertarian' . . . approaches to [health] behavior change" has been embraced by recent UK governments as part of a "growing resistance to state paternalism and its perceived propensity to breed dependency" (201). Prominent among such approaches are national social marketing campaigns that aim— though with only partial success, according to Crawshaw—to "construct liberal subjects who are positioned as reflexive health entrepreneurs, willing and able to manage their own wellbeing under the guidance of 'distant' experts" (Crawshaw 2012, 201). Brijnath and Antoniades (2016) similarly foreground the unabated government enthusiasm for self-management in Australia's increasingly neoliberal mental health system, noting that when Indian- and Anglo-Australian participants self-managed their depression they "appeared to . . . become neoliberal patients, releasing the government from its responsibilities" (6) while cautioning that patients' self-management understandings and practices tend to produce "risky health practices and poor health outcomes" (7). Examining "the recent resilience paradigm in the field of trauma" in the Israeli context, ethnographers Yankellevich and Goodman (2017, 61) argue that this popular therapeutic model entails paradoxes that both reproduce and challenge "the expanding bio-medical and neoliberal self-management paradigm in mental health" (71).

Other contemporary work on these phenomena has highlighted the ways in which local cultural and historical factors can transform meanings, enactments, and experiences related to biomedical management of mental illness. In an ethnography of depression in Japan, Kitanaka argues that "the re-Americanization of Japanese psychiatry" (2012, 53) ushered in with the introduction of the *DSM-III* in 2000 did not promote either the same ascendancy of an atomized "neurochemical self" or the technologies of socially decontextualized self-management as it did in the cases described above. Instead, it gave rise to a powerful hybrid narrative that allowed Japanese psychiatrists to articulate "how depression can be understood as both a biological and social disease" and to "[create] new understandings about local forms of oppression" (Kitanaka 2012, 79). Moreover, as Kitanaka notes, "the emergence of this critical awareness about depression in Japan is not an isolated local occurrence but part of the global movement happening concurrently in many nations to protest alienation in the workplace" (2012, 197; cf. Funahashi 2021; Molé 2012; Jolly and Saltmarsh 2009; Davis 2012 for European examples).

Coming at these issues from a different angle, still other scholars have contended that the concepts of neoliberalism and neoliberal subject-formation are analytically limited and that, as such, they should not be invoked as the automatic basis for understanding and critiquing every form (including certain therapeutic modalities and healthcare policies) of "governance and reflexive self-governance" (Cook 2016, 143; see also Reveley 2015; Hilgers 2010). In an examination of a series of parliamentary hearings on mindfulness in Westminster, UK, Cook found that "[m]indfulness as a political focus [was] being framed in multiple ways simultaneously, many of which [lay] beyond the limits of the analytic framework of neoliberalism" (2016, 143). Arguing against "the primary academic analysis of . . . mindfulness practice . . . [as] a neoliberal tool" (Cook 2016, 147) as put forth by Purser and Loy (2013), Žižek (2001), Binkley (2014), Ehrenreich (2009), and others, Cook concludes that this analysis "does not account for diversity in the motivations, experiences, and efforts of people practicing self-governance and the collaborative nature of the political processes by which it is promoted" (Cook 2016, 156). Similarly, Kirmayer—though more inclined than Cook to recognize the risk that mindfulness might be coopted in the interest of consumer capitalism or neoliberal personhood—urges readers to study "mindfulness and meditation in social context" (Kirmayer 2015, 462).

Although a more detailed account of the global circulations of Western psychiatry, neoliberalism, self-governance, "responsibilization," resilience, and adjacent concepts is beyond the scope of this book, I aim to respect the broad range of perspectives outlined above through two primary means: First, by focusing on self-management in the context of Chicago's particular history and sociology, I resist a universalizing description of the ways in which the phenomena under investigation interact; second, at a more granular level, I take even self-management in Chicago to be a collection of multiple, interconnected, often incommensurable projects that may lead, as Kirmayer writes, to "different forms of life, each with its own virtues and limitations" (2015, 461).

A Manageable Medical Condition: The Alignment of Mood Disorders with the Self-Management Paradigm in the United States

The confluence of shifting political interests and demographics among psychiatric patients, broad changes in state economy and mental health policy, and the rise of the biomedical model of psychiatry in the United States created the conditions of possibility for self-management to be regarded as an appropriate and even ideal form of treatment for mental illness. Yet the self-management approach has not been evenly applied to every category of mental illness and is by far most often recommended for the cluster of diagnoses classified as "mood disorders" in the American Psychiatric Association's *Diagnostic and Statistical Manual of Mental Disorders*.

Mood disorders, which include major depressive disorder (also called unipolar or clinical depression), bipolar disorder (formerly called manic depression), and dysthymic disorder (a chronic, mild depression), are the most frequently diagnosed conditions in the *DSM* (in the United States). Major depression—the most prevalent of the mood disorders—is defined as a period of time lasting at least two weeks marked by prolonged sadness, significant changes in appetite and sleep patterns, and feelings of irritability, anger, worry, agitation, anxiety, pessimism, indifference, worthlessness, guilt, inability to concentrate, indecisiveness, or anhedonia (DBSA 2017a). The lifetime prevalence of depression in the United States is 24% for women and 15% for men, and the World Health Organization recently named depression as the leading cause of disability among adults ages 15–44 (WHO 2008). Bipolar disorder or bipolar depression is characterized by alternations in mood between the "poles" of mania or hypomania and depression. It is equally common among men and women, and includes the symptoms of major depression as well as manic mood states defined by exaggerated self-confidence, excessive irritability, aggressive behavior, decreased need for sleep, grandiose thoughts, inflated sense of self-importance, racing thoughts, rapid speech, impulsiveness, reckless behavior, and—in severe cases—delusions or hallucinations (DBSA 2017b; American Psychiatric Association 2013). Bipolar disorder affects approximately 5.7 million American adults—2.6% of the population age 18 and older—each year (DBSA 2017c).

An examination of the historical construction of bipolar disorder—which at its extreme can produce symptoms that are indistinguishable from schizophrenic psychosis and yet is classified as a mood disorder, not a psychotic disorder—is illustrative of the ways in which mood disorders have come to be understood as comprising a distinct kind of mental illness that is particularly amenable to self-management techniques. Until the nineteenth century, "mania" was a broad term for madness in general, and "melancholia," a subtype of mania. In the early 1800s, French psychiatrist Jean-Étienne Dominique Esquirol, a student of Philippe Pinel, introduced the concept of "partial insanity" as a type of mania that resulted from a dysfunction in affect or volition rather than intellect (Lakoff 2005). He further specified melancholia as a distinct state characterized by sad affect. The two extremes of mania and melancholia were then brought together in the mid-nineteenth century under one concept of alternating, periodic, or "circular madness" (Lakoff 2005, 34; Martin 2007, 18). The emergence of this category of cyclic affective disturbance culminated in German psychiatrist Emil Kraepelin's radical and famous reorganization of all known mental illnesses in 1899 into two groups. Under Kraepelin's ontological scheme, *dementia praecox* (the forerunner of schizophrenia) designated diseases of the intellect marked by progressive mental deterioration and bearing an especially poor prognosis, while *manic depressive insanity* was a malady of the emotions and the will that could leave intelligence intact. Kraepelin's system "continues to operate with force in contemporary psychiatric taxonomies, shaping the division between cognitive and affective disorders" (Martin 2007, 18).

With the introduction of Kraepelin's system and the closely related "DSM-III revolution" (Young 1995; Spiegel 2005) in 1980, manic depression was re-termed "bipolar disorder" and subsequently divided into two broad subtypes: Bipolar 1, which requires a history of at least one manic or "mixed" episode;[9] and Bipolar 2, which is defined by a history of at least one milder "hypomanic" episode and the absence of full-blown mania. Both Bipolar 1 and 2 are thus characterized in contemporary American psychiatry by the occurrence of discrete pathological *mood* episodes—even though these moods may in turn have effects on the rationality of the diagnosed person's thoughts and behaviors.

The notion of mood disorders as distinct from—and more manageable than—thought disorders was underwritten by product developments and marketing strategies within the growing psychopharmacological industry. In particular, the distinction between schizophrenia and bipolar disorder was seemingly verified at around the time that the *DSM-III* was published, when lithium was found to have some specificity for bipolar disorder (Kirmayer and Gold 2012). Drug manufacturers seized upon such cases to advance their own economic interests; they "exaggerate[d] the specificity of medications," reinforcing a popular and inaccurate "neo-humoral" understanding of neurotransmitters as mapping onto specific functions or disorders (Kirmayer and Gold 2012, 311; Rose 2003). In the late 1980s, the first of a new class of psychotropic drugs acting on the serotonin system was developed and marketed as a tranquilizer. When the drug, Buspirone, failed as a tranquilizer in the marketplace, it was rebranded as an antidepressant (Healy 2006). The enormous success of associating Buspirone—followed by SSRIs, and other serotonergic drugs—with depressive disorders led to a rise in depression diagnoses and a sudden public discourse in the mid-1990s on depression as a major, but treatable, source of global disability (Healy 2006; see also Kitanaka 2012; Lakoff 2005).[10] In the case of bipolar depression, where SSRIs if used alone can induce mania, drugs that were originally developed as antipsychotics and anticonvulsants were rebranded as mood stabilizers, and they joined lithium in the ever-growing arsenal of medications available to bipolar patients. Drug treatment "cocktails" for bipolar disorder today are often elaborate and time-consuming projects that require ongoing monitoring and adjustment. This aspect of living with the disorder, together with the psychiatric notion of the bipolar patient as intellectually intact, has given rise to a conception of bipolar disorder as a mental illness extraordinarily well suited to the self-management modality.

As the psychopharmacological industry has grown, mood disorders have not been the only mental illnesses re-conceptualized in the United States as brain pathogens—albeit ones whose biomarkers have not been identified in most cases—comparable to physiological diseases. Indeed, the "thorough biologization of psychiatry" that began with the "decade of the brain" (Kirmayer and Gold 2012) left few if any psychiatric diagnostic categories untouched. Today, although there are some limited signs that scientists are beginning to revisit the social factors that cause mental illnesses (Luhrmann 2012b), the overwhelming trend in the United States is to look increasingly to brain chemistry and structure for mental illness etiologies and cures. Nonetheless, in conjunction with the other factors outlined above, the biomedicalization of mental illness in the United States has bolstered the conviction among policymakers and clinicians that patients with mood disorder diagnoses, like those with hypertension or diabetes, are *particularly* capable of (and empowered by) self-managing their own conditions.

That mood disorders should be identified as prime candidates for a treatment modality that envisions the patient as an autonomous actor who can objectify and rationally control their disease is problematic for two reasons: First, in imagining the mood disorder as entirely separable from (and therefore observable and modifiable by) the managing self, proponents of self-management overlook the fact that a hallmark of mood disorder diagnosis (especially bipolar disorder) is its calling into question of the patient's rationality (Martin 2007). Second, while the self-management paradigm focuses on an individual's relationship to their own disease—thereby largely effacing the role of social and economic context—depressive disorders are widely known to correlate with stressful life circumstances, and to have the most severe and persistent effects on those of lower socioeconomic status. The evidence that mood disorders constitute a *social* epidemic is often met with a strangely mismatched and highly *individualizing* discourse on mood disorders as biologically determined phenomena. Both national organizations (such as the National Institute of Mental Health [NIMH] and the Depression and Bipolar Support Alliance [DBSA]) and celebrity consumer advocates (such as Kay Redfield Jamison[11]) emphasize the biological in their efforts to decrease stigma, encourage individuals to seek treatment, and dispel the notion that mood disorders are signs of characterological weakness. For example, DBSA writes on its website:

> Depression is a treatable medical illness involving an imbalance of brain chemicals called neurotransmitters and neuropeptides. It's *not* a character flaw or a sign of personal weakness. Just like you can't "wish away" diabetes, heart disease, or any other physical illness, you can't make depression go away by trying to "snap out of it." (DBSA 2017a)

While aimed at downplaying stigma, this kind of response simultaneously renders the social causes of mood disorders invisible, justifies the disease self-management paradigm as an appropriate mood disorder treatment, and deflects a recognition of the possibility that self-management *itself* may require precisely the kinds of social and economic resources that are unavailable to individuals who are most at risk for mood disorders. The ways in which these paradoxes and ironies arise and play out "on the ground" is of central concern to this book.

Anthropological Theory and the Current Study

In tracing how logics of self-management get taken up and enacted across different sites and scales in the Chicago mental healthcare landscape—and how these enactments, in turn, both constitute and obfuscate sociopolitically disparate possibilities for patient subjectivity and agency—this ethnography engages with three strands of anthropological theory: literature on biomedical subjectivities; work on the relationships between ideology and therapeutic interventions; and linguistic anthropological theories of interactional positioning.

Clinical Subjectivities in Biomedical Psychiatry

Social scientists have long been interested in understanding how human subjectivity and experience are shaped by clinical psychiatric diagnosis and interactions with treatment paradigms (Kirschner 2015). Early interrogations of these effects critiqued what was viewed as the violence inherent in any act of mental illness classification (Szasz 1974; Scheff 1966; Goffman 1961). Departing from these unequivocal rejections of all mental illness designations, more recent conversations in critical medical anthropology have turned to a consideration of the *particular* modes of subjectivity that are conditioned or foreclosed by different ways of conceptualizing and treating mental illness, with an emphasis on the implications of the increasingly hegemonic biomedical model (Pickersgill et al. 2011; Jenkins 2011; Martin 2007; Callard et al. 2012; Dumit 2003; Ortega 2009; Buchman et al. 2013). Numerous researchers have raised concerns that biomedical psychiatry, which draws a sharp distinction between person and brain pathology, effaces complex temporal, phenomenological, and interpersonal aspects of the experience of living with mental illness (Carpenter-Song 2009; Choudhury et al. 2009; Sass 2007; Estroff 1989; Coleman 2008). Owing to such reductions, the biomedical model has been characterized by such scholars as figuring the mentally ill to be something less than fully human; according to this argument, although a conceptualization of mental illness as a disease extrinsic to selfhood renders those diagnosed "morally innocent" (Luhrmann 2000, 8), in so doing it denies patients the capacity for intentionality, and therefore dangerously precludes a culture of choice or responsibility. In contrast to this perspective, other social scientists have looked to the biomedicalization of mental illness as a site for the *recuperation* of accountable and agentive forms of subjectivity. Indeed, the emergent "somatic individual" or "neurochemical self" (Novas and

Rose 2000; Rose 2007; Fullagar 2009) of biomedical psychiatry has been (with varying degrees of optimism or dismay) described as epitomizing the ideal liberal subject: Here, the patient is seen as a "biological citizen" (Petryna 2004; Rose and Novas 2008), both empowered and obliged to deploy "techniques of the molecular self" to optimize their own brain (Rose 1999, 37).

This book builds on the above lineage by first recognizing that the ascendancy of biomedical psychiatry was a condition of possibility for the popularity of mood disorder self-management today, and then examining the forms of subjectivity that are brought into being by the practice of this particular psychiatric paradigm. As a clinical mode, it takes mood disorder self-management to be a historically distinct and relatively novel phenomenon: While the psychotherapeutic enterprise has always relied to some extent on the patient's willing participation in treatment (Foucault 1978), and psychological theories dating back to Freud's (1927) observing superego have posited models where one part of the self manages another, never before the contemporary moment have biomedical and neoliberal ideologies converged to produce a technology that explicitly names the responsibility to manage one's own mental illness as its principal therapeutic mechanism (i.e., the causal agent that mediates patient improvement) the way self-management does. As such, one contribution of this research is to provide a case study of the real-time practices and consequences of a therapy whose existence is indebted to the biomedical model of mental illness, to see how it compares to the theoretical positions outlined above. More important, this ethnography also contributes knowledge to a critical question that has been largely overlooked in medical/psychiatric anthropology: the role of political economy and local socioeconomic context in shaping the ways that biomedical psychiatry is taken up, practiced, and experienced in the United States. Studies of emergent biomedical subjectivities such as neurochemical or pharmaceutical selfhood often run the risk of treating their object as unitary and productive of only a single way of being in the world. Those works that do attend to the multiple ways in which biological psychiatry gets instantiated in different contexts have mainly done so by elaborating cross-cultural cases where a biomedical explanatory model or treatment is introduced into a milieu that does not share its foundational logics or categories (e.g., Lakoff 2005; Kitanaka 2012).

As a result, anthropological representations of the effects of biomedical models and treatments of mental illness on patient subjectivity in the United States are overly homogeneous, with particularly insufficient attention paid to the ways that these models and treatments are differently instantiated across socioeconomically disparate subcultures. The marginality of "class" as an analytic category in Americanist anthropology stands out in sharp and problematic contrast to its centrality in sociology and other social science disciplines (Ortner 2006). But while mental health research in fields such as health economics and epidemiology foregrounds the role of socioeconomic status in producing unequal outcomes, the methodologies of those disciplines attend less closely than anthropological ones to the subjective and intersubjective processes that mediate the relationships between psychiatry, economy, and mental health (Ramon 2007). Thus, an intervention that this book makes is to use ethnographic research methods to bring a consideration of race, class, and political economy into dialogue with critical questions in US medical/psychiatric anthropology about the real-time formation of new kinds of clinical subjectivities produced by biomedical psychiatry.

In deliberately bringing these sociopolitical factors into the domain of medical anthropology through the rubric of "subjectivity," I endorse Byron Good's assertion that the use of subjectivity as an analytic

> denotes new attention to hierarchy and exclusions, to violence and modes of governance, to new forms of "citizenship," and to subtle modes of internalized anxieties that link subjection and subjectivity. It indicates the importance of linking national and global economic and political processes to the most intimate forms of everyday experience. It places the political at the heart of the psychological, and the psychological at the heart of the political. (2012, 517)

Moreover, in order to understand and describe subjectivity in this way, I take seriously Good's guidance of the anthropologist's attentions toward

> that which is *not* said overtly, to that which is unspeakable and unspoken, that which appears at the margins of formal speech and everyday presentations of self, manifest in the Imaginary, in dissociated spaces and individual dream time, and in traces of the apparently forgotten, coded

in esoteric symbolic productions aimed at hiding as well as revealing. (Good 2012, 519)

My aim, in short, is to demonstrate how neoliberal and biomedical ideologies produce differentiated subjectivities along racialized and class lines vis-à-vis everyday instantiations of "self-management." In its consideration of clinicians, patients, policymakers, and others, this book thus serves to illuminate "that which is embedded so fully in everyday practices and assumptive worlds, shaped by contemporary assemblages of knowledge/power, that they become invisible to subjects, depending on their positions of power" (Good 2012, 519).

Therapeutic Paradigms and Their Ideologies

A second body of theoretical literature with which this book engages concerns the ways that psychotherapeutic treatments encode and enforce particular ideologies (Young 1993) about social relations—especially ones pertaining to the boundaries of selfhood and the meaning of intentional or agentive action. Nikolas Rose, drawing on Foucault's writings on governmentality and biopolitics (Foucault 1977; Foucault et al. 1988), has argued that the growth of the "psy" disciplines (psychology, psychiatry, psychotherapy, psychoanalysis, etc.) since the late nineteenth century "has been connected, in an important way, with transformations in forms of personhood—our conceptions of what persons are and how we should understand and act toward them, and our notions of what each of us is in ourselves, and how we can become what we want to be" (Rose 1996, 11). While Rose's analysis of the broad relationship between all of "psy" and our current regime of the self is useful, there are also crucial differences, unexamined by Rose, in the ways that selfhood and self-governance are envisioned across the various "intellectual and practical technologies of psychology" (11). For example, Alcoholics Anonymous's treatment system can be read as effecting a radical epistemological shift from a normative Western model of human action as delimited and purposive to a cybernetic model that locates selfhood and agency within a larger network of interacting human and environmental processes (Bateson 1972). According to this reading, the first two of AA's twelve steps—admitting powerlessness over alcohol and surrendering to a higher Power—contest and undermine hegemonic Western ideologies regarding "the division between Mind and Matter, or . . . between conscious will, or 'self,' and the remainder of the personality" (Bateson 1972, 319). Thus, participating in this "psy" treatment, which anthropologists might more readily characterize as one that demands conformity with a rigidly scripted confessional narrative (Cain 1991), can alternatively be viewed as a radical and ideologically subversive practice.

Similarly, E. Summerson Carr compares mainstream addiction rehabilitation programs with a newer therapy form called "Motivational Interviewing" to argue that the treatments espouse two distinct philosophies of language, which in turn have "far-reaching symbolic and material consequences" for personhood and agency (Carr 2013). Mainstream treatment, Carr contends, enforces the dominant language ideology of "inner reference" through its insistence upon the centrality of inner truth (and its denial) in clinicians' work (specifically what Carr describes as their "metalinguistic labor") with clients. The treatment serves as an "exercise in linguistic purification," and in so doing, it teaches people to "represent themselves in a manner that supports existing institutional and cultural orders" (Carr 2010, 15). Motivational interviewing, in contrast, draws on what Carr argues can be understood as a performative language ideology: "[W]hat counts in motivational interviewing is the semiotic linkage of clients' talk to future social action rather than to existing internal states" (Carr 2013, 179–180). Here (to some extent at least), clinicians and clients interactionally co-produce—and share responsibility for—the client's agency (or denial), and clients' utterances can constitute therapeutic change regardless of whether they denote an inner truth. In another study, Carr shows how a therapeutic discourse (in this case, case managers' talk about the issue of bed bugs in clients' homes) can be productive of an ecological/systems model of action and control, locating agency in the interstices of a network of human and nonhuman actors rather than in the clash of bounded, fully intentional individuals (Carr 2015; see also Latour 1987). As with Bateson's analysis of Alcoholics Anonymous, Carr's readings of motivational interviewing and bedbug management suggest that therapeutic paradigms at times have the potential to disavow and transcend—rather than simply to reaffirm—dominant ideologies of personhood and agentive action.

An article by Rebecca Lester further complicates this formulation by demonstrating the ways in which normative "economic and political commitments become imbricated in the self" (2017, 1) as constructed through a psychotherapeutic modality, even when that same modality enables clinicians and clients to articulate a nonnormative conceptualization of the self as multiple, processual, and dialogical. Lester's analysis centers on practitioners' uses of the newly popular psychotherapy technique of Internal Family Systems (IFS) in a US eating-disorders clinic. Lester argues that IFS—which "understands the self as a system of subpersonalities that constantly shift and interact" (2017, 5) and envisions a healthy self-system as one that is characterized by a sort of harmonious pluralism—permits clinicians to satisfy the divergent imperatives of managed care insurance providers and optimal client care. IFS offers a language for personifying a client's eating disorder ("Ed") as a "part" in the client's self-system—a part with its own agency that will never entirely disappear. At the same time, it teaches clients to "reorient their inner worlds as a sort of mini-congress, where various parts, each with their own diverse interests and motives, learn to work together for the good of the whole person" (Lester 2017, 10). As such, IFS presents a vision of pluralism and self-governance that is "a neoliberal ideal par excellence" (10), yet also contains an "incitement to multiplicity" that "refracts" a straightforward project of concurrent political and psychological subjectification and "complicates models of agency predicated on the assumption of a unified, singular actor" (9). In this way, Lester claims, the therapeutic modality of IFS provides a path for clinicians to navigate the paradox of having to produce "the right kinds of patients" for managed care when—by virtue of having a mental illness—those patients are inherently "the wrong kind of sick" (5).

The above works are part of a larger intellectual project concerning ways of constructing or conceptualizing "the self"—as a subjective formation and as actor or agent—in relation to its social environment. Such a project has, on the one hand, helped to identify beliefs about selfhood and agency that tend to be taken for granted in Western or liberal societies—these include dominant ideologies regarding the self as bounded (i.e., within the atomic individual), temporally continuous, coherent, introspective, and independent, and its agency as rational, active, conscious, and purposive (Geertz 1973; Shweder 1991; Sampson 1988; Markus and Kitayama 1991; Gershon 2011; Kirmayer 2007; Ewing 1990). On the other hand, it has provided ethnographic cases that *counter* prevailing assumptions that agentive selfhood need always be introspective, active, individualistic, or intentional (Ahearn 2001; see also Clarke et al. 2007; Bondi 2005): For example, Mahmood uses the apparently oxymoronic term "docile agent" to characterize the "conceptions of self, moral agency, and discipline that undergird the practices of [the Egyptian Islamic revival] nonliberal movement"—and to make the argument that such conceptions cannot be understood or interrogated when held in accordance to "normative liberal assumptions about freedom and agency" (Mahmood 2001, 203). Desjarlais (1994, 1997) similarly demonstrates through his ethnography of a homeless shelter in Boston that the meaning of agency is socioculturally specific even within the United States, and that the normative, middle-class, experience-based mode of being and acting in the world represents "only one, rather inward-looking arrangement of human agency among many" (Desjarlais 1994, 887).

Other scholars have moved away from the notion of agency as a limitless expression of individual free will by instead describing the ways in which agency is made available or constrained by local norms, discourses, and institutions (Cooper 2015); theorizing possibilities for tactical agency in relation to structures of power (Epstein 1996); providing accounts of how semi-agentive practices of social reproduction can end up destabilizing and transforming social structures (Sahlins 1981, 1985); or turning to dialogic approaches that "[locate] . . . agency in the interstices between people, rather than within individuals themselves" (Ahearn 2001, 129). This latter approach has been especially productive of "postmodern, poststructural, queer, or progressive understandings of subjectivity and social life" (Pitts-Taylor 2010, 639) that reject the individualist tradition of the rational agent in favor of new paradigms such as relational being (Gergen 2009), companion species (Haraway 2008), or moral responsibility in the face of discontinuous, unknowable selfhood (Butler 2005). Among these, of particular significance to medical/psychiatric anthropology are emergent conceptualizations of selfhood, responsibility, and agency in relation to the brain that go beyond biological determinism on the one hand, and neoliberal metaphors of infinite flexibility (Martin 1994) on the other. Such works have begun to develop or recuperate accounts of "the cybernetic brain" (Pickering 2010), affect transmission as a kind of neurological relationality (Brennan 2004; cf. Leys 2011, and Papoulias and Callard 2010), the brain as "acculturated" (Gergen 2010), and brain plasticity as the potential site of consciousness and political organization (Malabou 2008).

This book contributes to these theoretical questions by exploring the social and political economic conditions under which mood disorder self-management—a therapeutic form whose ideal type envisions a rational individual agent in direct control of their own diseased brain— offers patients either highly normative (and often unrealizable) or more radically refigured models of selfhood, agency, and responsibility. Following Carr, Bateson, and others, I am attentive to the subtle ways that ideologies of language, personhood, and social relations are encoded in the self-management paradigm, how such ideologies are transmitted to and interpreted by patients and clinicians, and what larger social and institutional orders the transmission of these ideologies serves. But this book also expands upon this intellectual project by considering the possibility that a single therapeutic paradigm may invoke and communicate multiple, heterogeneous ideologies of selfhood and agency, depending on the sociopolitical context in which it is instantiated. Following Malabou (loosely), I ask: If mood disorder self-management is neither inherently constitutive of neoliberal agency nor inherently suggestive of progressive or relational politics, then under what circumstances— and through what sorts of interactions (or non-interactions)—does it take on these characteristics? Put another way, this book asks when and how—if, indeed, ever—self-management may work to invert its own ideological premises and produce what Povinelli terms an involuntary "otherwise"—an alternative social project or way of being whose participants "seem to be structurally located within normative worlds in such a way that their everyday actions are heterotopic whether they intend them to be or not" (2011, 7).

Therapeutic Encounters as Interactional Positioning

In its analyses of various sorts of self-managerial enactments, encounters, and narrations, this book draws methodologically and theoretically on the linguistic anthropological concept of *interactional positioning.* According to this concept, interactional utterances

> position speakers and hearers because indexes in those utterances point out aspects of the context relevant to interpreting or reacting to them. Certain indexical values and not others become salient because speakers and hearers already presuppose various regularities that make some aspects of the context more salient. As the interaction proceeds, subsequent utterances establish the context that might have been relevant to interpreting prior utterances. (Wortham 2001, 46)

Thus, meaning in talk is produced through a dynamic, indeterminate, socially mediated, and emergent process that both refers back to and reaffirms or transforms the social identities of the speakers (Wortham 2001; Bakhtin 1981; Silverstein 2004).

At times, particularly when participants in an interaction occupy very unequal social positions, the alignments of the speakers and the positions that they voice may set up a sort of second, interactional-level text that powerfully indexes broader social issues. For example, in his analysis of a ninth-grade history class discussion, Wortham shows that "the relationship between disadvantaged and more privileged members of society plays an important role in the relationship between teachers and students in the classroom itself" (2001, 25). As the classroom discussion about a Spartan practice of abandoning unhealthy babies unfolds, the privileged white teacher characterizes the hypothetical Spartan mother in a way that "begins to sound like the contemporary American stereotype for some lower-class black welfare recipients" (Wortham 2001, 29). The students, most of whom are working-class and Black, in turn are interactionally positioned in alignment with the hypothetical unproductive Spartan baby. Wortham further develops this argument in subsequent ethnographic research, concluding that "subject matter, argument, evidence, and academic learning sometimes intertwine with and come to depend upon social identification, power relations, and interpersonal struggles in classrooms" (Wortham 2006, 2).

This book takes self-management enactments, like classrooms, to be sites in which social positionings and power inequalities are assembled, indexed, and crystallized through complex, dynamic interactions. It attends to the broader social discourses about self-responsibility and agency that are imposed upon subjects of particular socioeconomic statuses and racial categories, and interrogates how these discourses articulate with local instantiations of the self-management model. By bringing to bear the analytics of class and race, and the conceptual tools of linguistic anthropology, on the question of the forms of subjectivity brought into being by mood disorder self-management in the United States, the volume aims to unravel some of the subtle semiotic phenomena that may contribute to a situation in which mood-disorder self-management works on different populations in unequal ways.

Outline of the Book

This book consists of an introduction, a chapter situating the ethnography and ethnographer (chapter 1), five ethnographic chapters (chapters 2–6), and a conclusion. Each of the ethnographic chapters can be understood as highlighting a distinct aspect of self-management and its role in producing (or foreclosing) race- and class-stratified possibilities for agency and social relationships in the context of mental healthcare in Chicago.

Chapter 2, "Economies of Agency and the (Un)managed Self: Paradoxes of Self-Management in a Mood Disorders Support Group," looks closely at the mood disorders self-management paradigm—first as represented in patient-oriented clinical and popular literatures, and then as enacted and experienced in a support group for individuals diagnosed with depression and bipolar disorder. Drawing on a distinctly biomedical conceptualization of the isolability of personhood from pathology, the mood disorders self-management paradigm posits a stable and rational patient who can autonomously observe, anticipate, and preside over their own psychiatric disease. However, this chapter demonstrates, contrary to the paradigm's implicit promise, that the more that patients take on a project of autonomous self-management, the greater their struggle to delimit a rational, agentive self. In many instances, enactments of self-management lead patients to experience distress and uncertainty rather than any gain in control over their life. Moreover, the most "successful" instantiations of self-management are ones in which—contra the paradigm's vision—the patient is able to "distribute" agency and self-responsibility to actors and institutions outside of their "self." I make the case that by interrogating the structural conditions under which attempted enactments of neoliberal agency through self-management are productive of heterotopic, cybernetic models of agency, we may begin to appreciate the (otherwise effaced) role of political economy in shaping self-management's meanings and outcomes.

Having established, in chapter 2, the reasons for examining what it means to engage in mood disorder self-management across diverse sociopolitical contexts, chapters 3 and 4 turn to the role that therapists inadvertently play in constituting and naturalizing disparate clinical spaces with radically divergent expectations about patients' needs and responsibilities. Chapter 3, "'I've Put in My Time': Normative Trajectories and Structural Contradictions in the Helping Professions," focuses on the professional socialization and training of master's-level psychotherapists (i.e., social workers and mental health counselors) in the Chicago area. The chapter argues that therapists are bound within a broken system that simultaneously valorizes work with the poor, and renders such work unsustainable. Faced with irreconcilable economic and ethical imperatives, therapists attempt to preserve integrity and reduce ambivalence as they proceed along a normative career trajectory through acts of what I term *professional narrative self-management*. Their discursive strategies interactionally accomplish this self-preservation at the cost of erasing the structural contradictions in which both the therapists and their clients are caught.

Chapter 4, "Billable Services and the 'Therapeutic Fee': On the Work of Disavowal of Political Economy and Its Re-emergence in Clinical Practice," shows how therapists' discursive strategies for the self-management of political economy extend beyond the conceptualization and navigation of their own professional trajectories, and into their understandings of the relationship between billing practices and clients' needs. I argue that in both agency and private practice settings, therapists deploy situated strategies for disavowing economic considerations by shifting to a moral register that aligns local billing logics with notions of "therapeutic appropriateness." In so doing, therapists inadvertently articulate and legitimate a class-differentiated *moral economy of mental healthcare* that reasserts precisely the market-based logics that they seek to transcend. This moral economy ultimately helps to constitute two moments in the therapist's normative professional life course—agency work and private practice—as two distinct and non-overlapping clinical spaces, and to naturalize disparate therapeutic temporalities, relationships, and self-management practices as appropriate to each of these spaces.

Chapter 5, "'If You Close My Clinic, I Will Die': Structural Subordination and 'Unwilling' Radicalism in a Grassroots Mental Health Consumer Protest Movement," analyzes the case of a publicly abandoned group of psychiatric patients-turned-activists—the Mental Health Coalition (MHC)—as a kind of perverse endpoint to the logic of self-management, in which we encounter consumers who are literally forced to self-manage by virtue of having had their supports and mental health services taken away from them. The chapter begins with an examination of the ways in which race- and class-based tensions have shaped how MHC members are apprehended in the Chicago consumer activism scene. While the MHC has garnered sufficient recognition to dialogue with city officials about budgetary or political matters, I argue that structural barriers render ineffective attempts on the Coalition's part to speak in the rational bureaucratic register of the Chicago politicians and prompt various efforts on the part of coalition members at a kind of linguistic self-management. At the same time, MHC members' use of the rhetorically effective strategies available to them is read as overly confrontational and unruly by consumer coalitions engaged in similar activism projects on Chicago's more affluent and Caucasian North Side. I argue that the politics of the MHC must be understood in terms of these multiple marginalizations, and that the Coalition's project—as oriented toward a desire for basic inclusion within the state psychiatric apparatus rather than toward a will to self-determination—represents an emergent form of "unwilling" (Clark et al. 2007) radicalism and unwanted self-management of the structurally subordinated.

Chapter 5 also analyzes a policy conflict that arose between the MHC and a North Side consumer activist group. Initially pursuing the common cause of restoring public mental health services across the city of Chicago, the groups diverged when the slightly more affluent of the two shifted its energies to the establishment of a new psychotherapy clinic funded by—and only serving—residents of its own neighborhood. I argue that this project, described by its developers as one that "place[s] communities back at the forefront of mental health by allowing them to initiate, fund, and oversee their own mental health services," ruptured the potential for solidarity between the two consumer groups by extending the self-managerial logics of privatization, competition, and self-governance from the state and city to the community level: As "the community" was refigured by the North Side group as a self-interested entrepreneur that achieves empowerment by competing for scarce resources, a sense of common purpose between the two sets of marginalized consumers became inaccessible, while preexisting structural distinctions were magnified. Further, by being drawn into an ethos of competition and the "narcissism of small differences" (Freud 1930), North Side coalition members unwittingly participated in the erosion of public services, and in a micro-level reproduction of the very structural inequalities to which they were victim.[12]

Chapter 6, "Use of the Self: Boundary Maintenance, Subjectivity, and Cybernetic Entanglement," explores how class-stratified boundaries around various aspects of selfhood are constructed, maintained, or opened up in therapeutic encounters. Through an analysis of two terms of art frequently invoked at the Chicago School for Psychoanalytic Psychotherapy (CSPP)—"use of the self" and "enactment"—I argue that therapists in private practice settings envision and produce the self as affectively porous and intersubjectively connected, but that these same concepts demand the rigid enforcement of boundaries between the individual and their physical surroundings. Thus, middle-class patients are afforded access to *some* key features of what I describe as a cybernetic model of selfhood and agency that is premised on ongoing social support—but the private practice model may be limited in its ability to accommodate a cybernetic conceptualization of the interconnectivity of self and material world. Agency settings, on the other hand, could be interpreted as mobilizing a "use of the self" in precisely the cybernetic sense of self as continuous with a material world that CSPP therapists, in their studious avoidance of enactment, foreclose. I consider, in light of this analysis, the reasons why cybernetic modes of being and the normalization of distributed agency remain less attainable for working-class clients than for middle-class patients. Finally, I explore the potential ways in which management of boundaries around selfhood could be reconceived, in both private practice and agency settings, so as to account for the individual as cybernetically embedded in a system of historical, political, and structural forces.

The book concludes with a reflection on the conditions of possibility for collectively creating an alternative to a mental healthcare system imbued with logics of self-management. It grapples with the question: How can the project of thinking about an outside to self-management be carried out in such a way that it does not become a self-managerial exercise in itself? The conclusion offers the cultivation of critical reflexivity and structural competency (Hansen and Metzl 2016) in clinical training as a potential avenue for achieving this goal.

1

Sites and Situations in an Ethnography of Home

Sympathy, Complicity, and the Field of Power

Situating This Ethnography

This book is a multi-sited clinical ethnography (Calabrese 2013; Good et al. 1982) of psychotherapeutic self-management as enacted and understood within diverse social scenes across the political economic landscape of contemporary Chicago, Illinois. While many of the theoretical and empirical problems that it engages can be generalized beyond the city of Chicago to the United States more broadly, an objective of the research design was to select fieldsites that foregrounded significant sociological and political economic aspects of the mental healthcare situation in this *particular* place and historic moment. The purpose of my grounding the fieldwork in such sites was not, ultimately, to produce a Chicago case study, but rather to tease out the relationships between place-specific regimes of municipal governance, technologies of self-governance, and the production of clinical subjectivities and communities: By tracing self-management's migrations and refigurations in relation to local public health policy shifts—and by theorizing those refigurations in the context of long-standing structural configurations particular to Chicago—this book is thus written in the tradition of a line of community studies research in the anthropology of the United States that aims to "go beyond a case-study approach to raise analytical questions of broader interest" (Cattelino 2010, 278). Following Gregory (1998, 11; in Cattelino 2010), who asserts that "community describes not a static, place-based social collective but the power-laden field of social relations whose meanings, structures, and frontiers are continually produced, contested, and reworked in relation to a complex range of sociopolitical attachments and antagonisms," this book undertakes to show how—in conjunction with broader neoliberal and biomedical ideologies—the sociopolitical conditions of contemporary Chicago compel self-management practices that in turn constitute and maintain disparate communities.

The bulk of the research for this book was carried out in Chicago and the surrounding suburbs between 2013 and 2015, with some follow-up interviews occurring into the summer of 2016. The study is set in the wake of a budget crisis that prompted newly elected Mayor of Chicago Rahm Emanuel, in 2011, to put in motion a strategic plan that pivoted on the dismantling and privatization of the city's once-robust system of community mental health clinics. The main fieldsites in this ethnography include the Chicago School for Psychoanalytic Psychotherapy (CSPP) introduced in the preface, two community mental health agencies (pseudonymously referred to throughout the book as Wellness Behavioral Health [WBH] and RecoveryNet/Community Recovery Center [CRC]), and the Mental Health Coalition (MHC)—a grassroots mental health activist movement rooted in Chicago's South Side.

The period of data collection for this book overlaps with my own course of training and employment at several Chicago-based clinical institutions including CSPP, WBH, and CRC. Although holding a clinical credential and engaging in clinical practice in the field are not requirements of medical anthropological research in general, they were central to the design of this project in ways that are detailed in the discussion of clinical ethnography that follows this section.[1] Likewise, although my clinical credential was not a necessary condition for my participation in the Mental Health Coalition, it helped initially to position me as a legible type of ally to this set of informants.[2] In addition, my clinical training afforded me access to a shared vocabulary for discussing psychiatric categories and treatments with my informants in moments when such topics were raised, and lent me a small but helpful degree of authority when I accompanied Mental Health Coalition members to Community Mental Health Advisory Board meetings with Chicago Department of Public Health officials.

Situating the Ethnographer: Reflexive Work at the Intersection of First-Instance Americanist Anthropology and Clinical Ethnography

There are two forms of auto-ethnographic reflexivity, drawing on two distinct (yet overlapping) anthropological traditions, at work in this book. The first of these concerns the fact that this project focuses exclusively on physical spaces, ideologies, policies, and professional trajectories contained within or emblematic of the contemporary United States. It is a study firmly grounded in this ethnographer's own country of origin and residence—indeed, it is set in the city and at times the very neighborhoods in which I had been dwelling for several years prior to the start of fieldwork. Moreover, this domestic study represents my first large-scale independent research undertaking; thus, it was not conducted subsequent to—or in any sort of implicit dialogue with—a significant history of fieldwork outside of the United States. These characteristics locate me squarely within what anthropologist Faye Ginsburg describes as

> an emerging generation of ethnographers who launched their research in the United States over the last two decades, hoping both to understand and contribute to the efforts of people in local communities—organized along a range of vectors—to transform their worlds through collective action. Increasingly, these are anthropologists who have decided to work in the United States as their first commitment rather than as a second project after a first fieldwork stint "elsewhere." (Ginsburg 2006, 488)

Engaging in this sort of domestic project—a project for which Jessica Cattelino proposes the designation "first-instance Americanist anthropology" (2010, 281)—entails a set of strategies, concerns, and opportunities that are continuous with, yet distinct from, those of anthropological studies conducted further afield. Because first-instance Americanist anthropologists, almost by definition, possess prior and ongoing commitments to the social worlds that they investigate, they often inhabit multiple roles or rely analytically on personal invest-ments in ways that make their relationships to informants qualitatively different from those of ethnographers whose fieldsites are abroad. "Although anthropologists have often committed themselves to ongoing support for communities they have worked with abroad," Ginsburg explains, "as researchers 'working at home,' we are far more complicit in the worlds we study as citizens who have a stake and a say in the cultural policies shaping our own and our informant's lives; and as writers whose work will enter into their discursive world as well as that of the academy" (2006, 489).[3]

To the extent that seemed ethical, I tried when conducting my research to embrace, rather than deny, this sort of reflexive understanding of and complicity in some of the circumstances that my research subjects were navigating. By the time that I began participant observation among members of the Mental Health Coalition, for instance, I was already sympathetic to the Coalition's cause through casual interactions with MHC members who, in collaboration with "Occupy Chicago" protesters that I knew, had camped out for several months near my university in the vacant lot of what had formerly been the Chicago Department of Public Health's Woodlawn Mental Health Center. And although the Coalition introduced me to the *particular* problem of the city clinic closures, I (like many Chicago residents with my political and sociological profile) had already formed my own set of opinions about the broader trend of defunding and/or privatizing Chicago city services—a trend whose growing list of victims included low-income housing, public schools, toll roads, public transportation, and even parking meters (Perlstein 2015b). When I attended rallies, vigils, town halls, and press conferences with the MHC—or when, at the Coalition leader's request, I gave a speech on "Mental Health and the 2015 Election" to an invited audience of Chicago mayoral and aldermanic candidates at an MHC event—I was giving voice to my *own* vision of a just and humane Chicago as much as that of my informants. In this regard, my role in the MHC fits Ginsburg's description of many US anthropologists who "are simultaneously studying communities and working on behalf of them, either as at least partial members or as sympathetic fellow travelers" (Ginsburg 2006, 491). I do not mean to minimize the vast and at times insurmountable sociological divides between myself and my MHC informants; I merely aim to point out that when I worked for and with this group, my modes of doing so were fueled by prior political commitments and concerns that aligned me with the Coalition as something more akin to a "fellow traveler" than a detached onlooker or supportive outsider.

Related to this notion of working on behalf of a community under study, the second mode of reflexivity with which this book engages concerns my identity as a clinician in general, and more specifically my status as a clinical intern and then an employee in some of my ethnographic fieldsites. Joseph Calabrese, a medical anthropologist and psychologist trained in the department where I earned my doctorate, defines "clinical ethnography" as

> culturally and clinically informed self-reflective immersion in local worlds of suffering, healing, and well-being to produce data that are of clinical, as well as anthropological, value. Empathic skills and self-awareness are emphasized in this approach because they are understood as indispensable to both clinical understanding and cultural understanding. (2013, 51–52; see also Good et al. 1982)

Similarly, my aim in carrying out, writing up, and publishing this research is to apply my own subjectivity and self-awareness to the end of producing generative insights for both anthropological theory and clinical mental health practice. Drawing from Davydd Greenwood's approach to participatory action research (PAR) as a process and a goal (Greenwood et al. 1993)—and putting some of the tenets of PAR into dialogue with the tradition of clinical ethnography—I have tried to allow my experiences and clinical interactions "on the ground" at CRC and WBH to shape my research questions and theoretical formulations in this book. For example, because my position as a community support worker at CRC included meeting with clients in their homes or public places with the objective of teaching them how to function independently "in the community," I was able to ground some of my theorization of mental health treatment disparities in my clients' reflections on the strengths and limitations of this service delivery model. Thus, when an African American client who lived in an area with heavy gang activity explained that he felt unsafe receiving services in his neighborhood, and requested that instead we meet 18 miles away from his home—or when a working-class client remarked that it was insulting to hold our therapy sessions at a Starbucks or McDonald's rather than in a private office—I not only modified my clinical practices, but also took these moments as significant data points regarding the beliefs held by clinicians versus clients about appropriate therapeutic care that were in play at CRC. Conversely, my role as clinician-ethnographer at times afforded me the opportunity to direct my anthropological findings toward interventions that could effect tangible improvements in the quality of my clients' daily lives: During my fieldwork at CRC, for example, a heated debate unfolded as to whether the agency should continue to provide clients with access to a cafeteria and free meals. After talking about the issue with many of my clients and attending their town hall meeting, I was invited by a senior manager at RecoveryNet to present my research and make recommendations. We discussed the heterogeneous meanings of concepts such as "community" and "recovery," the possibility that self-responsibility and autonomy could be partial or distributed, and the notion that providing working-class clients with certain forms of social or material support was not necessarily incompatible with promoting their independence or self-determination. Our conversation led the RecoveryNet manager to postpone plans to close the cafeteria, and to ask me for additional readings about how issues of race and class intersect with mental health consumer recovery projects.

By leaving room in this book to acknowledge my personal and political attachments to my research object, and by reflecting on and accommodating the usage of my clinical skills in the course of ethnographic data collection, I hope to continue the efforts of Americanist anthropologist predecessors (e.g., Myerhoff 1980; cited in Ginsburg 2006) whose self-conscious research among their own communities helped to "[break] a dichotomous deadlock . . . in which work [is] either 'scientific' (and therefore significant primarily to a community of scholars, but not necessarily of more general interest) or 'applied' (and therefore meant to be of practical use to the community being studied, but assumed to be of lesser intellectual value)" (Ginsburg 2006, 489). I thus offer myself, throughout this book, as a sort of special case of a "boundary object" (Star and Griesemer 1989)—one who existentially "inhabit[s] several intersecting social worlds" (393) while working to expand and enrich the overlapping areas between those worlds.

Racialized Geographies of Health in Chicago

This book is and is not about Chicago. The stories that it tells—about the process of becoming a psychotherapist and making impossible choices, about inequalities in mental health policy and treatment, about structural racism and class frictions, about our need for self-determination without social abandonment—are more far-reaching. They point out paradoxes and struggles that were happening, at a certain historic moment, in many places and in many forms all at once. And those paradoxes and struggles, of course, persist and drive new stories imbued with the particularities of their places and time. Yet when it came time to write this book, I found that the book could not be *not* about Chicago. I could not bring myself to situate my ethnography "in a large urban area in the Midwestern United States" as I had once imagined I might do. There were, it turned out, too many qualities of the place itself that deserved a place in the stories. While a comprehensive overview of the history and sociology of Chicago is beyond the scope of this work, some attention to Chicago's distinctive relationship to the phenomena of racialized geography, healthcare disparities, and social activism is needed in order to understand how a study of mood disorder self-management and clinical practice eventually led this ethnographer to the heart of a struggle between the Chicago Department of Public Health and a working-class Black mental health consumer activist movement.

I first arrived in Chicago in 2006, in the last years of the neoliberal Mayor Richard M. Daley administration (1989–2011). I had rented an apartment, sight unseen, at 53rd Street and South Ellis Avenue, just on the border between Hyde Park and Englewood, in a class and racial transition zone between the white bourgeois cloisters of the University of Chicago and the working-class Black neighborhoods that constituted much of the city's South Side. I soon found that the university was itself a site of struggle over race, class, and labor. Its president, Robert Zimmer, was the highest paid in the nation, receiving over $3.4 million in 2011, and at the institution he served, capitalism verged on theology. The campus chapel was dedicated to the memory of John D. Rockefeller, while just down the block, a gothic theological seminary was transformed into an institute dedicated to the legacy of neoliberal economist Milton

Friedman. The surrounding neighborhood had been maintained as an affluent and segregated space, subject to university-backed "slum clearance" in the 1950s and, later, university-funded gentrification projects (Bradley 2021; Karlin 2013). The streets were patrolled by the university's private police force, which was frequently accused of police brutality and racial profiling, while campus service workers, who were predominantly working-class people of color, faced harsh kinds of labor discipline and union-busting. The campus security guards were outsourced in 2009, only to be offered their jobs back at $11 per hour, reportedly less than half their old wage. Asked on a cold winter night how the job was going, one security guard replied: "On nights like this, some people just walk off the job: 'Fuck this.' They go home. They're not getting health benefits. The pay is low" (anonymous student labor organizer notes; personal correspondence). Naturally, the university prided itself on its contributions to the local community, boasting of its status as the "largest employer on the South Side" and its capacities for "creating economic opportunity" in surrounding communities of color.[4]

Similar struggles and dynamics had played out for decades at the university in the domain of healthcare. The University of Chicago Medical Center (UCMC), founded in 1927, had strategically isolated itself from its local neighbors outside of the strictly defined geographical boundaries of Hyde Park, and had denied care to Black patients until 1945.[5] During the 1970s, "when most medical schools saw widespread success in making community arrangements with other types of hospitals, including community hospitals and veterans' hospitals, the UCMC attempted, but failed, to create lasting partnerships with other Chicago hospitals" (Karlin 2013, 527). By 2005, the University of Chicago found itself serving as the only tertiary care center on the South Side of Chicago, which also lacked an adult level 1 trauma center.[6] Without connections to a network of community care facilities, the UCMC faced what its CEO Dr. James L. Madara described in a controversial commentary published in the *Journal of the American Medical Association* as an unsustainable level of financial stress stemming from the burden of serving as the default provider of routine primary care to "dense populations of economically marginalized and low-income individuals" (Hill and Madara 2005). In order to fulfill its mission as an academic medical center "to educate and train physicians, to perform novel medical research, and to treat the sickest and most debilitated patients," Madara argued that UCMC would need a mechanism for redistributing lower-cost, routine-care patients to community hospitals (Karlin 2013, 523, citing Hill and Madara 2005). To accomplish this, the UCMC developed the Urban Health Initiative (UHI)—"a series of projects seeking to stem the tide of poor patients by forging new alliances and service agreements for the provision of health care on the South Side" that was led by Michelle Obama until the 2008 presidential campaign (Karlin 2013, 528). While the university boasts that the UHI "[improves] health and access to quality care on the South Side of Chicago" (UChicagoMedicine n.d.), critics—particularly in the program's early years—accused the University of Chicago of using the UHI to improve its own finances by dumping its poor Black patients on neighboring institutions (Novak and Fusco 2008).

In its exploitation of race and class divides, and its capacity to rationalize these as contributions to the common good, the university was emblematic of Chicago itself, a city fast transitioning away from its industrial past to a postmodern "knowledge economy," based on higher education, medicine, culture, tourism, gentrification, and the exaltation of affluence. Stark class and racial divides themselves were nothing new to the city, as Upton Sinclair's *The Jungle* (1906) or St. Clair Drake and Horace R. Cayton's *Black Metropolis* (1945) attest. Yet the city's political economy developed new forms of precarity and social abandonment by the close of the twentieth century. In the wake of deindustrialization, South and West Side communities suffered from massive depopulation and economic disinvestment. Steel mills closed, and public housing projects were torn down, along with hospitals, schools, and even subway lines (Walley 2012). In such environments, new kinds of professional and political subjectivities continued to be forged, delicately sustained and reproduced through various forms of self-management.

Overview of the Fieldsites

This book moves about a variety of spaces, tracing the structures, policies, and discursive processes through which self-responsibility and agency are differentially envisioned and instantiated across the mental healthcare landscape of contemporary Chicago. On first pass, one might be tempted to formulate the study as a *comparative* ethnography that asks, fundamentally, what the technology of self-management looks like "in action" (Latour 1987) in a mood disorders support group versus a psychotherapeutic training institution versus a nonprofit community mental health organization versus a consumer activist coalition. While such a framing would capture some aspects of this research, it would fail to represent a central aim of the project, which is to demonstrate how these seemingly disconnected—even incommensurable—sites are in fact interrelated nodes located within a common *social space* or *field of power* (Bourdieu 1989). As Bourdieu notes, "[t]he groups that must be constructed in order to objectivize the positions they occupy hide those positions" (16). Indeed, a project about self-management that evaluated only, for example, "the psychoanalytic training institution" or "the agency" as a self-contained object—or even a study that attempted to make a side-by-side comparison of these as separate entities—would overlook the significant implications of the positions of power that each site/group occupies in relation to the others. Moreover, such an analysis could not adequately theorize the roles of those social actors who move between—and through their own embodied and discursive maneuvers, help to construct and reproduce—these disparate nodes in the field of power: In this book, for example, therapists are considered in terms of the ways in which they are compelled by material, ideological, and structural forces to advance along a professional trajectory that begins in the agency and culminates in private practice. Following the circulation of these therapists allows for an understanding of the politics undergirding how they—as human commodities of sorts—accrue and bestow professional or moral value (Appadurai 1988). Thus, I would insist that this book's strategy be thought of as "multi-sited"—rather than "comparative"—in the sense of multi-sited as a mode of ethnographic research that

> moves out from the single site and local situations of conventional ethnographic research to examine the circulation of cultural meanings, objects, and identities in diffuse time-space. This mode defines for itself an object of study that cannot be accounted for ethnographically by remaining focused on a single site of intensive investigation. It develops instead a strategy or design of research that acknowledges macrotheoretical concepts

and narratives of the world system but does not rely on them for the contextual architecture framing a set of subjects. This mobile ethnography takes unexpected trajectories in tracing a cultural formation across and within multiple sites of activity that destabilize that distinction, for example, between lifeworld and system, by which much ethnography has been conceived. Just as this mode investigates and ethnographically constructs the lifeworlds of variously situated subjects, it also ethnographically constructs aspects of the system itself through the associations and connections it suggests among sites. (Marcus 1995, 96)

Put another way, this book represents an effort to harness what Cattelino identifies as the power of anthropology "to name spatial and cultural units where they might otherwise remain invisible or disconnected" (2010, 278). Its goal is to guide readers into and between a set of Chicago lifeworlds, persuading them in the process that these lifeworlds are bound together by a logic of self-management enacted at multiple scales, by diverse actors, and in various contexts. If self-management works to perform a kind of political economic mystification whereby class distinctions are reinforced yet their conditions and contexts are obscured (Moore et al. 2015), then this ethnography's purpose is to construct and render visible the very system in which self-management is embedded.

To that end, this book focuses on four sociopolitically disparate yet interconnected "sites": a therapeutic training institution, two agencies, and a grassroots activist group. A brief description of each site is provided below.[7]

The Chicago School for Psychoanalytic Psychotherapy (CSPP)

CSPP is a clinical training center that occupies one floor of a larger educational institution in the downtown Chicago "Loop." It offers doctoral and master's degrees in clinical mental health counseling and social work, nondegree programs, clinical consultation, and continuing education units. Tuition rates at CSPP at the time that I conducted research were similar to national averages for the field (Mulvey 2011), at around $20,000 per year for the PhD program and $30,000 per year for the master's program. The school offers onsite and "distance learning" options, both designed to accommodate the schedules of students and instructors who are employed elsewhere during regular business hours. Students in the doctoral program at CSPP are required to already hold clinical master's degrees, and to be engaged in clinical practice and supervision while they complete four years of coursework and write their dissertations. Dissertation projects are typically grounded in this ongoing clinical practice experience. Upon receiving their doctoral degrees, students' capabilities (from a professional and legal standpoint) to engage in clinical practice do not fundamentally change. However, the credential may open doors to new roles in a variety of institutional settings, or it may enable the graduate to earn a higher income as a private practitioner.

The master's program, which is significantly newer than CSPP's doctoral training, attracts students of a broad range of ages and backgrounds who wish to begin (often second or third) careers as psychotherapists. The MA program comprises four semesters of full-time coursework on topics including clinical theory, assessment and practice techniques, life course development, and professional ethics. The courses are taken concurrently with two yearlong, unpaid clinical practica. The first year's practicum is typically sixteen hours per week, while the practicum undertaken in the second year is a more intensive twenty-four hours per week. Only the second-year practicum is required by the state of Illinois for licensure. CSPP provides psychoanalytic clinical consultation on students' practica work. CSPP endeavors to assist master's students with finding practicum opportunities at psychoanalytically oriented sites that align with the student's experiences and career goals; as a new and small program, however, the school's network of field placements was relatively limited during the time of my research, and students often struggled to secure these positions. At the end of the master's program, CSPP students are eligible to apply to take the Illinois state counseling licensure (LPC, or Licensed Professional Counselor) examination. As with any master's-level program in counseling, students at CSPP must complete 2,000–3,000 hours of supervised clinical work after they graduate before they are eligible to sit for the examination for *clinical* licensure (i.e., LCPC, or Licensed Clinical Professional Counselor)—the precondition for "hanging a shingle" and establishing one's own private psychotherapy practice.

CSPP is a small operation, with modest-sized student cohorts and a slightly nonstandard, though functional, accreditation status. The school's recruitment efforts are ongoing, quite visible, and at times aggressive. Staff turnover is high; although I was not privy to any details, I often received the impression that disagreements among the school's leadership were regular and disruptive. A powerful board of trustees, which includes many clinicians who are well connected within the Chicago psychoanalytic scene—appears to hold sway over major administrative decisions.

The faculty of CSPP consists almost entirely of experienced clinicians who maintain private and/or group psychotherapy practices alongside their adjunct teaching appointments. The vast majority of the instructors are Caucasian; slightly more than 50% are women, and two-thirds hold clinical doctoral degrees, while the remainder have terminal master's degrees. Course teaching is compensated (as of 2017) at about $2,000 per eighteen-week semester, and therefore does not constitute a primary source of income for the instructors; many choose to teach for noneconomic reasons such as diversification of their work activities, intellectual fulfillment, or prestige. Others—particularly younger faculty members or those who are in the process of working toward a PhD—do rely financially on the supplemental income that they earn from CSPP.

Consistent with the orientation of the school, most of the faculty members at CSPP have been trained in a psychoanalytic tradition, and many incorporate elements of this approach into their own clinical work. All are required by the school to include psychoanalytic thought or technique in their course offerings. Taking cues from psychoanalytic theories of transference and parallel process, many of the instructors at CSPP draw pedagogical attention to interpersonal dynamics in the classroom as a central element of their teaching technique. It is a tacit (and occasionally explicit) expectation of the program that students "work on themselves"—whether in private psychotherapy or through other means—while receiving clinical training, and that they perform a willingness to show emotional vulnerability and interrogate their own psychodynamic processes in the classroom. During my time at CSPP, one student was put on probation and ultimately expelled from the program for nebulous reasons having to do with their alleged failure to achieve sufficient self-awareness and personal growth.

As indicated earlier, this book incorporates a large auto-ethnographic component that includes my own course of clinical training, which was undertaken concurrently with some of my anthropological fieldwork. My full training, leading to my licensure as a Professional Counselor in the state of Illinois, ultimately comprised coursework and internships tied to four separate clinical educational programs at three schools in the Chicago area. While the entity that I refer to as CSPP is largely inspired by one of these programs in particular, in certain parts of the book I amalgamate details or characters from across my clinical training, and present these under the description of CSPP. This is done for purposes of increasing anonymity, as well as to broaden my representation of clinical training and private practice clinicians.

In this ethnography, I rely on interactions that I had with CSPP instructors (both in the context of interviews and in the classroom) to make claims about the notions of patient selfhood, agency, and self-management that are produced and affirmed in private psychotherapeutic practice. In particular, I argue that in private practice settings—and *not* in agencies—patients are afforded access to a model of *cybernetic* or *distributed* agency based on a presumption of their therapeutically appropriate need for enduring and unmediated relational support from their therapist. In interviews with CSPP instructors, I was able to deduce some of these findings by listening to these therapists narrate their own clinical career paths and describe their approaches to working with patients at different points along that professional trajectory. And in classes, my instructors would at times present transcripts or process notes from their sessions with patients, which helped to give me a sense of how their clinical encounters unfolded in real time.[8] While these data provided something of a proxy for observing actual private psychotherapy sessions, they of course cannot be viewed as a true substitute for such observations. The virtual impossibility of my gaining access to private therapy sessions, compared to the ease with which I was able to conduct and witness therapeutic work in agency settings, speaks to the class disparities in the nature of the therapeutic relationship that this book delineates.

Wellness Behavioral Health (WBH)

WBH is an outpatient community mental health agency that offers individual, family, and group therapy as well as a psychosocial rehabilitation (PSR) program and case management services.[9] The facility is located on the western outskirts of the city of Chicago and comprises three separate sites: Two are adjacent buildings near an interstate highway in a predominantly white (Italian/Irish/German), lower-middle-class suburb. The third site is located in a somewhat more working-class, mainly Hispanic and Italian-American village in Cook County that is a short drive from the two adjacent buildings.

Of those two buildings, one—which employees referred to as the "Wellness Center"—contains slightly more attractive, clean, and comfortable institutional furnishings. The Wellness Center houses the offices or cubicles of many of the full-time staff clinicians at WBH. The small portion of WBH clients who have private health insurance—as opposed to Medicaid—usually receive their therapeutic services by licensed staff clinicians in this nicer building. The building is also the site of an underutilized play therapy room for children, and of several conference rooms that are used for group work. With one notable exception, the staff therapists here do not have their own psychotherapy rooms; instead, several generic spaces for therapy sessions—each identically appointed with two vinyl couches, a few chairs, a simple coffee table, and a white noise machine—are available for staff to use interchangeably. Since therapists are mobile, they must have with them an agency-issued laptop computer and malfunction-prone electronic signature pad when they meet with clients in the therapy rooms. These technologies are used during sessions to facilitate therapists' completion of progress reports, or to update clients' consent forms and treatment plans. In contrast to the depersonalized spaces of the agency therapy rooms,[10] staff clinicians in this building often decorate their own cubicles with family photos, inspirational quotations, toys, or pieces of art.

Next door to the Wellness Center is a more run-down building with poor air circulation, harsh lighting, outdated technology, and a dearth of comfortable seating. This site is where several unpaid student interns (myself included) and some permanent WBH clinical staff work, and where hard copies of client paperwork are filed. In this building, clients are seen for sessions in therapists' own offices. A bulky, old laptop computer generally serves as the centerpiece of the office/therapy room. Depending on their inclinations and resources, some therapists make efforts to decorate their offices with lamps, books, games, or pictures drawn by their younger clients.

The third site is home to the majority of the student interns at WBH, who share one common workspace and have access to several therapy rooms. It also contains the offices of approximately eight staff therapists, a twenty-four-hour crisis hotline, the PSR program, a large kitchen and function room, and a meeting room for interns' weekly group supervision sessions. This is the largest of the three buildings, and often the liveliest due to the stream of activity associated with the presence of PSR clients in the building throughout the day.

Wellness Behavioral Health is part of a larger behavioral health service network in the state of Illinois. That network, in turn, exists under the umbrella organization Wellness Health Care—a complex system of affiliated entities that own and operate an assortment of healthcare services including hospitals, nursing homes, diagnostic centers, hospice, physician practices, home care providers, and a college of nursing. Wellness Health Care has in excess of 20,000 employees, 4,000 of whom are medical professionals. The three sites that make up WBH were formerly part of a different, smaller healthcare network, and were only acquired by Wellness Health Care a few years before my research began. Wellness Health Care is a Catholic institution and, as such, employees are subject to the Ethical and Religious Directives (ERD) for Catholic Health Care Services. I was aware of one clinician who incorporated Catholic-influenced "spiritual" guidance into his therapeutic work, but for the most part the religious affiliation of the organization did not play a role in my experiences as a clinician or ethnographer at WBH, and is therefore not thematized in the book. Although Wellness Health Care/WBH is not one of the community mental health providers that was initially awarded funding by the Chicago Department of Public Health as part of its plan of mental healthcare reform in 2012 (City of Chicago 2012), it has collaborated with the city of Chicago on mental health–related trainings, and its client population includes individuals who had been treated in city clinics prior to closures.

Wellness Behavioral Health is one of several agencies where I worked and received (individual and group) supervision as an unpaid intern during my clinical training. My WBH internship required a formal application and interview process. I was hired for approximately ten months along with nine other interns who were also enrolled in various master's degree programs in counseling or social work. All of the interns in my cohort were women, ranging in age from mid-twenties to mid-forties. Eighty percent of the cohort was white and 20% was Black. The majority of the interns were from the Midwest and planned to stay in the Chicago area after they completed their graduate studies. On three-year follow-up after my internship ended, four of the interns in my cohort had secured full-time clinical positions at WBH or another Wellness Health Care facility.

Clients came to WBH from throughout the Chicagoland area, though many lived in or near the neighborhoods where the outpatient facilities were located. They encompassed a diverse array of sociological positions, but generally were more working-class than the modal resident of the surrounding communities. The majority of WBH clients received health benefits from "straight Medicaid" or from a Medicaid managed care plan such as IlliniCare Health, Aetna Better Health, Meridian, or CountyCare.[11] These plans generally operated on a fee-for-service basis, wherein WBH would submit claims to the state for reimbursement of each billable unit of service provided to clients, according to regulations and rates set by Illinois Healthcare and Family Services (HFS).[12] Some clients came to WBH without any health insurance; if they met a set of diagnostic and bureaucratic criteria, these clients could fall under the Illinois Department of Human Services/Division of Mental Health's Eligibility Group 2—the "Non-Medicaid Target Population"—and qualify for a limited amount of state-funded care (Illinois Department of Human Services 2017). Interns at WBH were allowed to conduct intakes and provide therapeutic services and case management only to those clients who received Medicaid or were uninsured. As previously mentioned, WBH clients with private, non-Medicaid insurance received services from paid staff members (who also had Medicaid clients on their caseloads).

RecoveryNet/Community Recovery Center (CRC)

As noted earlier, RecoveryNet is a large community mental health organization with several dozen programs in more than a hundred locations across Chicago, the surrounding suburbs, and a wide swath of adjacent counties. The organization was founded in the era of deinstitutionalization in the late 1950s, just a few years before John F. Kennedy, in his last act as president, signed the Mental Retardation and Community Mental Health Centers Construction Act ordering state and county mental hospitals to release many of their patients for treatment in the community (Foley 1975; Myers 2015).[13] At the time of its creation, RecoveryNet was one of a small number of pioneering institutions across the nation whose aim was to help patients released from hospitalization find a community and participate in social activities. RecoveryNet began as a small agency, but rapidly expanded in its first decade to offer individual and group therapy, vocational support, residential programs, homeless outreach, and other services.

A few decades later, in 2004, President Bush's *New Freedom Commission* issued a recommendation that the American mental healthcare system move toward a recovery-oriented model. Building on the logic of deinstitutionalization, this recovery model—according to its proponents—would reduce the fiscal burden of the mentally ill on the United States' economy by producing independent and empowered citizens "in recovery" and capable of (re)entering the work force:

> The "traditional" mental health system, the [*New Freedom Commission*] found, did not offer enough independence, empowerment, and hope for service users to transform their everyday lives. The traditional model accentuated principles of rehabilitation: stabilize the illness, reduce the negative impacts of illness, and help clients avoid rehospitalization. In contrast, the so-called recovery model accentuated the positive . . . It suggested that people's goals should include being reintegrated into a community of one's own choosing in a way that was meaningful to them. (Myers 2015)

The recovery model articulated well with RecoveryNet's vision, and was embraced by the agency as its organizational philosophy.

My ethnographic fieldwork and clinical employment involved interactions with staff and clients at a number of RecoveryNet sites and programs, including the CST shadowing experience described in the introduction. However, the bulk of my time with RecoveryNet—a period of about nine months that began after I graduated with my master's degree in counseling from CSPP—was spent at a site that I refer to as Community Recovery Center (CRC). CRC is one of the oldest programs within RecoveryNet. It was originally located in an old converted mansion in an affluent Chicago neighborhood. Clients who receive services through CRC reside throughout Chicago, particularly in the far North and Northwest parts of the city. A large portion of CRC clients live in psychiatric care nursing homes, single room occupancy (SRO) buildings, homeless shelters, halfway houses, and other low-income or assisted living arrangements. Historically, CRC clients were predominantly white; fewer struggled with dual diagnoses (i.e., severe and chronic mental illness as well as substance abuse disorders) or had criminal records than do those in the current CRC client population. Among CRC "old-timers," who have been using the facility for many years or even decades, there are at times perceptible undercurrents of race- and class-based hostilities toward the agency's newer clients, and there is a frequently recited lament that CRC is not as "safe" or "comfortable" of a space as it used to be. The shift in the demographics of the CRC client population is related to the fact that RecoveryNet is a major "community partner" of the Chicago Department of Public Health. RecoveryNet now operates some mental healthcare facilities that were previously run by the city, and its programs—CRC included—have absorbed a substantial influx of former city clinic clients.

CRC was designed—and to some extent still operates—in accordance with the "clubhouse model" of community mental healthcare. The clubhouse model originated at Fountain House in New York in the late 1940s in response to early phases of deinstitutionalization. It is "based on the idea that members [i.e., clients] and staff work side-by-side to fulfill the responsibilities of maintaining the clubhouse. The model posits that through shared activities centered around kitchen, clerical, and maintenance duties, members derive value and purpose from the sense that their contribution is needed to sustain the clubhouse community" (Spitzmueller 2016, 43). During the time of my research, RecoveryNet's

CRC facility retained some of these communal features: One floor of the building contained an industrial cafeteria, a lounge area with a television, a game room, a common social space with round banquet-style tables, and a dining room with picnic tables and a piano. Historically and during my data collection period, CRC clients have been welcome to spend their days relaxing or socializing at the center, and to partake of free meals prepared by clients who hold staff positions within RecoveryNet. More recently, CRC has been relocated to a somewhat less affluent (but still middle-class) area, and has undergone major administrative shifts such that many of the center's clubhouse elements have been abandoned.

At the time of my research, CRC offered two broad categories of service: Psychosocial Rehabilitation (PSR) and Community Support Individual (CSI). While there was overlap between the two categories on occasion, in general the clinical staff at CRC comprised one PSR team that engaged in informal therapeutic interactions and other programming with clients in the center, and two CSI teams that were expected to conduct at least 60% of their work with clients outside of the building "in the community." While at CRC, I was employed on a part-time basis as a clinician on a six-person CSI team. The team leader was a Licensed Clinical Social Worker, while the other members of the team were in the process of accruing the supervised clinical hours required for eligibility to sit for the clinical licensing examination. The team was racially and sociologically diverse, creative, and highly synergistic in terms of the personalities and clinical orientations of its members. Unlike the RecoveryNet CST program that I had shadowed, therapists on my CSI team at CRC each had their own set of clients. Each therapist received individual supervision once per week from the team leader. The team also convened weekly as a group to support one another and discuss particularly challenging cases. Apart from these meetings, it was typical to go a couple of days at a time without seeing other members of the clinical team, due to the large quantities of time that staff spent outside in the field. Driving around Chicago in one's own automobile—either alone or with client passengers—could easily fill three or four hours of some workdays. Members of my team adapted to this feature of the job by taking measures to turn their vehicles into comfortable work environments equipped with bottles of water, snacks, music collections, and even scented candles.

I maintained a caseload of about twenty adult clients at CRC, and attempted to meet with each of them on at least a biweekly basis. All of my clients had previously been working with another clinician on my team or with a former CRC therapist; unless otherwise indicated, I tried to continue, with each client, the sorts of activities and interactions that the client was accustomed to doing with their previous therapist. Examples of my typical client sessions include trips to the grocery store, medical appointments, home visits, walks in the neighborhood, visits to social security offices, and meetings in fast food restaurants, coffee shops, or at CRC. The content of sessions varied from one client to another, but often involved my assisting the client with practical matters (e.g., job and housing searches, Social Security Disability Insurance applications, appointment scheduling) or "checking in" with the client on their overall functioning and progress toward personal goals (e.g., exercise, nutrition, engaging in social activity, making and keeping to a budget). One of my clients insisted on a regimented routine in which we would meet each week at CRC, walk together to a nearby Starbucks, complete a self-management worksheet (the client was indifferent to the substance of the worksheet), and play one game of gin rummy. Another client preferred to serve me tea at his home while watching classic movies and talking about his life. A few clients only got in touch with me at the beginning of the month, when I was authorized through Recovery-Net to cash and disburse their social security checks. One client stated explicitly that he wanted to engage in private therapy-type introspective and trauma-focused work, albeit in the challenging setting of a coffee shop (cf. Altman 2013).

The Mental Health Coalition (MHC)

The Mental Health Coalition is an activist movement led by consumers of public mental health services in the city of Chicago. The central aims of the Coalition are to preserve and improve Chicago's free public mental health services, organize for racial justice, and fight for the human right to healthcare. The MHC was created by an umbrella community organization founded in 2004 with the mission of developing leadership among working-class and low-income Black residents of the South Side of Chicago.

At the time of the MHC's inception, its umbrella organization was in the midst of a successful campaign against the displacement of more than six hundred working-class African American tenants from their low-income housing. When, following a loss of funding, the Chicago Department of Public Health announced plans in 2009 to close four of its twelve city-run clinics that served mentally ill communities of color, the organization's key tenant leaders argued that the continued success of its campaign against housing displacement required that the organization fight to save the mental health services that keep South Side communities stable.[14] Drawing inspiration from the grassroots strategy that had been effective in its housing campaign, the umbrella group organized consumers of the mental health clinics that were threatened with closure and trained them to take on the City of Chicago in its own protest movement.

The umbrella organization's nascent coalition of mental health consumer activists (together with advocates including the American Federation of State, County, and Municipal Employees [AFSCME] Council 31—the union representing city clinic staff) was victorious, in the short-term at least: Their actions led Mayor Daley to halt his plan to close the four city clinics and investigate the causes of the city's loss of $1.2 million of state funding for its mental health centers.[15] Energized by this early success and by the continued threat of cuts to public mental health services in Chicago, the umbrella organization and its clinic consumer activists inaugurated the Mental Health Coalition (MHC), an ongoing community outreach and political advocacy program.

Chicago's public mental health centers were not out of trouble for long. Immediately following his election in 2011, Mayor Rahm Emanuel released a budget proposal that included the closure of six city clinics— four located on Chicago's South Side—in 2012.[16] This time around, the CDPH did not claim that its hand had been forced by budget shortfalls; instead, it framed the closures as a component of a multipronged strategy of mental healthcare "reform," in which psychiatric services for the poor would be "expanded" and "enhanced" through the city's investment of $500,000 in partnerships with private community mental health providers, while the remaining six city clinics would be "consolidated" to more efficiently and effectively serve Chicago's uninsured clients (City of Chicago 2012). In spite of the Mental Health Coalition's vigorous protests, all six closures went into effect within the year.

Throughout the period of my research, and (with some notable changes) to this day, the Mental Health Coalition has campaigned relentlessly to restore and improve what it views as a critical *public* mental health safety net distinct from federally qualified health centers (FQHCs) and other private community mental health providers in Chicago.[17] At hearings, town halls, rallies, sit-ins, press conferences, meetings, letter-writing campaigns, and other events, the MHC aims to push back against the city's narrative of progress and reform by bringing to the public's attention the stories of city clinic consumers who either fell through the cracks entirely in their "transition" to community partners, or who now receive inadequate mental healthcare. It also tries to counter the city of Chicago's arguments about the economic necessity of mental healthcare privatization by drafting budgets, recommending ways to make the city clinics more profitable, and by publicizing the relatively low cost of maintaining the clinics in comparison with other expenditures that the city chooses to prioritize. Since 2012, the MHC has garnered widespread positive media coverage of its cause. It has succeeded in raising the CDPH's awareness of mental health–related issues affecting working-class communities of color, and has played a role in persuading the city of Chicago to begin accepting insurance at its remaining public clinics.[18] As of mid-2023, more than a decade after Emanuel's devastating inaugural act, the MHC had not achieved its primary goal of reversing the tide of mental healthcare privatization in Chicago: Indeed, in December 2016, the CDPH quietly moved its staff out of one of the six remaining public city clinics (Roseland) and transferred management of the mental health services at that facility to a new private partner (Cook County Health and Hospitals System [CCHHS] and Centers). Furthermore, in the time period between 2012 and 2020, four distinct Chicago communities that had once been served by the city clinics voted to establish their own, self-funded Expanded Mental Health Services Programs (EMHSPs) (Coalition to Save Our Mental Health Centers n.d.).[19] Two additional EMHSPs—one of which will, ironically, serve the Mental Health Coalition's own Woodlawn neighborhood—are currently underway (Coalition n.d.). But in spite of these ongoing neoliberal developments, recent political events in Chicago have sparked cautious optimism among community organizers that a victory for the MHC could finally be on the horizon: On April 4, 2023, former public school teacher and union organizer Brandon Johnson won the Chicago mayoral runoff election, following a campaign in which he pledged to reverse Emanuel's clinic closures. Johnson reiterated his intentions in an "inauguration applause line about finding a bunch of ways to make sure Chicagoans get the mental health care they need, 'including reopening our mental health care centers across the city of Chicago'" (Byrne 2023). True to his word, a press release in May of 2024 announced Mayor Johnson's plan to reopen the shuttered Roseland mental health clinic on the far South Side of Chicago by the end of the year, as well as to "expand clinical services at an additional two City-run locations" (City of Chicago Office of the Mayor 2024).

Consistent with the demographics of the city clinics and the South Side of Chicago, most of the consumer members of the MHC are poor and African American.[20] Consumer members' experiences with political activism vary, but many—including some of the Coalition's most outspoken leaders—had never been involved in a protest movement prior to the city clinic closures. Other members of the MHC include current and former clinical employees of the Chicago mental health centers, representatives from AFSCME and the Illinois Nurses Association, political organizers affiliated with the South Side community and/or the University of Chicago, and leaders of the Illinois Single-Payer Coalition. Of this latter group, there are a number of individuals who themselves identify as mental health service users, but who had not been receiving those services at a city clinic. Because of the involvement of these different parties in the MHC, the Coalition's larger events were often strikingly diverse in terms of the race and class identities of attendees, while still "segregated" in the sense that a disproportionate number of the white, middleclass members of the MHC are professional allies rather than city clinic consumers. At the time of my research, I was the only identified MHC member who was also an ethnographer of the group; however, during my research the MHC was approached by (and agreed to work with) a documentary film team, a journalist who was launching an online newspaper focused on issues affecting Black men, and other media outlets.

My fieldwork with the Mental Health Coalition throughout 2014 and 2015 consisted primarily of my attendance at the Coalition's biweekly organizing meetings in Woodlawn, and my participation in political actions, monthly Community Mental Health Advisory Board meetings at the Chicago Department of Public Health, and many other MHC events. I also conducted a small number of interviews with both consumer and advocate members of the Coalition. Because my engagement with the MHC centered on the forms and consequences of self-management brought into being in the *absence* of sufficient clinical care, I did not necessarily encounter or analyze MHC consumer members qua patients, nor did they interact with one another principally vis-à-vis psychiatric categories. MHC meetings were focused on brainstorming, community organizing, and political event planning; interactions were decidedly *not* in the genre of a clinical support or self-help group. That said, at certain moments, the existence of (treated or untreated) mental illness was a felt presence within the group. MHC members tended to be unusually understanding about each other's structural and psychiatric vulnerabilities; they tolerated the occasional disruptive outbursts that occurred during meetings, checked in on those members who seemed to be struggling with symptoms, and at times even collected money to support a member dealing with a personal crisis. It was tacitly recognized within the group that a member—even a leader of the Coalition—might experience periods when they were less communicative, reliable, or present if they became overwhelmed by mental illness or other life problems.

2

Economies of Agency and the (Un)managed Self

Paradoxes of Self-Management in a Mood Disorders Support Group

I neither willed with my whole will nor was I wholly unwilling. And so I was at war with myself and torn apart by myself. And this strife was against my will; yet it did not show the presence of another mind, but the punishment of my own.
—Augustine, *Confessions and Enchiridion*

A Scene of Self-Management

In a donated basement of a private psychotherapy center, assembled members of an organization for people living with mood disorders are talking casually before the official start of their weekly support group meeting.[1] Predominantly in their twenties and thirties, they commute from all over the city, and although as usual there are a few new faces in the room, the group "regulars" look forward to this time to catch up with what for many have become their closest or only friends.[2] Several people arrive in work clothes; others may mention later during the meeting that this is the first time all day, or all week, that they have gotten dressed and left the house. With few exceptions the presentation of members and the tone of discussion in the space of the support group room are notably "normal"; the diagnosed conditions of major depression and bipolar disorder that unite the members of the group and occasion their presence in this basement are referenced and rationally analyzed far more often than they are enacted. The irony of the situation doesn't escape the group. On this holiday season evening, when a bipolar woman arrives from a crowded store late and flustered,[3] announcing that "people are *crazy* this time of year," another member doesn't miss a beat in delivering the response: "Yeah, kind of makes *us* less special!"

As the meeting gets underway, people raise and discuss issues ranging from the everyday to the existential. The only criterion, invoked weekly by the leader who recites a list of support group rules, is that the discussion relates in some way to depression or bipolar disorder.[4] Members are encouraged to manage the discussion among themselves, and to intervene if they feel that their peers are veering too far off topic.

On this particular evening, the group lands on the subject of psychiatric hospitalization, an experience familiar to many, but not all, of those present. Jessie, a bipolar woman in her mid-twenties wearing a T-shirt that reads "I wish my lawn was emo so it would cut itself," poses a question in her usual bored-yet-slightly amused tone:

> So, how come some of you are always getting hospitalized, and I've never been? I mean, my aunt tried to make me go once because I was cutting myself, but I was cutting *responsibly*. It's my coping strategy, and I knew I wasn't trying to kill myself, and I told them that at the hospital, so they didn't admit me. I told them "I'm not going to *kill* myself; I just want to lay in bed for a week," and that's what I did. So how do you *decide* if you need to be hospitalized? How do I know if *I* need to go to the hospital?

Tricia, a bipolar woman in her late thirties, responds with an anecdote:

> Well for me, getting hospitalized is the way I reset myself. I think of it like my two-year tune-up; that's about how often I need to go, and I can usually tell when I start showing signs that it's time for a tune-up. The most recent time, I knew for a couple of weeks that I needed to go, and I kept telling my boyfriend to take me, but he'd say "oh, I don't feel like it tonight," or "next week; we have plans this weekend." I got so frustrated that while I was shaving my legs, I took the razor—I don't cut often anymore, but when I cut, I *know* it's time for me to go to the hospital—and I did, and then I showed my boyfriend and was like "look—*I'm cutting—I need to be hospitalized.*" So he finally took me. I could have just driven myself, but I wanted to *be hospitalized*, you know?

The foregoing narrative may seem an unexpected place to begin this chapter: a (mostly) clinician-free mood disorders support group. While subsequent chapters of this book are concerned with specificities related

to therapist socialization and discourse production—and the complex relationships between these phenomena and the therapeutic management
of mental illness for disparate class populations—this chapter analyzes
a scene of therapeutic self-management that is as decoupled as possible
from a single, defining clinical or sociological context. The individuals
introduced in this chapter, though by and large limited in their access to
material resources and social supports, are not collectively considered as
embodying the experiences of mood disorder self-management as constructed within a particular sort of class-determined clinical milieu (e.g.,
the agency or the private psychotherapy practice). Nor do they necessarily share the sociopolitical identities and circumstances of the Mental
Health Coalition, whose members' self-management I treat as emergent
from the conjuncture of political activism and public abandonment. Instead, this chapter's informants are approached in a manner that takes
up the self-management paradigm at its face value—as a purportedly
context-indifferent clinical technology that any patient can learn and
practice on their own.

There are several reasons for beginning an exploration of the political economy of mood disorder self-management here. The first is
chronological: The support group described in this chapter was the
site of my earliest research, and it served as my point of entry into the
paradoxes—and later, the heterogeneities—of self-management. Before
I became a clinical trainee myself, received professional instruction on
the implementation of self-management approaches with community
mental health clients, or observed other therapists explicitly or tacitly
conveying their class-differentiated expectations about client autonomy
and self-responsibility, I learned about the existence of self-management
as a clinical treatment modality through the efforts and accounts of the
support group members discussed below. Moreover, it was only by virtue of my early acquaintanceship with the support group's self-managers
that I became attuned to the critical role of those structural and social
contexts that the self-management paradigm so effectively conceals, as I
reflected on the unarticulated conditions that seemed to predict whether
members' self-management practices would lead to empowerment
or despair. By providing a close reading of the forms of selfhood and
agency envisioned within the clinical self-management paradigm as an
ideal type—and then documenting the variety of workaround behaviors,

outside resources, and participating actors and institutions required to even *approximate* the self-management technology as envisioned—this chapter opens up questions central to the book regarding the bearing of the patient's sociopolitical status and access to resources on the very meaning of mood disorder self-management: If a successful implementation of the self-management protocol always necessitates relationships beyond the one between self and disease foregrounded in the clinical literature, then what are the consequences of situating self-management within a context that privileges ongoing interpersonal support versus one that emphasizes the primacy of the goal of independence? Findings from this chapter support my argument, substantiated in subsequent chapters of this book, that the meaning and outcome of self-management is not stable across contexts (Moore et al. 2015); that it is a self-defeating clinical modality in the absence of resources that allow for the social distribution of agency and self-control; and that silently embedded within the clinical practice of the self-management paradigm is a class-stratified *political economy of agency* that asks those with fewer resources to exercise an impossible degree of autonomy while it affords those of greater means access to a more *ecological* or *cybernetic* model of self-control (Bateson 1972; Pickering 2010).

Jessie's question above about hospitalization and Tricia's story about cutting illustrate a complex and often contradictory model of selfhood, mental illness, rationality, and agency that is the broader focus of this chapter. Jessie does not simply wonder why she has never been hospitalized. Instead, she asks how one *knows* and *decides* whether one needs to be. Her very questions disrupt the logic of psychiatric hospitalization for bipolar disorder as it is popularly imagined, whereby a floridly manic or suicidally depressed patient, decidedly out of control, is brought to an institution by someone more capable of rational judgment. Likewise, Tricia's response reveals some surprising spaces of negotiation and indeterminacy between self-knowledge, self-control, and rational decision-making. In this chapter, I argue that Jessie and Tricia model a form of discontinuous selfhood and distributed agency produced at the intersection of their experiences living with a condition that calls their rationality into question, and their engagement with the self-management therapeutic modality which entails extremely rational practices of calculation, prediction, and self-surveillance.[5] In so doing, they render particularly visible more universal contradictions and dilemmas contained within the premises of neoliberal selfhood, and offer insight into the often-disavowed political economic conditions of possibility for the distribution of managerial selfhood.

As Emily Martin (2007) has eloquently described, "being known as a manic-depressive [or bipolar] person throws one's rationality into question" (5). Such a designation carries high stakes for the diagnosed, both in terms of its practical implications and its foreclosure of claims to foundational aspects of personhood in Western society. While the ontological and legal status of the mentally ill has shifted, through various disciplining practices and technologies, from little more than beasts in the seventeenth and eighteenth centuries to potentially recuperable citizens by the nineteenth (Scull 1989; Foucault 1967), Martin argues that a vastly overdrawn yet powerful divide still demarcates and degrades those classified as irrational:

> [A] diagnosis of major mental illness, in practice, if not in law, often disqualifies a person from high-security clearance, from employment of various kinds, from political office, from insurance coverage, and from college enrollment. Some kind of terrible abyss is still thought to divide "normal people" from the "mentally ill." (Martin 2007, 87)

Martin's seminal ethnographic research on mania shows that within this imagined abyss, there exists a wide range of complex social experiences that blur the boundaries between rational and irrational. Deliberate enactments of mania that Martin observes, for example, effectively index the diagnosed person's volition and awareness of their putative irrationality, thus illustrating that they in fact possess key attributes of rationality. Likewise, clinicians and rational bureaucratic organizations can be viewed as acting *irrationally* when they elect to place a mentally ill person in a managerial role (Martin 2007, 95).

This chapter examines a related but distinct dimension of the relationship between bipolar disorder and rational selfhood: the injunction that certain types of people who have been designated as chronically mentally ill, particularly those diagnosed with bipolar disorder, undertake a project of vigilant self-management as the pivotal component of their treatment regime. Rooted in a biomedical distinction between person and disease, the very term "self-management," when applied to bipolar disorder, contains an unintended dual meaning which foregrounds the difficulty that people with this diagnosis face in locating themselves in the space between rationality and irrationality: While meant to emphasize the diagnosed person's central role in taking responsibility for the everyday management of their *disease*—management of bipolar disorder *by* the self—the term is suggestive of a slippage; the management *of* a self. This ambiguity is borne out in the experiences and practices of bipolar individuals such as many of the individuals discussed in this chapter, for whom participation in a weekly mood disorder support group discussion is a component of their conscious self-management efforts. Whereas Martin draws our attention to the forms of rationality that are obscured by psychiatric classification, I ask what possibilities for subjectivity and agency are conditioned or foreclosed by a biomedical paradigm that seems to simultaneously confer and deny rational selfhood to bipolar patients.

Self-management approaches to the treatment of bipolar disorder have been widely lauded in the clinical literature as empowering the patient, who is often in this context referred to as a "consumer,"[6] to regain control of their life (Depp et al. 2009). But the practices and modes of thinking envisioned within this therapeutic modality would hardly include or predict those described by Jessie and Tricia above. This is because the paradigm of self-management engages in two forms of reification that are unsustainable in ways that become particularly apparent in the case of bipolar disorder.[7] First, the paradigm posits a stable and rational managing self who can observe, measure, anticipate, and preside over a disease separable from the self. Such an imagined subject draws upon broader notions of a kind of compulsorily free *homo economicus* who satisfies the demand of neoliberal government for "active individuals seeking to 'enterprise themselves,' to maximize their quality of life through acts of choice" (Rose 1996, 57). Never fully realizable, this choosing self is experienced as especially elusive for people diagnosed with bipolar disorder, who on the one hand are enjoined to take on a hypervigilant form of rational self-surveillance, but on the other hand in order to do so must constantly second-guess the rationality of their every thought and feeling. Contrary to the discourse's implicit promise, it seems, the more that bipolar patients take on a project of self-management, the greater the ambiguity generated around delimiting a rational, agentive self. Second, the reification of bipolar disorder as an isolable "disease" to be managed fails to adequately describe the ways in which it is experienced as neither a fixed object nor apart from the self, but rather as a temporal formation that expresses or realizes the self in a particular, if pathological, way.

Agency, Responsibility, and the Biomedical Subject

Contemporary psychiatric taxonomies and treatment modalities in the United States are increasingly driven by a biomedical model that presumes the isolability of personhood from pathology and focuses on the latter as the object of intervention. This model, humanist anthropologists have long argued, carries consequences for "the way doctors perceive patients, the way society perceives patients, and the way patients perceive themselves" (Luhrmann 2000, 23), often doing violence to the patient's complex psychological experiences and identity. In her foundational ethnography of the ways in which two competing conceptions (psychoanalytic and biomedical) of personhood and mental illness play out in American psychiatric education and practice, anthropologist Tanya Luhrmann claims that the biomedical model results in the sacrifice of "a respect for the difficulty of human life" (290). The "popularized, vulgarized medical model," she writes, invites a moral instinct of viewing the mentally ill as "not as human, not quite as alive, as we are" because it sees them as having been "struck by something that came in from the outside. It was not under control in the first place, and it remains no more under control than a doctor can control it" (284–285). Furthermore, in rendering patients blameless for their psychiatric diseases, this model simultaneously denies patients the capacity for intentionality and effectiveness. Ultimately, Luhrmann worries, the danger of biomedically derived epistemologies is that they preclude the maintenance of a desperately needed "culture of responsibility"—in which, despite constraints of illness and suffering, individuals are compelled to "choose to live good and productive lives"—and instead encourage fatalism and unaccountability (290–291).

More recently, however, medical anthropologists and science studies scholars have begun to interrogate and re-envision the possibilities for subjectivity, responsibility, and agency conditioned by the biomedical paradigm (Schüll 2006; Sunder Rajan 2005; Lakoff 2005; Rose 1996, 1999, 2003, 2007). Examining modes of selfhood that are emerging from new medical technologies, these researchers have proposed that we are entering an age of such actors and models of being as the genomic "sovereign consumer"/ "patient-in-waiting" (Sunder Rajan 2005) and the modulating "homo-addictus" (Schüll 2006), and of psychiatric taxonomies that are based not on broad disease categories but on specific medication response profiles (Lakoff 2005).

Nikolas Rose in particular has written extensively on the implications of what he views as a contemporary shift to "somatic" or "molecular" (as opposed to psychological) selfhood, motivated by the biomedical psychiatric gaze and its related technologies for intervention upon madness. In contrast with Luhrmann's view, Rose argues that through this gaze, varieties of normality "[become] open not to fatalism but to choice," individuation, explanation, and manipulation (Rose 1999, 11–12). To be a somatic individual, Rose claims, "is to code one's hopes and fears in terms of [the] biomedical body, and to try to reform, cure or improve oneself by acting on that body" (Rose 2003, 54). For Rose, the somatic subject is afforded a new type of agency and moral responsibility by means of "the application of what one might term techniques of the molecular self" (1999, 37).

According to Rose, the technologies of the psychological sciences in general, and especially those of the emergent somatic individual, are deeply tied to and appear to constitute the free embodied subject of liberal democracy:

> The modern liberal self is "obliged to be free," to construe all aspects of its life as the outcome of choices made among a number of options . . . The technologies of psychology gain their social power in liberal democracies because they share this ethic of competent autonomous selfhood, and because they promise to sustain, respect, and restore selfhood to citizens of such polities. They constitute technologies of individuality for the production and regulation of the individual who is "free to choose." (1996, 100)

The restoration/subjectification that Rose envisions these technologies as potentiating is distinctly liberal in its linkage of "the notion of self-realization with individual autonomy, wherein the process of real-izing oneself is equated with the ability to realize the desires of one's 'true will'" (Mahmood 2005, 11). Applied to the neurochemical self-management of mental illness, Rose's perspective would seem to suggest—as does the clinical literature for bipolar patients—that learning and engaging in this set of practices will instantiate the ideal neo-liberal subject: "an entrepreneur managing his or her own life . . . that calculates rationally and acts responsibly" (Maasen and Sutter 2007, 7).

The Reified Managing Self

In the practices and technologies advocated in the literature on bipo-lar disorder self-management, the self is established as separable from disease and recognizable through its properties of coherence and conti-nuity. The managed disease, in turn, is figured as calculable, visualizable, and thus able to be ordered, predicted, and tamed by the rational man-ager. *The Bipolar Disorder Survival Guide* (Miklowitz 2002), a resource that was regularly referenced during conversations between members of the support group, speaks directly in the second person to the presumed diagnosed reader. Written by a clinical psychologist who was inspired by the coping strategies he witnessed in a bipolar support group as a predoctoral intern, the *Guide* is a particularly insightful and sensitive example of the self-management workbook genre. But while the text lends credence to the distinct set of questions and difficulties faced by those managing a mood disorder, and takes seriously the role of social support as a component of self-management, it nonetheless draws upon and reifies the notion of a true and autonomous choosing self who can learn to control their disease through rational practices. The language of governance is present from the beginning of the *Guide*: "It is my sincere hope," the preface reads, "that after reading [this book] you will feel less alone in your struggles, realize that there are effective treatments avail-able, and *have at your fingertips strategies to prevent mood swings from ruling your life*" (Miklowitz 2002, ix, emphasis added).

A chapter of *The Bipolar Disorder Survival Guide* titled "Is It an Illness or Is It Me?" begins to demonstrate how the self-management paradigm, when applied to mental illness, imagines and seeks to instantiate a sepa-rable, stable, and transparent self. Likening the experience of adjusting to a chronic mood disorder diagnosis in some ways to that of patients who live with physiological conditions such as diabetes or hypertension, the text proceeds to acknowledge that "bipolar disorder has its own particularities" (Miklowitz 2002, 55). These "particularities" are encapsulated by two questions to the reader which, while rhetorical-sounding, are meant to be read literally and answered through strategies offered in the *Guide*:

> How do you know what is really your illness and what is your "self" or your personality (your habits, attitudes, and styles of relating to others; the way you are most of the time)? How do you train yourself to know the difference between you when you're well and you when you're ill, and not fool yourself into thinking that changes in mood, energy, or activity are just "how I've always been"? (55)

According to the model developed in the *Guide*, the distinction between self and illness is real, complete, and always already existent. The task of the diagnosed reader is to cultivate "the ability to *recognize* these differences" (Miklowitz 2002, 55, emphasis added). This recognition is important not only for effective disease management, but also because it "can contribute to a more stable sense of who you are" (55). An example of the type of unproblematic self-management work that ostensibly can be accomplished through appropriate differentiation of person and disease is provided through the case of the hypothetical patient "Maureen," who is able to see and act upon her pathology while leaving her real self intact: "Maureen . . . knew she had always been extraverted but realized she needed to visit her doctor when she began staying up late to call people—all over the country—to whom she hadn't spoken in years. The requirement of an increased dosage of lithium did not interfere with her appreciation of others" (55). In contrast, those who do not fully and correctly delineate the stable and true self run the risk of not realizing their full potential or letting the disease take control, as alluded to in the book's preface:

> [S]ome people begin thinking of themselves as if they were nothing more than a diagnostic label or a set of dysfunctional molecules . . . They usually accept the need for medications but unnecessarily limit themselves

and avoid taking advantage of opportunities that they actually could handle. (Miklowitz 2002, 56)

> You may start to think that you can accomplish little with your life, believing "All I am is bipolar, and I can't change. It's all biochemical and I can't take responsibility for myself." This way of thinking may lead you to avoid going back to work, withdraw from social relationships, and rely more and more on the caretaking of your family members . . . I disagree with this way of characterizing bipolar disorder. Many—in fact, most—of my patients are productive people who have successful interpersonal relationships. They have adjusted to the necessity of taking medications, but they *don't feel controlled by their illness* or its treatments. (Miklowitz 2002, 66, emphasis added)

In boldface type, the *Guide* succinctly lays out the relationship that drives the self-management model: "Bipolar disorder is something that you have, but it is not who you are" (Miklowitz 2002, 56).

To help readers identify who they really are, the text provides a "Self-Administered Checklist" tool called "What's Me and What's My Illness?" consisting of two columns: "your personality traits" on the left and "your manic or depressive symptoms" on the right. "Spirited," "boisterous," and "talkative" are among the left column options; "full of energy" and "overly goal-driven" among the right. "Erratic" and "indecisive" are personality traits; "wired" and "highly distractible," illness symptoms. "What's me" or the real personality, the workbook explains, "hang[s] together" coherently and stably across time; it is "the cluster of traits that describe you throughout your life" (Miklowitz 2002, 63).

This notion of the real, isolable, and enduring self is also pervasive in *bp*, a bipolar disorder lifestyle magazine heavily sponsored by full-page psychopharmaceutical advertisements. Although a recurrent narrative in the magazine articles is that of the celebrity who bravely fights stigma by telling the public about their personal experiences with mental illness, *bp* does *not* endorse a view of bipolar disorder as a culture or identity to be embraced. Instead, it generally retains the biomedically derived distinctions described above: Bipolar disorder is a brain disease to be treated and self-managed without shame, in the service of liberating the "real" person to the fullest extent possible. An article about author and mental health advocate Ross Szabo, for example, concludes with the following quotation by the celebrity: "For me, I've wanted to find out what is bipolar disorder and what is me . . . I try never to use the disorder to get out of anything or as an excuse, but to use it as a challenge to understand who I really am, how my brain works" (Roberts 2010, 40).

Similarly, an exchange between readers in the "Letters" section of *bp* magazine reveals the apparent stakes of semantics in the representation of the separable self. The Spring 2007 issue of *bp* published a letter with the following criticism:

> As a psychiatrist who receives your magazine, I am appalled by a phrase that recurs throughout your magazine: "he/she has bipolar." In many years of practice, I have never heard a mental health professional use this terminology. Someone is bipolar, or has bipolar disorder. To use your terminology makes the writer (and by extension, the magazine) sound uneducated. Patients who imitate this usage will sound uneducated too—surely not your intention.[8]

A subsequent issue of the magazine featured three letters, all written by mental health professionals (one of whom was also herself diagnosed), in response to the psychiatrist's criticism. All three took offense at the suggestion that it would ever be preferable to say that someone *is*, rather than *has*, bipolar, with or without the with word "disorder" attached:

> I learned in medical school nearly 20 years ago that it is completely inappropriate to refer to an individual as "being" their disease, as if that sums them up.[9]

> To call someone bipolar is dehumanizing. I am not bipolar. I do not identify with my disorder. I am a woman who has bipolar disorder. I am also a mental health professional who has bipolar disorder.[10]

> [The phrase "I am bipolar"] is tantamount to saying, "I embody the illness"—not unlike someone saying "I am cancer" or "I am diabetes." It is not healthy for one's self-esteem, coming to terms with yourself, or making forward progress.[11]

As these examples from the clinical literature illustrate, the managing self of biomedical discourse is predicated on a distinct notion of authentic selfhood as something that is and must be delineated and distanced from the disease. According to this logic, there exists a subtle but actual boundary between the real person—who is characterized by coherence and stability, or continuity across time—and disease manifestations that may assume the appearance of personhood and "fool" the untrained patient. Thus, when the *Guide* describes learning to know "the difference between you when you're well and you when you're ill," as in the example of Maureen, the implication is that in fact even when ill, the real self retains the ability to rationally assess and act upon the disease. Proper self-management, then, as a "technology of the self" (Foucault et al. 1988), entails a transparent self that is fully knowable and recognizable to itself.[12]

The self as envisioned in this model not only is autonomous from bipolar disorder, but also must characterize and locate the disease in a particular way. Conceptualizing bipolar disorder as a biological imbalance is necessary but not sufficient; one also must avoid conflating the managing self with this "set of dysfunctional molecules," and instead position the rational self in a relationship of direct control over the neurochemical. For this reason, the possessive phrasing of "I have bipolar [disorder]" is viewed as more accurate and favorable than "I am bipolar." Although medical anthropologists have noted that persistent and severe psychiatric disorders are often—and sometimes to better effect—subjectively experienced as "I *am* illnesses" (Estroff 1989; see also Strauss 1989), the discursive insistence upon the "I *have*" formulation seen above firmly divides and structures the relationship between manager and object managed.[13]

Disciplining the Disease

In examining the relationship between disease and management as envisioned within the self-management model, we can see that the discourse of bipolar self-management treats the disease to be managed as though it were a stable object whose internal logic is discoverable by a calculating subject through rational processes. The paradigm thus reifies both disease and rational manager.

Daily Mood Chart							
Day	**1**	**2**	**3**	**4**	**5**	**...**	
High Mood	+3						
	+2						
	+1						
Normal							
Low Mood	-1						
	-2						
	-3						
Hours Slept							
Anxiety							
Irritability							
Medication							
Alcohol/Drugs							
Physical Exercise							
Unusual Stressors							
Documentation of stressors:							

Figure 2.1. An example of one of the many mood-charting tools that can be found on the internet (MoodSurfing 2017). Reprinted with permission from Peter Forster.

The self-management literature strongly encourages bipolar consumers to "take control" of their disorders through various forms of recordkeeping, with units of surveillance and scrutiny ranging from hour-to-hour fluctuations to one's entire life history. The simplest versions of such tools suggest that the patient rate their mood, on paper or in a web application, one or several times per day using an ordinal scale (−3 to +3, −5 to +5, 1 to 20, etc.) with full-blown mania at one extreme and major depression at the other. Many mood-charting tools are quite a bit more extensive, with fields to record and cross-reference information such as medication types and dosages, hours of sleep, symptoms of anxiety, physical activity, and menstrual cycle in addition to mood levels (e.g., figure 2.1). *The Bipolar Disorder Survival Guide* explains that mood charting is critical to maintaining wellness because "becoming aware of even subtle changes in your mood and activity levels will help you recognize if you are having a mood disorder relapse and determine whether you should contact your doctor to see if a change in medication would be helpful" (Miklowitz 2002, 154). Moreover, coordinating all of the other information on the chart with the mood level is said to help the patient identify "environmental triggers" that cause mood cycling. This combination of recognition and causal identification promises to instantiate the proper relationship between rational actor and neurochemical object of management: "Identifying mood triggers is an important step in gaining control over your moods" (155).

The Bipolar Workbook (Basco 2006), following a technique developed by a clinician at the National Institute of Mental Health (NIMH), advises bipolar self-managers to also create a "life chart" plotting time, labeled with ages and major life events, along one axis, and corresponding episodes of mania or depression along the other. Once this history is charted, consumers can fill in additional information about times in which they drank alcohol excessively or used street drugs, periods of hospitalization (and medications taken there), and other psychological events. Life charting, *The Bipolar Workbook* explains, reveals to the manager "your common patterns" which in turn enables "you [to be] in a better place to predict when the next episode is likely to occur so that you can take precautions to keep it from happening" (Basco 2006, 41). Besides this predictive and preemptive function, discerning patterns also serves to impart clarity and order to the disease:

> If you're like many other people who have bipolar disorder, you may struggle with so many daily ups and downs that you find it hard to see discrete periods of depression and mania. When your life of ups and downs seems like a blur, you can get the sense that you have no control over it. Looking more closely at the patterns can give you ideas for how you might take control over this illness rather than feeling out of control. (41)

Rational management techniques such as mood and life charting are "borrowed directly from the neoliberal arsenal of tools with which consumers/clients can plan their own futures and govern their lives, their consumption, their health, and their risks" (Valverde 1998, 175; see also Schüll 2006, 230). Based on what Weber described as a "specifically modern calculating attitude" (Weber 1978, 86), they imagine and seek to constitute a self-surveilling accountable subject who can measure and control these risks through rational processes. Thus, the self as posited by self-management discourse is not only coherent, continuous over time, and separable from the disease, but is also taken to be a fully rational actor—a "calculating individual" (Miller 2001, 380) whose conduct is governed through "technologies of the self" (Foucault 1978; Foucault et al. 1988; see also Strathern 2000), and who is the subject "simultaneously of liberty and of responsibility" (Rose 1996, 12).

As the rationales for charting in the clinical literature illustrate, self-management discourse also imagines and reifies the bipolar disorder "disease" as a fixed object that can be isolated, ordered, predicted, and disciplined. By engaging in rational practices, the manager is envisioned as capable of uncovering the true hidden logic or patterns of the disorder, partitioning what only appears to be random into discrete and controllable rationally organized entities.

Sociologists and philosophers of science have noted that quantification practices such as charting and accounting "[accord] a specific type of visibility to events and processes, and in so doing [help] transform them" (Miller 2001, 382; see also Dean 1999; Poovey 1998). This idea, along with the concept of *inscriptions*, is helpful in understanding the way in which bipolar disorder appears to become a governable object in the self-management literature. Inscriptions, as invoked by Latour (1987), are the readable output produced by scientific instruments and technologies, which subsequently become the basis for scientific texts. Moreover, as Rose elaborates, inscriptions differ from *phenomena* in that

> inscriptions must render ephemeral phenomena into stable forms, which can be repeatedly examined and accumulated over time. Phenomena are frequently stuck in time and space, and inconvenient for the application of the scientist's labor; inscriptions should be easily transportable so that they can be concentrated and utilized in laboratories, clinics, and other centers of accounting, calculation, and administration. (1996, 108)

In purporting to convert seemingly "blurry" or chaotic mood phenomena into true discrete and quantifiable inscriptions or "episodes" to be read and acted upon, self-management inscribes the biomedical divide between agentive rational person and static disease.

When we look at the practices and paradoxes that emerge as people diagnosed with bipolar disorder attempt to take on projects of vigilant self-management, we find that many of the very acts and utterances that self-management entails paradoxically constitute the patient as a subject *unlike* the kind that the paradigm envisions and promises. Yet there are forms of agency that, under certain circumstances, these bipolar self-managers are able to claim and model.

Unfolding Diseases, Elusive Selves: (Dis)locating the Agent and Disease in Self-Management Practices

"Do you want me to tell my war story?"

Kevin, a bright, attractive young member of the support group, asked me this facetiously at the start of an interview. Yet in a way, his phrasing is apt. While there are many, often long and circuitous, paths by which a person might ultimately wind up with a diagnosis of bipolar disorder, the diagnostic criterion for the disease's classic form (Bipolar 1) is a history of a single manic episode. Moreover, regardless of their particular clinical subtype classification, every member of the support group seemed to have a "war story" that began with a psychiatric incident and marked a turn in the way that the person talked about and experienced their present and future self. In Kevin's case, his first and only manic episode had occurred during college six years prior to our interview. He recounted writing a letter to President Bush detailing a plan to end all religious wars, hearing auditory hallucinations, and eventually spending nine days in a psych ward. Since then, Kevin had moved back closer to his parents, changed his career plans, and reoriented his life around managing his mental illness. He was taking a cocktail of 20 mg of Abilify (an antipsychotic), 1,200 mg of Trileptal (an anticonvulsant used as a mood stabilizer), and 40 mg per day of Adderall (an amphetamine), and was diligent about medication adherence. Although Kevin had never before or since experienced anything similar to his "war story" episode, when I asked whether he thought he could ever become manic again, the response was unhesitant: "Oh yeah, if I stop taking my medicine I'll become manic within like a week." Moments later, he frowned and added: "I've been doing really well, but the medication can just stop working . . . At my job [working with severely mentally ill people] I often think 'this is me; I can relate.' But sometimes it's 'this will be me again,' like I'm just waiting for the shit storm to come. That makes me anxious."

For Kevin and other group members with whom I spoke, having a diagnosis of bipolar disorder and choosing to try to manage it entails the inculcation of a particular identity and anticipated life trajectory; a shift in ways of talking about, acting upon, and experiencing the self.[14] This subjectivity emerges out of—but is, paradoxically, contrary to the self envisioned by—the biomedical self-management paradigm. As we have seen, self-management imagines a fully rational, continuous, and recognizable self who can calculate and act upon a fixed and isolable disease. Here, however, we see that acting on the "disease" generates ambiguities regarding its location and boundaries, and that enacting expertise in self-management constitutes and indexes the self as discontinuous and uncertain.

Specificities and Ambiguities in Neurochemical Self-Management

As is common practice in many types of support groups, the official start of each meeting I attended was marked by a ritual of introductions (Cain 1991; Martin 2007). The group's peer leader, a friendly and rather giddy man in his mid-thirties who often described his personal "baseline mood" as slightly hypomanic, enjoyed startling everyone at the appointed time by loudly and abruptly interrupting casual conversation. A typical pass around the room might begin:

> Hi! I'm Warren! I have bipolar disorder, OCD, and anxiety, which are all kind of the same thing! I was thinking this week about how it's funny never to know what you're going to be like the next day. Like, what's it gonna be? Will I be depressed or manic?
>
> I'm Tricia, I have bipolar 2, anxiety, and ADHD which is probably caused by the other two. I've had an okay week, but I'm concerned today because apparently Abilify is causing me neurological damage, according to some test results. I can't feel it, but my psychiatrist noticed some subtle differences in my movements and behaviors.
>
> James. Bipolar, um, PTSD, and a bunch of other shit. We just raised my dosage of Trileptal today and I'm feeling totally drugged out. It's causing dizziness, drowsiness, blurred vision—but it's doing what it's

supposed to do. I can read and concentrate now for the first time in years.

As these introductory statements indicate, gaining direct access to and control of the disease via drugs, or even delineating the psychiatric disease categories that are being treated, is far from unproblematic for bipolar self-managers. Indeed, in many cases the effort to do so only makes more apparent the elusiveness of the managing self and the impossibility of isolating pathology from experience in time or space.

Rose (2003) argues that one of the principal processes by which individuals in the contemporary United States have become "neurochemical selves" is the spread of the biomedical presupposition of specificity, which has become central to the research and campaigns of the pharmaceutical industry. Tracing this way of thinking to the development of selective serotonin reuptake inhibitors (SSRIs) in the 1960s, Rose claims that the presupposition was initially made up of three parts:

> First, it was premised on the neuroscientific belief that these drugs could, and ideally should have a specificity of target. Second, it was premised on the clinical belief that doctors or patients could specifically diagnose each array of changes in mood, will, desire, affect as a discrete condition. Third, it was based on the neuroscientific belief that specific configurations in neurotransmitter systems underlay specific moods, desires, and affect. (2003, 55)

When subsequent research proved incorrect the theory that there was one kind of receptor for each neurotransmitter, the presupposition was not abandoned, but rather elaborated with *further* specificity: "It was now argued that each of these subtypes of receptors had a specific function, that anomalies in each type were related to specific psychiatric symptoms, and that they could be ameliorated by drugs designed specifically to affect them" (Rose 2003, 55).

This logic of increasing specificity and accuracy of target has been influential in the treatment of bipolar disorder. Whereas the disorder was once treated only with lithium, bipolar patients today work closely with their psychiatrists to develop and constantly tweak a "cocktail" of sophisticated psychotropic medications, each chosen to act on a specific aspect of the disease. At meetings, it was not uncommon for group members to bring up issues related to their sometimes very elaborate cocktails. Many carried a chart or list at all times, detailing their prescriptions and dosages in case of an emergency. Most considered lithium to be too crude and dangerous, and would only think about using it as a last resort.

But while these pharmaceutical cocktails seem, as Rose argues, to "offer the promise of the calculated modification and augmentation of specific aspects of selfhood through acts of choice" (2003, 59), their specificity often produced an experience of diminished agency or even randomness for members of the support group. This occurred for a variety of reasons. Lapses in health insurance coverage, changes in provider policies, periods of hospitalization, or simply clinician turnover at the community mental health centers where some members received services led to switches in doctors, prescriptions, and sometimes diagnoses. Even those who were treated by the same psychiatrist for a long period of time became familiar with endless medication adjustments or overhauls, which came to feel, members reported, more like arbitrary guesswork than systematically calculated modulations or informed acts of choice. New drugs often caused new side effects, followed by more drugs to treat those side effects, and so forth. Over the years, members lost track of why particular changes in their treatment regimes had been made, and during group discussions they sometimes questioned whether their current cocktails were redundant or suboptimal. Furthermore, at times the drugs seemed to have agencies of their own that defied a relationship of rational management by the somatic individual. Like Kevin, many of the group members had experienced or worried that a medication they relied upon might suddenly become ineffective. Others, like Tricia and James, had to weigh the benefits of a medication against risky or debilitating side effects, either all-too-perceptible or dangerously invisible to them.

Not only did neurospecificity fail to produce an experience of rational disease management, but the process of determining which moods and thoughts needed to be pharmaceutically acted upon also proved to be less than straightforward for group members. One week during introductions, for example, Christine wondered aloud whether she needed to make an appointment for a medication adjustment. "I think I'm a little hypomanic today," she described, "but maybe I'm just excited because I got a call about a job interview. It's hard to tell." More confusingly, Kevin explained that not being in the mood to go see his therapist was often a sign that he was becoming symptomatic (and therefore that he *needed* the therapy). Faced with the task of having to constantly export the experiential to the neurochemical, and the suspicion that nearly anything could be a symptom, group members struggled in their attempts to locate the managing self and an ordinary, asymptomatic position from which to manage.

As the rational manager became more elusive and indeterminate, so did the disease. The quotations in the beginning of this section demonstrate that support group members did not necessarily perceive themselves as targeting or modifying specific psychiatric disorders, let alone particular symptoms or neurotransmitters, through their self-management practices. Instead, they casually conflated categories that psychiatry would hold to be distinct, such as Warren's equation of bipolar and obsessive–compulsive disorders. This conflation was especially notable on several occasions when the subject of schizophrenia would arise in the support group discussion. Although schizophrenia and bipolar disorder are among what clinicians in the United States consider to be the "big three" severe mental illnesses (Luhrmann 2000, 13), the diseases are classified as ontologically discrete (i.e., as disorders of thought versus mood, respectively), and a diagnosis of bipolar disorder is generally associated with a superior prognosis (Lakoff 2005; Benabarre et al. 2001).[15] Nonetheless, given the overlaps in symptom presentation and treatments, bipolar group members at times experienced the diseases as continuous and themselves as at risk of slipping into the schizophrenia category. Tricia, for example, described an incident in which she'd found a man urinating on her lawn during a dinner party she was hosting. Explaining to the group that she had felt more empathy toward the man than did her friends, Tricia said: "He was probably schizophrenic and off his meds, which could be me. There but for the grace of medicine I'm not schizophrenic."

Occasionally, a member of the support group would attempt to invoke the comparison between bipolar disorder and diabetes or hypertension in a manner that was aligned with the clinical self-management discourse; that is, as a metaphor for unproblematic disease management in which the locations of rational self and disease are ostensibly fixed and non-overlapping. However, such attempts usually led to commentary on the inadequacy or unsustainability of the envisioned biomedical relationship. These emergent critiques foregrounded members' experiences of bipolar disorder as an unfolding temporal formation that moves with and through the self, rather than a measurable or targetable object. For James, these intangible and dynamic qualities of the "disease" produced an inability to ever know with certainty that one was sick or well:

> I've heard a lot of people in the group compare depression and bipolar to diabetes, and I don't find that very helpful. I mean it's useful for sort of justifying it to quote unquote normal people but in a lot of ways it's not useful. Diabetes is fairly controlled. You know, you take your blood test and you take your insulin and you have a special diet and you're gonna be fine for a fairly long period of time. And if you don't you're gonna die. And mood disorders aren't like that. For one thing, there's no blood test. There's no way of absolutely knowing how sick you are at any given point. And there's no way of regulating your diet and regulating your meds to the point where you're gonna be fine.

For Tricia, the problem was also a communicative one: In the absence of a visible sign, she had difficulty expressing to others her experience of bipolar as "shifting back and forth" as a disease:

> Now James has a shake, so they're gonna notice that right away. But particularly [with] bipolar—I mean depression you *look* depressed, real mania you're acting kinda crazy, you really are. But bipolar, when you're not high, like completely suicidal or completely manic, when you're just shifting back and forth—it's very hard to explain to people. You know, [they say] "I don't understand why you can't brush your teeth or get out of bed." Or "you look fine, why can't you get out of the house?" It's very hard to explain to 'em. Part of me wishes I had a little brand on my head that said you know "don't ask me anymore. This is what I am."

Thus, the experience of bipolar disorder as temporally unfolding phenomena intertwined with selfhood defied attempts to neatly extricate manager from disease, or to fix the disease in space and time. Moreover, management practices designed to effect a relationship of governance through neurochemical specificities had the unintended consequence of producing new ambiguities.

The Paradox of Enacting Self-Management Expertise

Of all the support group members, James's story was the one that hit me closest to home. Once a PhD student like myself at the time, he had dropped out of graduate school in the middle of writing his dissertation after a frightening psychotic break. Since then, he mostly stayed at home, living a circumscribed life of simple routines and supporting himself on the tight budget of his monthly disability check. Our interview ran nearly twice as long as any of the others I had conducted, and when I apologized for taking up so much of his time, James replied wryly: "I'm on disability; I have nowhere else to be. And hey, we're talking about me—there could not be a better subject!"

When he is not too debilitated by the neurological damage his medications cause, James is eloquent, articulate, and unusually scholarly. He immediately intuits some of the theoretical implications of my research, and seems to enjoy having the opportunity to converse in academic jargon; upon learning that I am an anthropologist, James nods knowingly and asks whether I am studying the ways in which bipolar disorder is both socially constructed and real. Group members joke that James is the "anger expert" because of his sarcastic humor and the homicidal fantasies that he admits to having. But according to James, he is far less angry and more responsible now than he ever was in the past. "Seven years ago," he tells me, "when I chose to go on medication, I chose to live. And I take that very seriously. I want to live." At the support group, James conveys his commitment to a lifelong project of vigilant self-management by calling himself "a professional bipolar" whose "job is to do a good job being alive and getting up every day." But choosing to act responsibly and rationally in spite of the disorder is complicated because, as James puts it, "bipolar alone is not sufficient to explain every behavior that you do—but neither is it *not* the explanation for everything that you do."

For support group members such as James who make a choice to engage in self-management, the act of consistently attending support group meetings is both a management practice in itself and an occasion in which self-management expertise—a type of "second order indexicality"—can be discursively enacted (Silverstein 2003; see also Carr 2010a, 2010b; Agha 2007; Wortham 2001). However, this expression of expertise entails a paradox: Whereas self-management discourse imagines a rational, transparent, coherent, and continuous self, the types of statements that one must make to index oneself as a responsible self-manager constitute a model and experience of selfhood as unreliable, fragmented, and discontinuous.

One of the principal ways that support group members could discursively practice expert self-management was by interrogating their own thoughts and emotions for possible errors in rationality (which in turn would ostensibly allow them to determine whether they were symptomatic and modify their symptoms with medication). Thus, during meetings it was common for someone to discuss their current mood with detachment and suspicion, even if the mood seemed to have a reasonable antecedent: "I've been kind of in a funk because someone broke into my apartment and my computer was stolen," Kevin remarked one day. "Other people might get upset if that happened too, though. I'm gonna give myself a couple days' leeway to see if this is depression or a normal emotion." Another time, a bipolar man received a parking ticket that everyone in the room agreed was unfair. "I'm feeling really angry about it," he said calmly, "which makes me wonder if maybe I'm hypomanic."

These practices of hyperrational self-interrogation did not instantiate the isolable, "real," agentive, and enduring self envisioned in the clinical self-management literature. Instead, they blurred self and disease, and divided the managing subject into fragmented selves marked by uncertainty and distress. James described to me how his self-management practice of scrutinizing in therapy—and often modifying with medication—any out-of-the-ordinary thoughts, left him unable to recognize or find himself:

> A few weeks ago, it occurred to me that I could do a project: I could write a paper. On my own. You know just—I had an idea and it seemed interesting and it would give me something to do. And as I, you know, as I've gotten more medicated, that idea has kind of slipped away from me. So is that me losing a thread of mania? Or is that the drugs completely, you

know, just sort of squashing me flat? And I don't know: Would another person in my situation—I'm on disability—would another person want to do some work? Or would they be okay with basically doing nothing? Which is mostly what I do with my day, is nothing. And I don't know.

What is striking about James's narrative is the multiple uses of "I" and "me" that emerge as true choosing self and disease elude definition or delimitation. These personal pronouns, or shifters (Jakobson 1971; Benveniste 1971), index and simultaneously constitute James as a collection of disjointed speaking subjects. Self-management as articulated here leaves James uncertain as to whether he is the person who is interested in work and "could do a project"—in which case, management leaves him flattened—or the person who remains after extricating himself from a harmful and irrational inclination. Neither can James determine whether a piece of himself has "slipped away" or he has agentively facilitated the removal of "a thread of mania." By expressing his distrust of his desire to engage in a possibly irrational activity that "other people" might not choose, James aligns himself with the type of proper manager envisioned in the clinical workbooks, and interactionally attempts to persuade his interlocutor of his competence as a self-manager. In the end, however, this enactment of rational self-management does not free James to act and choose; it perpetuates his life of "doing nothing."

Not only did engaging in self-management produce an experience of uncertainty and fragmentation within the present managing self, but it also led group members to narrate and view themselves as unreliable and discontinuous over time. In contrast to the knowable self— who uses rational calculation and prediction to delineate a continuous person separate from their pathology—presupposed by the discourse, support group members were compelled to imagine an unpredictable and irrational future self through their self-management practices. As Tricia described it, a future unmanaged state of depression or mania was something that she anticipated but could not predict or control, regardless of medication compliance:

One of the most frustrating things about bipolarity—I think anybody would say this—is you don't know—you can't be depended on. That's the thing that bothers me the most. Um I can be, like right now I feel pretty normal, and meet you here we'll have lunch; it will be fine. But then one day, or one moment, I will just suddenly shut down. Brushing my teeth is just *too much* for me to manage. It doesn't matter how much medicine I take. There's gonna be days—I've accepted it now—that my pink night-gown is going to be my friend [laughs] for the next few days!

Scrutinizing herself and her disease in the manner required of proper self-managers leads Tricia to accept as certain *not* that she will remain a true, continuous, choosing self over time, but that she will become a different kind of self regardless of her efforts.

In response to this type of experience of the self, many group members took on a conscious self-management practice of not committing to any future plans. Christine, for example, explained her rationale and strategy for managing her social life as: "I might be fine or manic today, but tomorrow I may be suicidal. My friends will call and ask me 'are we still on for Wednesday?' and I'll say 'ask me tomorrow.'" Similarly, some of the group members who had once held full-time jobs now felt that they could not resume employment on the basis of their imagined future irrationality. James hoped that he would someday work again, but made a habit of talking to his therapist any time he "got these feelings like I could actually start working." Nor did he envision a time in the future where he would ever become a fully self-controlled employee. In spite of his intelligence and over-qualification for many jobs, James claimed, it was difficult to apply for work knowing that "you'll occasionally [have] paranoid delusions that coworkers will poison you. I'll have months when I don't feel like getting out of bed. And I'll occasionally go to work and feel slightly homicidal."

To describe the way in which being a responsible self-manager meant never fully trusting the rationality of the present self, and anticipating the appearance of an unmanaged irrational self at some unknown time in the future, support group members developed a term that I did not encounter in any of the clinical literature: *tentativeness*. As invoked by the group on several occasions, tentativeness referred both to the literal practice of avoiding commitment to future plans that would require a reliable, continuous self, and to a cultivated stance of uncertainty and suspicion toward one's own thoughts and emotions at any given moment. Tentativeness thus described a distinct disposition in relation to risk—one that required an acknowledgment of the management of *future* uncertainty by an uncertain *present* self. Discursively enacting tentativeness by expressing awareness of one's own uncontrollability and skepticism toward the legitimacy of one's own emotional experiences indexed members' expertise at self-management by demonstrating a kind of vigilance. It also bespoke a rational regimentation of the bipolar disease/self through members' voicing of a scientific register, using the language of hypothesis testing, comparison with a norm, and deductive reasoning to scrutinize themselves for bipolar symptoms. But at the same time, as seen above, "doing" recognizable expert self-management by embodying tentativeness undermined the implicit promise of the therapeutic paradigm by foregrounding the unlocatability of an isolable, stable, and continuous managing self.

In his exegesis of Wittgenstein's philosophical works on solipsism through an analysis of the phenomenological reality described by a patient, Louis Sass provides an account of schizophrenic "double bookkeeping," or ability to "live in two parallel but separate worlds: consensual reality and the realm of their hallucinations and delusions" (Sass 1994; in Martin 2007, 55). These two worlds, Sass shows, are differentiable to persons with schizophrenia "according to their felt ontological status" (1994, 43), enabling patients who are "profoundly preoccupied with their delusions" to "nevertheless treat these same beliefs with what seems a certain distance or irony" (21). Sass argues that this extreme self-awareness is a widely overlooked but in fact fundamental characteristic of mental illness:

> Madness, on my reading, is neither the psyche's return to its primordial condition, nor the malfunctioning of reason, nor even some inspired alternative to human reason. It is, to be sure, a self-deceiving condition, but *one that is generated from within rationality itself rather than by the loss of rationality.* The parallels between Wittgenstein and Schreber reveal not a primitive or Dionysian condition but something akin to Wittgenstein's notion of a disease of the intellect, born at the highest pitches of self-consciousness and alienation. Madness, in this view, is the endpoint of the trajectory consciousness follows when it separates from the body and the passions, and from the social and practical world, and turns in upon itself. (1994, 12, emphasis added)

To the extent that successful self-management, as described in this section, requires that consumers enact constant rational self-surveillance, it similarly helped to constitute bipolar group members as elusive subjects *through*—rather than in spite of—their rational practices. As James described, the kind of self-awareness that managing his "disease" demanded produced an experience of heightened fear and lack of control:

> They always say that as long as you know that you're crazy, that you're not *actually* crazy, but that's not true. Sometimes the more you know that you're crazy the more fucking scary it is because you *know* the things you're thinking are not *real*. You know the things that you're thinking aren't true. And that's a lot scarier than just sort of living your way through the delusions. I mean because [for example:] you're scared of things. You're scared of going out in public, but whatever. But who cares? But if you *know* that your fear of going out in public is irrational, then that's how much you know you're out of control. That's how much you know that your disability is ruining your life. Or running your life.

Distributed Agency and the (Un)manageable Self

Having considered the ways in which the choosing self and disease are envisioned and reified within self-management discourse, and the paradoxical subjectivities that emerge as bipolar patients attempt to locate themselves within and properly enact this paradigm, it is useful to return to Tricia's hospitalization narrative. How are we to conceptualize a managing self who agentively "knows" and "decides" that she needs to visit the hospital, yet desires—and then orchestrates—the passive experience of "being hospitalized"? What kind of relationship between self-control and unmanageability is constituted, as "hospitalization" becomes a drawn-out process of negotiation and scheduling, while its necessity remains a foregone conclusion? And what are the implications of Tricia's final act, if the distinction between readable disease sign and self-management practice collapses, and cutting becomes a form of calculated—albeit not clinically sanctioned—rational choice? As we will see, under some circumstances, bipolar self-managers are able to claim certain kinds of *provisional* and *distributed* agency, exemplified by unexpected and contradictory practices such as Tricia's. These forms of agency bear consideration because, although they are produced through the very technologies of self-surveillance and rational calculation that characterize ideal neoliberal personhood, they are constitutive of a *heterotopic* (Foucault 1984) model of selfhood and choice that poses challenges to the presumed self-knowledge and integrity of choosing subjects. They also are significant because their availability hinges upon the consumer's degree of access to institutional and social support structures that reach beyond the self-disease dyad; for this reason, reflecting on the conditions of possibility for distributing agency through mood disorder self-management helps to reveal the role of sociopolitical and economic contexts in shaping self-management's heterogeneous meanings and practices. The import of such contexts has been widely neglected by clinicians and in policy initiatives that focus on self-management as individualized activity (Moore et al. 2015).

"What Goes Down, Comes Back Up": Agency as a Passive, Partial, or Provisional Project

One genre of self-management narrative that support group members sometimes told was that of a particularly difficult day or moment that the member was able to overcome *not* by acting upon themself or the disease, but by waiting. Reflecting on such incidents, group members would remark that even when, for example, they felt suicidal, they knew that "the good thing about bipolar is—what goes down, comes back up" and they could, therefore, count on bipolar disorder itself to bring about the change in mood that they desired but could not willfully produce. This sort of wisdom did a great deal of work to carve out a space of partial agency for the bipolar patient, and to shift the paradigm from one in which the disease could only either control or be controlled to a more fluid and distributed conceptualization of agentive management. In claiming such knowledge about the nature of bipolar disorder, members could thus recuperate a form of choice—though one unlike that of the envisioned somatic self—via the very quality of temporally unfolding vicissitudes that rendered the disease and the manager inextricable.

Confronted phenomenologically with the limitations of the ideology of direct and complete self-governance, support group members at times elaborated complex alternative models of self and agency. Tricia, for instance, took pains to parse her own repertoire of possible behaviors and actions into those that were predictable and under her full control, and those that were not. Recounting a time in which she had defaulted on her credit card payments because of hypomanic compulsive shopping, relied on her parents' financial support to rescue her from debt, and then immediately made the same mistake again, Tricia theorized her excessive spending as made up of both unmanageable and deliberate, reasonable, or even therapeutic components:

> I guess it's a release. It's something you can't control and yet in some ways it makes me feel normal, 'cause normal people go and spend money. I don't spend it on like . . . a whole bar. I go and buy a shower curtain. And you know what? You probably need the things to go with the shower curtain. And you know? The toilet paper's piled up in the corner; we probably need the thing to hold the toilet paper so let's spend fifty dollars on it. So they're *sensible* things, which is kind of weird. But they're—they add up, you know?

Choosing/succumbing to this kind of lapse in self-management, however, did not completely place Tricia outside of the project of vigilance and awareness. Instead, Tricia positioned herself in a provisionally agentive relationship with her bipolarity, through which she could coordinate with or work around those disordered behaviors that eluded full managerial regimentation. When asked whether she ever stopped herself from compulsively buying something, Tricia replied that she typically did not attempt to do so,

> but I'm pretty good about saving the receipts. That's usually my way of curing it . . . You know, I'll keep one thing and then I'll take the rest back. I've gotten pretty good about that; probably drive Target and Joanne's crazy but—I really don't do it every week—but it is a constant in my life that I have to be aware of.

Tricia's "cure" thus draws upon technologies of the self that are central to clinical self-management discourse, such as the cultivation of attentiveness in order to recognize regularities and modify imbalances. In so doing, however, she is able to articulate a claim to rational choice and responsibility as a self who can only ever be *incompletely* managed.

Another way in which some bipolar group members modeled a distributed form of agency was through a discourse of "faking it" and the consequences therein. Faking it—or performing mood stability in spite of one's "actual" state of hypomania or depression—was a powerful self-disciplining technique with real and often far-reaching effects for the consumer. Described at times as a painful mask that one could put on for the sake of "holding it together" for a particularly significant event, faking it could also refer to a more sustained strategy for functioning that was nonetheless experienced as less authentic than something felt to underlie it. One woman in the support group, for example, recounted how after a month-long psychiatric hospitalization, she had summoned the strength to return to work and "fake" her way to success in her corporate career:

> I told myself, "they're all expecting me to fail. I'm not going to. I'm smarter than these people and I'm going to prove them wrong by showing them just how well I can do here." Whenever I am feeling bad or disconnected from my coworkers, I tell myself that the joke is on them; they have *no idea* what I'm really thinking or feeling.

When discussed in these terms, faking it indeed began to sound not unlike a realizable instantiation of the clinical self-management ideal, in which the sovereign self transcends the isolable disease through constant micro-acts of self-surveillance and rational choice. Yet most of the time, such narratives were immediately followed by an acknowledgment that faking it was a tenuous and risky endeavor because the "disease," never truly or permanently contained, would ultimately exert its own agency with a force proportional to that with which the manager had suppressed it. Thus, those who were able to perform stability at a given time or place reported experiences of uncontrollable rage or immobilizing sadness, often redirected toward family members or spouses, which they attributed to a sort of calculus of managerial rebalancing. Tricia, for example, recounted an incident in which she returned home after controlling herself for several days during a family emergency:

I walked in the back door and [my boyfriend] hadn't cleaned out the lit-ter box, and I completely went berserk. Like he could have been sleeping with someone else, you know what I mean? Like, in the bed! So it's like I sometimes can steel myself but then it's gonna be a nightmare. Then it's cutting and it might be hospitalization.

In this more distributed model of agency, self-management and choice came to refer not only to the kinds of technologies of the self imagined to be enactable in the biomedical paradigm, but also to the cultivation of an intuition about when and to what degree to *defer* management. This intuition was based on a reflexive understanding of self-governance as fundamentally multifaceted, partial, and distributed temporally as well as across various human and nonhuman actors.

Managing the Fragmented and Unreliable Self

In addition to taking up rational choice and self-surveillance in order to model a form of agency other than that of the reified choosing subject, bipolar self-managers also articulated a model of responsibility based on a nontransparent self. As discussed earlier, engaging in expert self-management enactments paradoxically required that group members index and become acutely aware of their unreliability as predictable or continuous selves. As such, their claims to agentive action (or non-action) emerged neither from what Foucault et al. (1988) described as the modern moral imperative to know oneself entirely, nor from an unproblematic notion of somatic individuality, but instead out of a rec-ognition of self-knowledge as inherently limited. In this manner, Tricia explained that while she experienced many of her own behaviors as *reactions*—outside of the purview of her ability to choose or even antic-ipate them—suicide was something that she could subject to rational choice and control with certainty:

I have always said: I'm not suicidal. I'm not. I said at this point, as much money and time as I've spent on this, I'd kick my own ass if I fail. It's pointless. It's not something [my parents] should worry about. But they do. I may have ideation, but I'm not gonna do it. And I know I won't . . . I can't predict how I'm gonna react—you know be it panic attacks or hiding or [laughs] you know, not bathing for several days—but I *know* I'm not gonna die. *That* I know.

In place of the absolutely locatable and knowable self envisioned in clinical discourse, then, Tricia's formulation enables her to possess a piece of expert self-knowledge and intentionality while simultaneously denying the possibility or necessity of full transparency.

Under the experienced conditions of shifting "disease" and elusive managerial selfhood, even the charting technologies emblematic of the self-management paradigm for mental illness could be repurposed in ways that foregrounded the fragmentation and distribution of the imagined singular and agentive self. For example, Tricia found it helpful to follow a self-management protocol of assessing her mood four times per day on a scale of one to twenty. But with such finely gradated intervals, she often claimed that it was difficult to discern for herself whether "I am a fourteen or a seventeen right now," or even at times to know "with a mixed episode if I'm really bad or sorta bad or just a little less than normal." These ambiguities did not lead Tricia to abandon the management technique altogether, but rather facilitated a shift in the practice, rendering calculation of self and disease an intersubjective and distributive project. Specifically, Tricia stated that within moments of hearing her voice on the telephone, her mother could provide a read of her true mood level: "I can say 'hello' and she can tell me with an amazing amount of accuracy where I am on a scale of one to twenty." By diligently tracking her mother's instantaneous impressions of her depression or mania each day, Tricia in some ways instantiated the biomedical relationship of responsible choosing subject disciplining isolable "disease," yet did so through a displacement of the boundaries of the free embodied individual.

Tricia similarly talked about a list of "how to let your boyfriend know what he should look for" that she had half-jokingly developed with her therapist. Functioning as a sort of algorithm for quantifying and interpreting her observable and presumably symptomatic behaviors, Tricia's list, she felt, was her method of imparting her own self-management expertise to her nonperceptive boyfriend: "I've deliberately set that up. My boyfriend's got, you know, 'here are your visible steps, 'cause you obviously can't spot it otherwise.'" While thus maintaining a form of authority, Tricia simultaneously models, through the list, a gradual expansion of the boundaries of agentive self-management from within the single actor to between the couple:

How to let your boyfriend know what he should look for:
    If you stay in your pajamas one day, it's nothing to worry about; you're having a bad day.
    If you stay in your pajamas two days, it's time to ask, "honey, are you okay?"
    If you stay in your pajamas for three days, then you ask, "maybe you should call your therapist?"
    Four days, you call the therapist for her.

Even Tricia's language in her narration (above) of the how-to list itself reflects the shifting and multilayered aspects of agentive action emergent through her self-management practice. What begins as a set of instructions by, to, and about herself ("how to let *your* boyfriend know; *you're* having a bad day") gives way to a blurring of the positions of manager, actor, and observed (If *you* stay in your pajamas for three days, then *you* ask "maybe *you* should call your therapist?"), and finally produces a full relocation of agency and self-control ("*you* call the therapist for her").

Hospitalization, Revisited

Thus, a close examination of the kinds of subjectivity enacted by bipolar self-managers foregrounds a significant destabilization of—but not complete departure from—the reified notion of agentive selfhood upon which the therapeutic modality is based. It suggests, more broadly, that the choosing subject of liberal democracies may be less of a contained and transparent self-modulating or maximizing rational actor, and more of a never-fully knowable or controllable, "shifting" (Ewing 1990) self whose agency resides in the negotiated spaces between action and inaction, and is distributed beyond the body of the individual. Framed as such, the exchange between Jessie and Tricia about knowing and deciding that one must "be hospitalized" begins to gain intelligibility: It points to the elusive and paradoxical aspects of self-surveillance and control, and foregrounds the ways in which conscious self-management makes visible its own limits. By cutting, Tricia acts agentively, in collaboration with her boyfriend, to the end of *being hospitalized* passively. "Hospitalization" thus stands in for an act of self-management, a form of intersubjective agency, and a refusal to inhabit the position of choosing subject. That Tricia's act of cutting herself serves, in her narrative, both as an index of her unmanageability and as a recuperation of a form of agency, compels us to consider a model of self-management in which the patient does not act upon an isolable and static disease, but rather around and through shifting phenomena that overlap with personhood.

Conclusion

In *The Birth of the Clinic*, Foucault (1973) traces the origins of the contemporary biomedical model, in which disease is reconfigured as discrete bodily lesion, to the work of Bichat and other French anatomists in the late eighteenth century. For Foucault, this ontological shift is closely related to the emergence of a mode of inquiry that he terms the "anatomo-clinical gaze," the basis of which lies not in the experiences and symptoms of living patients, but in the dissection of the corpse. This medical gaze is multisensorial but ultimately guided by the "figure of the visible invisible" (Foucault 1973, 170): "Multi-sensory perception is merely a way of anticipating the triumph of the gaze that is represented by the autopsy; the ear and hand [of the clinician] are merely temporary, substitute organs until such time as death brings to truth the luminous presence of the visible" (165).

Inverting Foucault's title to describe a turn that he calls "the death of the clinic," Nikolas Rose asserts that in the contemporary age of the brain, "[t]he clinical gaze has been supplemented, if not supplanted, by [a] molecular gaze, which is itself enmeshed in a 'molecular' style of thought about life itself" (Rose 2007, 12). In this new style of thought, Rose argues, bodies are no longer envisioned and acted upon primarily at the "molar" level of organs, tissues, and lesions. Rather, they are molecularized; technologies of visualization are overshadowed by technologies of mobilization and optimization, and "our somatic, corporeal neurochemical individuality has become opened up to choice, prudence, and responsibility" (8).

Contrary to Rose's claims, however, my findings suggest that the paradigm of clinical self-management does not escape, and indeed relies upon, the notion of the culprit object or lesion in its formulations of the managing self and that which is managed.[16] Bipolar self-managers are promised in the clinical literature that by inhabiting the anatomo-clinical gaze and turning it in upon themselves, they too will render the invisible visible, locating, bringing to light, and cutting apart the bipolar "disease" from the true rational self. It is the failure of bipolar phenomena to conform, through self-management enactments, to a figuration as fixed structural condition that at times brings about provisional styles of agentive selfhood.

I have argued that the relationship between selfhood and disease entity envisioned as enactable in the self-management literature for bipolar consumers—which relies more broadly on contemporary notions of the transparent choosing subject—is unsustainable in a way that draws particular attention to the limitations of somatic selfhood. As bipolar consumers cultivate and perform what is taken as expertise and responsible behavior within the self-management paradigm, they must, paradoxically, index and increasingly recognize themselves as uncertain, discontinuous, unreliable, and never fully knowable. Furthermore, their efforts to predict, calculate, and discipline the bipolar "disease," while valuable, ultimately foreground the absence of a singular agentive subject and the inextricability of bipolar phenomena from the expression of the managing self. As a result, bipolar self-management is sometimes productive of what we might consider to be a more nuanced and realistic model of agency as distributed across multiple actors and technologies, yet as always provisional and incomplete.

The condition of being putatively irrational by virtue of a psychiatric diagnosis, but simultaneously compelled to perform constant rational self-surveillance, positions some of the bipolar self-managers in this chapter to draw our attention to the unexpected forms of agency that are possible within this paradoxical space. However, these contradictions of governmentality, and the ways that its technologies both presume and elude rationality and transparency, extend beyond mentally ill subjects. My findings here thus contribute to a growing recognition within anthropology of the ways in which mental illnesses and treatment modalities do not exist outside of, but rather co-constitute and articulate with, conditions of modernity (Carr 2011; Martin 2007; Schüll 2006; Molé 2008). The dilemma of self-control—of, as Saint Augustine (1955) confessed, being a self that is torn apart by itself—is not a new one; yet, it is a dilemma that seems particularly relevant at a moment in which we are both pressed by social and political economic forces to manage our selves to an intense, unprecedented degree, and simultaneously (or perhaps, therefore) potentially more aware than ever of the impossibility of this management. Indeed, the widespread use of psychoactive medication epitomizes this concurrent dilemma and possibility: We now have a technical means by which we can manage our selves, but those very means also communicate the fact of our necessarily incomplete autonomy.[17]

The model of agency and selfhood that is elaborated by Tricia and some of the other bipolar self-managers in this chapter can be characterized as *ecological* or *cybernetic*, in the Batesonian (Bateson 1972) sense of subordinating the importance of intimate self-knowledge or bounded individual coherence, and foregrounding the distribution of control—including self-control—across a network of complementary human and nonhuman actors (see also Latour 1987). Such a model invites consideration of the forms of moral responsibility and choice that are available to the discontinuous and never entirely knowable subject. Judith Butler (2001, 2005) writes extensively on these possibilities, arguing that the inherent nonsingularity of the self accounts for the unattainability of full transparency and is simultaneously the precondition for questions of responsibility:

> I want to suggest that the very meaning of responsibility . . . cannot be tied to the conceit of transparency. Indeed, to take responsibility for oneself is to avow the limits of any self-understanding and to establish this limit not only as a condition for the subject, but as the predicament of the human community itself . . . I cannot think the question of responsibility alone, in isolation from the Other, or if I do, I have taken myself out of the mode of address that frames the problem of responsibility from the start. (Butler 2001, 37–38)

In a different manner, philosopher Annemarie Mol proposes a related shift in considering issues of responsible and good action from a "politics of who" to a "politics of what" (2002), or from a "logic of choice" to a "logic of care" (Mol 2008). The ideal of choice, Mol argues, "carries a whole world with it: a specific mode of organizing action and interaction; of understanding bodies, people and daily lives; of dealing with knowledge and technologies" (7). Viewing action through the lens of choice, encoded in the language of market rationality and rights of citizenship, then, obscures as many possibilities as it liberates for patients. According to Mol, "in care practices patients are not passive at all. They are active. However, they do not primarily figure as subjects of choice, but as the subjects of all kinds of activities" (7). A characterization of bipolar self-management as agentive action that complicates and exceeds the relationships presupposed by the figures of the somatic consumer and reified disease offers a productive site for an interrogation of the modern subject of choice.

The story of bipolar self-management with which we have engaged is one in which the limitations of the clinical modality—and, more broadly, of neurochemical selfhood and neoliberal agency (Gershon 2011)—are brought out *through* its practice. In other words, rather than focusing on the ways in which self-management practices themselves resist, undermine, or contradict the clinical discourse, I wish to draw attention to the unexpected forms of agency that are embedded within, and emerge directly out of, its embodiment in certain contexts. In this regard, Povinelli's notion of an "otherwise"—an alternative social project or way of being whose participants "seem to be structurally located within normative worlds in such a way that their everyday actions are heterotopic whether they intend them to be or not" (Povinelli 2011, 7)—is useful: If expert enactments of clinical self-management are never productive of the forms of subjectivity and agency that the paradigm posits, then under what conditions do they lead to the sorts of workable or even empowering alternative models described in this section—and when do these enactments, instead, call into being the world of inescapable self-doubt and distressing paralysis described by James? It is the contention of this book, elaborated in the next several chapters, that clinical self-management is a heterogeneous mode that differentially produces and forecloses various possibilities for agentive selfhood based on the socioeconomic context in which it is set. More specifically, these class-stratified versions of self-management reflect ideologically and help to reinforce a *moral and political economy of agency*, in which those with access to fewer resources are made to aspire to an impossible-to-attain degree of autonomous self-control, while those of greater means are thought to benefit more from forms of self-management that involve the distribution of agency across external supports. As we will find in the next chapters, an intertwined system of policy-driven economic constraints and professional norms and strategies constitutes and naturalizes a mental healthcare landscape in which self-management as livable, heterotopic otherwise is sanctioned for some patients and denied others.

3

"I've Put in My Time"

Normative Trajectories and Structural Contradictions in the Helping Professions

How a Rescuer Lets Go

The day I learn that my practicum supervisor, Abigail, is resigning from Wellness Behavioral Health (WBH)—and from community mental health altogether—begins like many others: First, a dark morning commute from Hyde Park to the agency.[1] I am running late for a therapy session, anxiously glancing at the clock while navigating the rush hour traffic on Lake Shore Drive. I consider calling the office so that the receptionist can tell my client—if he even shows up today—that I am on my way; optimistically decide to hold off for ten more minutes and see how much more of the distance I have traversed by then. A radio newscaster issues ominous words about a winter storm on its way, which I am dismayed to realize will be in full force at 8:30 pm when I begin my drive home. Leaving work early is not an option today, because this evening is the introductory session of an adolescent girls' "coping skills" group that I have been told I must co-facilitate with a staff therapist in spite of our unresolved ideological differences. The requirement that I co-lead this group is not rooted in a consideration of either the clients' best interests or my professional development; rather, it is because my presence in the group, by virtue of my status as a student intern, brings down the client co-pay rate, thereby increasing the group's enrollment. It is going to be a long day.

At last I arrive—only six minutes late; not so bad—at the parking lot of the agency's dilapidated clinic in a working-class suburb on the outskirts of the West Side of Chicago. I rush past a hot dog stand, sidestepping puddles and patches of dirty ice while attempting to clear my mind and shift into counselor mode. My first scheduled therapy session of the day is with a boy and his foster father, with whom I have been meeting since the fall in spite of my lack of formal training (up until now) in family therapy. I push back encroaching worries about whether I am actually helping any of my clients, along with the counter-worry that even if (by some accident, surely) I *am*, any progress we make will be lost when a new counseling intern takes my place in a few months. I remind myself that supposedly everyone, not just the clinical ethnographer, feels like an imposter during therapy practicum; that according to our group supervisor, many of the agency's clients *enjoy* working with interns because what we lack in experience we make up for in energy and enthusiasm; that I just need to *get out of my head*, as Abigail is fond of telling me.

Now in front of the building, I burst through the double glass doors—onto which are mounted a framed copy of the mission statement of the now-defunct health network that was acquired by WBH—and into the clinic's waiting area. Seven empty vinyl armchairs stare back at me. Either my client is a no-show today or he is running even later than I am.

Relieved, I cross the waiting area and enter my office—a large but uncomfortable and windowless space that I have attempted to brighten through the addition of a halogen lamp and an upholstered IKEA chair. I sit down at my desk with the intention of catching up on some progress notes from earlier in the week while I can still recall what transpired during those therapy sessions.[2] But first, I open my work email. As usual, I delete the majority of my new messages without reading or even opening them; WBH is a mammoth organization, with dozens of programs and facilities, and very few of the circulated communications are directly relevant to my job.[3] I come across an email announcing a Wellness employee's resignation (subject line: "WBH staff Continuing her Career Path"), replete with that genre's familiar tropes of evolution and professional growth, and nearly hit the "delete" button before noticing Abigail's name. The email reads:

Hi Everyone,
I wanted to let you know that Abigail Miller has resigned. Abigail has been with the organization for 10 years now and during that time she has really grown into the clinician she is today. Abigail started out work-

ing in the shelter program we had at WBH as a case manager and then evolved over time into taking a full time clinician position in which she has many years of training and experience working with our trauma clients. She has been a great resource to her colleagues when working with trauma patients as well as a supervisor to students over the years. Abigail is a Licensed Marriage and Family Therapist (LMFT) as well as a Licensed Clinical Professional (LCPC). She currently works part time and has a private practice as well. Abigail plans to continue to pursue her private practice and also hopes to teach courses at the College level. We are so happy for her and wish her well as she continues her career path helping others and teaching the next generation of therapists. We appreciate the many years of service that Abigail has provided to so many clients over the years. She will truly be missed.

I had always felt grateful to have been the only student intern my year at this WBH clinic, out of ten interns in total, assigned to work under Abigail. Whereas most of my colleagues' supervisors were just a couple of years out of clinical training themselves, significantly younger than me, and disinterested in—if not outright hostile toward—the psychoanalytic styles of therapeutic intervention that I had been taught to use, Abigail was in her late forties and had an air of wisdom refined over the course of her decade of experience as a therapist. In an agency where so many of the staff clinicians provided short-term, manualized treatments focused on cognitive and behavioral modification, Abigail had carved out a niche at WBH conducting intensive, years-long introspective relational work with severely traumatized clients using her own spin on an integrative therapeutic modality previously unknown to me called Internal Family Systems (IFS). Abigail was good at what she did, and everyone at WBH knew as much: She was regarded with a kind of reverence by the younger clinicians, and essentially was given free rein by her superiors at the agency—who undoubtedly realized that a therapist of Abigail's caliber was a steal at her $25 per hour salary—to run her own show. As my supervisor, Abigail respected and understood my critical anthropological engagement with psychotherapeutic paradigms and practices; at the same time, she tried to "keep [me] honest" by letting me know when she thought I was using my intellect (or what she frequently referred to as my "academic part," adapting the terminology of IFS) as a way to shield myself from a deeper empathic connection with my clients. Together, we had drafted and signed a "Supervision Learning Agreement" stating that through her judicious attention to our moments of "parallel process" in supervision,[4] Abigail would help me understand the "use of the self" in a therapeutic relationship and to experience therapeutic transformation firsthand, which we hoped would lead me to genuinely "buy in" to the therapy process. On many occasions, Abigail had voiced her commitment to training me (our plan had been to co-facilitate Abigail's well-regarded trauma therapy group in the spring), to treating her clients, and more broadly to working at Wellness Behavioral Health. Despite—and perhaps also because of—her unconventionally long tenure as an agency therapist, I had in no way seen the resignation coming.

Later that day, Abigail and I meet to "process" the news. Abigail apologizes for the impersonal manner in which I had to learn of her resignation plans. She explains that the all-staff email was not supposed to go out until after she had gotten a chance to speak to me personally, and that, in the interest of "making this very clean," she had not even discussed her departure in advance with other senior clinicians. She then offers, with a certain urgency, the following account of her decision to leave community mental health:

> It's not like I just burned out one day. Over the past ten years, I've burned out and then had second and third and fourth winds! You know, I'm a socialist at heart . . . and I put far more time into community mental health than most clinicians with my level of skill and experience. Two years ago, I realized I needed to cut back and I switched from full-time to two days per week. And that helped, but eventually it wasn't enough . . . I'm 48 now, and I've put too many of my other interests on hold for too long. In community mental health, no one is going to say "you seem overworked; let me reduce your workload." They *can't* . . . Honestly, a lot of people just do the two years [of supervised agency work] until they get their license, and then they escape after that. I wasn't like that, probably in part because of my childhood. I was always ignoring my own needs to take care of my mother—I'm a rescuer! But recently, I realized that I could do one day a week of private practice in [a middle-class suburb near WBH], in addition to the three days a week in [another affluent suburb near Abigail's

home and far from the agency]. Realized I was *willing* to do that, and that I could actually give some of my clients the *option* [of continuing to work with Abigail as their therapist]. And that's when I finally felt like I could let go. I mean, it will *cost* them—they'll have to save and be empowered and really work for this—but when I realized that I could slide [the fee], and that was something I was *willing* to do—at least for now; I don't know if that will be sustainable long-term—then I started to seriously think about doing this.

Listening to Abigail's narrative, I was struck at the time by its intense degree of ambivalence, particularly as this stood in contrast to her typically confident self-presentation. Questions lingered in my mind for months following her departure: Abigail had offered several plausible explanations for her desire to leave WBH—she was exhausted, chronically overworked, and wanted more time to pursue her other interests. Why, I wondered, in spite of the sufficiency of these reasons and the apparent support of her employer, had Abigail seemed intent, in her account, on calling into question her own agency in the decision by working to demonstrate that she was ultimately overcome—almost against her own will—with a need to leave her workplace? Why had she spoken with pride of her unusually lengthy commitment to community mental health, implying that this commitment could be read as an expression of her core socialist values, only to recast the same commitment, moments later, as a symptom of her dysfunctional childhood? Perhaps most curiously, what was the performative significance of Abigail's inclusion in her narrative of the bargain that she had to make with herself before she could give herself permission to become a private practice clinician—a bargain whose long-term sustainability was uncertain by her own admission?

This chapter explores the above questions by situating the everyday struggles of agency work within an analysis of the normative professional trajectory of psychotherapists in the Chicago area.[5] I make the case that therapists are bound within a structurally contradictory profession that prescribes upward mobility on one hand, and a selfless commitment to helping the underprivileged on the other. A profound sense of unease, born out of these divergent imperatives, is instilled in therapists early in their professional socialization process, and remains with them—close to the surface at some moments and all-but-imperceptible at others—as they move along a career path that normatively begins in an agency (working with the poor) and culminates in private practice (providing services predominantly to the middle class). We will see that therapists' career paths—and in particular the progressive distancing of therapists from working-class populations over the course of their careers—are propelled by powerful political economic and institutional forces, exerted incrementally on mundane aspects of the therapist's everyday existence, that often coalesce to render agency work materially and affectively unsustainable. Indeed, it is the accumulation of these routine manifestations of structural contradiction that helps to produce the thanklessness and exhaustion that characterize agency work and that animates the normative turn to private practice.

But while therapists may look to private practice for a resolution to the unarticulated structural contradictions that they experience, they instead discover that the same tensions persist and reverberate across the professional life course. Furthermore, therapists' feelings of ambivalence regarding their own professional desires and frustrations, and regarding the gradual convergence of their own and their patients' class statuses, lead them to formulate their professional trajectories in overly individualizing terms that minimize or occlude the role of these enduring structural contradictions. This strategy of internalizing structural constraints in the form of personal ambivalence, and of dealing with that ambivalence through what I will term "professional narrative self-management," enables therapists to hold on to a sense of partial agency and integrity under compromised, frustrating, and at times heart-wrenching circumstances. The price of this self-preservation, however, is that therapists lose access to a language for recognizing and critiquing the structural conditions that simultaneously inculcate, valorize, exploit, obstruct, and penalize their will to help the mentally ill poor. Furthermore, therapists' discursive strategies for the disavowal of political economy extend beyond the conceptualization and navigation of their professional trajectories, and into therapists' understandings of the relationship between their billing practices and their clients' therapeutic needs. In that context, therapists' strategies of disavowal ultimately help to constitute two moments in the therapist's normative professional life course—agency work and private practice—as distinct and non-overlapping clinical spaces, and to naturalize disparate classes of clients and forms of treatment as "therapeutically appropriate" to each of these clinical spaces.

"Not in It for the Money": Professional Socialization into Contradiction

The psychotherapists that I encountered in my research—most of whom held master's-level degrees in either counseling or social work[6]—were structurally compelled to advance along a normative career trajectory that began with a few years of work in an agency setting and culminated in the establishment of a full-time private practice.[7] Only through adherence to this trajectory, and in particular to its proscription against providing direct services to agency clients for much longer than the two years necessary to become eligible for clinical licensure (a prerequisite for independent practice), could the therapists—whose educational debt was often substantial and whose credentials carried the lowest status in the mental health professional hierarchy (Wolfson 1999; Ehrenreich 1985)—hope to accrue even a modest amount of monetary reward or disciplinary respect.[8] At the same time, however, my therapist informants were professionally socialized to envision themselves, and the work that they did, as selfless, unmotivated by profit, and grounded in a commitment to serving the underprivileged. In this regard, engaging long term in the very work at an agency that marked a therapist as unsuccessful paradoxically indexed and performed the therapist's dedication to their professional mission. Leaving agency work for private practice, in turn, provoked ambivalence even if it was understood by the therapist to be sanctioned, for it was tantamount to a shift in the therapist's clinical attention from the poor to the middle class, and could be read as evincing the therapist's self-interested aspiration to raise their own class status.[9] To further complicate matters, therapists in agency settings often had to contend with bureaucratic constraints on their clinical practices so intrusive as to constantly risk frustrating the therapist's ability to see their work as worthwhile or fulfilling (Brodwin 2011, 2013; Hopper 2001; Ware et al. 2000).

Structural Dissonance and Frustrated Expectations
in Therapist Training

From the moment they matriculate (if not earlier) at a two-year master's degree program in counseling or clinical social work, future therapists are interpellated—and learn to narrate themselves—as self-sacrificing, socially conscious care workers or "helping professionals." Over the course of their educational training and concurrent 1–2 years of unpaid agency-based clinical internships, they are socialized to equate this identity with, among other things, a willingness to prioritize the needs of others over their own (Buch 2013) and to embrace the credo of "not being in this line of work for the money." Therapy students are indirectly informed, through their graduate schools' promotional materials and mission statements, that theirs are higher-order values than personal gain or material comfort. School documents describe curricula "focused on . . . social justice issues," declare a dedication to "working toward a more just and humane society through . . . service to the community," and reference the profession's "historic commitment to serve oppressed, disadvantaged and at risk members of our society." Students repeatedly hear from instructors in the classroom, and from clinical supervisors at their practicum sites, that they are not the sorts of people who are motivated by wealth and that, had they wanted to make money, they would have chosen a different profession. They joke nervously with one another about not caring that the starting salary they will earn in a clinical position after graduation will be lower than what they were making in the jobs they held before starting graduate school, and about the $30,000 or more in loans that they are amassing and will never be able to repay (Yoon 2012; Mulvey 2011; Whitaker 2008).

Social work and counseling trainees also come to understand that staying true to the ethos of their professions comes at a cost in social as well as economic capital. In their coursework, they read and discuss classic essays encouraging them to take pride in, and keep alive, the indispensable yet marginal and delegitimized forms of "practice-based" knowledge that they are said to be uniquely positioned to acquire through work "on the ground" with the indigent. One such essay, read by a number of my informants at various institutions, asserts that "[h]idden beneath the trappings of scientific respectability and social approval are the heartlines of the [social work] profession. . . . Because the material lodged in these rich veins is not the official coin of the realm, it forms the guilty knowledge of social work" (Weick 2015, 35). The essay passionately advises social workers to "speak and honor . . . the wisdom that has formed the basis of our guilty knowledge" (39); to resist, as a field, the temptation to emulate higher-status clinical disciplines such as psychology, "whose stature is equated with research productivity" (35). To be sure, this is not the only—or even, in many current-day counseling and social work programs, the predominant—narrative of professional identity imparted to psychotherapy students; in many programs, counselors and social workers are in fact encouraged to become well-versed in "evidence-based" practices and theories so as to gain access to a wider range of clinical work settings outside of agencies (Howard et al. 2003). Nonetheless, the experience of classroom training seems to prepare therapy students to enter the clinical workforce with an attachment—albeit an ambivalent one—to the mission of doing low-status work (Borenzweig 1981).

But alongside this cultivation of a sense of pride in working with clients of lower social and economic status—and thereby in relegating their own status to a correspondingly low position relative to other mental health professionals—master's-level social work and counseling trainees and entry-level clinicians are socialized to view agency work as a time-limited career stage "in the trenches" that one must endure before joining the higher status therapy ranks, rather than as a lifelong obligation. According to this understanding of the clinician's professional trajectory, beginning therapists are expected to "put in [their] time" (as it is sometimes described) at an agency for approximately 2–3 years, or for as long as it takes to accumulate the number of supervised hours they need to be eligible to sit for their field's clinical licensing examination,[10] after which point it is assumed and normatively demanded that they either move up to a supervisory position or leave agency work altogether.

While this norm is seldom explicitly voiced in the classroom, social work and counseling instructors—many of whom work primarily as private practice therapists and teach on the side[11]—tend to draw on their professional experiences as clinicians when explaining psychotherapeutic theories or intervention techniques, even typing and distributing de-identified transcripts of therapy sessions with their current patients to illustrate course concepts or to engage students in psychotherapeutic role-playing exercises. Such pedagogy works to set up trainees' expectations of the roles that they will, or should, inhabit as clinicians—expectations that then radically fail to map onto the realities of their professional duties at a therapy internship or in an entry-level clinical position. Upon arriving in agency settings, therapists rapidly discover that their day-to-day work with clients entails an assortment of not traditionally psychotherapeutic—and at times tedious or physically unpleasant—tasks colloquially (if not always in billing code terminology) glossed "case management," including helping clients schedule medical appointments or buy groceries, waiting in long lines with clients at the social security office, or assisting clients with low-income housing applications. As a new clinician at Community Recovery Center (CRC), for example, I was asked to inspect a client's home for bedbugs on one occasion, and in another instance was required—in spite of my squeamishness—to accompany a client to a surgical procedure in which small holes were burned into the client's iris with a laser. Such activities, while usually viewed by trainees and new therapists as worthwhile and essential to the maintenance of clients' mental health,[12] are not particularly glamorous or professionally rewarding by even modest standards. Moreover, the centrality of case management to the therapist's role as an agency clinician—coupled with the overwhelming paperwork burden generated by the compulsory mental health assessments, financial interviews, treatment plan updates, service notes, and case file audits that come to define the job for many therapists—is often difficult for therapists to reconcile with the type of work that they had believed they were being trained to perform on the basis of the clinical material presented to them in their graduate programs.

Allusions to this mismatch between therapeutic training and agency work in practice featured regularly in trainees' weekly group supervision sessions at WBH. Notably, over the course of the internship year, the quality of trainees' comments about the mismatch—as well as their stance toward it—gradually shifted as confusion and disappointment gave way to instrumentalism and nonchalance. For example, Denise—a personable and dynamic young intern who had arrived at WBH eager to practice the substance abuse counseling and cognitive-behavioral therapy techniques she had learned in her Clinical Mental Health Counseling program—expressed frustration throughout the fall and winter about the unexpected domination of case management activities in her client sessions. Presenting in group supervision one week on her attempts at psychotherapeutic work with a chronically depressed, divorced, former alcoholic client,[13] Denise began with a lament that in spite of her client's intelligence and insight, his overwhelming case management needs left no opening for the kinds of clinical interventions that were more compelling to Denise:

DENISE: I feel like there's *so much* [psychologically] interesting stuff going on with him, and right now all I'm doing is like "well, I think we should make a chore goal. What would you like to do? You want to apply to jobs? Ok, how many jobs do you want to apply to this week?" You know, so like, just little by little, picking off . . .

SUPERVISOR: So small victories along the way?

DENISE: I guess that's exactly right . . . I mean, I think a job would help him because it would kind of cut the boredom which would then reduce his loneliness. And that's another thing too, because he wanted to come [to therapy] weekly but he doesn't have funding— he's self-pay—and being cognizant of his financial trouble I said I think it might be better to just do biweekly for a little bit. 'Cause he didn't know about CountyCare, so then we had to do all the County-Care stuff. And so then we started applying to that because he didn't have health insurance—it's a lot for me! I literally don't know, it's sort of overwhelming, so that's why I'm trying to do these small goals. I mean I want to help him work on like journaling and stuff like that, because he's really smart. That's the thing, I wouldn't expect him to work at a clothing store or something, but it's like we need to find any job he can get. But then there's transportation: he has to take like two buses, three buses to get here. And then his *bike* was stolen recently. So he comes and it's like "I'm sorry I'm late; my bike was stolen and I had to walk four miles to get here from the last bus stop." And it's like, that's the thing, it's almost as overwhelming right now for me as it is for him.

SUPERVISOR: So, you can request specific donations from [the agency]. And then there's also—I know in the past, and I don't know if we have the money right now—but sometimes we've helped somebody, you know, find an apartment and pay for a deposit and furnish it.

There's also a form to fill out for any families that you have that you feel, maybe around the holidays, that they need some additional help. Like maybe to buy presents for the children or even just have a meal. They're really generous; families adopt the people we identify, and then usually they also send a card.

A discussion of the resources that Denise (and the rest of the interns) could access on behalf of clients for charitable donations and employment assistance ensued for the remainder of the group supervision meeting. At the end, our supervisor informed Denise that she was doing a good job with a tough case, and advised Denise about updates that she could make to her client's documented diagnoses that might enable him to qualify for Illinois state non-Medicaid funding for mental health services. Denise's clear weariness of getting swept along in an endless sea of practical problems to resolve—performatively conjured through her frenzied and self-interrupting case description, yet reframed by the supervisor as the achievement of "small victories along the way"—was never addressed. It was, I later realized, as though the group—in its obsessive and time-consuming efforts to collectively manage Denise's case—could not help but re-enact the very impossibility of attending to cognitive and psychic processes that had been so demoralizing to Denise when working with this client. As the meeting ended and we walked out of group supervision together, Denise muttered her common refrain to me: "Case management is the worst! This isn't why I went to school to become a counselor. I may as well go back to my old job [as a kindergarten teacher's assistant] if I have to do case management."

By the end of the internship year, Denise and the other interns were not necessarily any fonder of case management tasks than they had previously been, but the ways that they made sense of the imposition of this type of work on their therapeutic aspirations had transformed significantly. No longer taken aback or viscerally overwhelmed by the many distractions of agency work to their vision of professional fulfillment, therapy interns instead remarked that they were not bothered by the disjuncture, and that they were just trying to satisfy the requirements of the internship before moving on to the next step in their clinical careers. Case management, in this new formulation, became a tolerable short-term hurdle to overcome rather than a final professional destination with which to reckon. In Denise's case, so confident was she that case management could be compartmentalized to the internship experience and avoided afterward that, as a newly minted Licensed Professional Counselor, she declined any psychotherapy job offers that she suspected of "secretly" involving case management responsibilities. In this way, what began as a form of structural dissonance that emerged out of the tenacious and frustrating contradictions of clinical training was ultimately reworked by therapists as an unproblematic temporal process.

Interestingly, just as the normativity of this professional timeline was never fully articulated in the clinical training classroom, it was also circumvented in the context of formal group supervision interactions at WBH. Thus, when Denise and other interns reflected at the end of the year on their newfound association of case management with temporary, early-career work, the group supervisor—perhaps motivated by her own exceptional status as a long-term agency therapist—hastened to recast the distinction between case management and private practice therapy as a matter of choice and personal preference that was indifferent to career stage: "There's people who get bored by, you know, the worried well," she told the group. "And not that—I mean, [private practice patients] do have real problems—you know, but it's *different*. It's completely different. So it's figuring out where your strengths lie and what's the better fit for you." While the supervisor's comments offer a counternarrative to the therapy interns' normalization of the notion of "putting in time" at an agency and subsequently moving on to something more fulfilling, both accounts work to efface the structural conditions that lead the majority of therapists to experience case management—and, by extension, work with poor clients in agency settings—as disappointing, unfulfilling, and overwhelming—in the first instance by nullifying these tensions through the introduction of a temporal mechanism, and in the second by positing an individualized, nonstructurally induced cause of one's potential aversion to agency work.

Managing Contradiction in the Daily Flows of Agency Work

While generally left unnamed and at times even actively contested, the norm of exodus from the agency is deeply entrenched in its institutional processes, and comes to feel both desirable and inevitable to many psychotherapists (even as they might simultaneously feel guilty or ashamed for leaving as described previously): Many agencies (such as WBH) can only afford to keep their doors open either by relying on the unpaid labor of student interns, who must complete around twenty-one hours per week of clinical work during their second year of training as a requirement for graduation, or by taking advantage of the limited job options available to new, unlicensed clinicians to hire them at extremely low salaries.[14] In the latter case, as a supplement to the low wages, unlicensed employees are sometimes given an hour a week of supervision by a qualified licensed clinician at the agency. This service is apprehended by new therapists as a valuable commodity, as its increasingly common alternative requires the already-indebted counselor or social worker to pay a weekly out-of-pocket rate, comparable to the cost of a private psychotherapy session, for supervision from an independent clinician (Ungar and Costanzo 2007; Wilkinson and Suh 2012). Obviously, the tradeoff of receiving "free" clinical supervision in lieu of higher wages is no longer appealing or rational to a therapist once their licensure requirements have been met, at which point the agency salary may begin to feel prohibitively low.

Employment arrangements between new therapists and agencies are thus mutually beneficial, but they are structured in such a way as to indirectly communicate and validate the built-in assumption of their short duration. Supervisors often carry this message further by tacitly or explicitly acknowledging that the agency will exploit the therapist's labor during the limited period of time that they are able to do so. In other words, supervisors presume and effectively ensure that the therapist will "burn out" on agency work by placing unsustainable, exhausting, and at times physically degrading expectations on the therapist, typically rationalized through a discourse on the agency's own financial precarity. For example, therapists at CRC were incentivized with a small cash bonus to meet a productivity requirement that consisted of billing five hours per day of direct client services for state reimbursement. Each morning, therapists received an email with a bar graph depicting their own productivity from the previous day (and the week-to-date) and comparing it to the productivity of the other therapists on their team. The productivity standard was known by both therapists and supervisors to be unachievable within a 7.5-hour workday given that most days included several hours of (unbillable) time driving to and from the office to visit clients in the field, and taking into account the high volume of service notes and other forms of unbillable paperwork—the quality of which was regularly audited—that the therapist needed to produce on a daily basis. Nonetheless, supervisors seemed to realize that they could count on therapists to overwork themselves to whatever extent was needed to meet the billing requirement. One senior clinician explained that the reason the agency hired master's-level therapists like me was not only for our advanced training and clinical skills, but also because the agency was not required to compensate us for the many hours of overtime work that it implicitly relied on us to undertake. While one might not need to have a master's degree to do the job well, the supervisor added, a bachelor's-level employee holding the same position would, according to agency policy, have to get paid by the hour (rather than receive a fixed salary). Given the very high likelihood that the employee would routinely need to work more than forty hours per week, the supervisor concluded, a worker without a master's degree could potentially become too expensive for the agency to keep on its payroll.

To stay at, and often above, 100% productivity, many therapists remained at the agency after hours to do paperwork, ate lunch in their cars, and took work home over the weekends. One therapist, whose billable productivity was high but who tended to fall behind on his paperwork, liked to catch up by taking "staycation days"—that is, by using his paid time off of work to write service notes at home to avoid effecting a decline in his billing numbers.[15] Therapists were somewhat enticed to take on these uncompensated hours of labor by the prospect of the biannual productivity bonus, in spite of the fact that the bonus amounted to significantly less than equivalent pay for the overtime hours that they worked. More fundamentally, they were motivated by a normative pressure to perform their commitment to care work and their disregard for financial compensation.

Much of the time, agency work proceeded felicitously and therapists did not seem to struggle with ambivalence about the competing imperatives to feel good about doing uncompensated, low-level labor on one hand, and to seek higher status work with better remuneration on the other. But on occasion, some event or experience would break the flow of a therapist's everyday strategies for managing these contradictions, prompting ambivalence to rise to the surface. At CRC, a major winter storm was the cause for one such break. During the storm, therapists drove through dangerous weather conditions to keep their scheduled home and community visits with clients. The next morning, they found in their inboxes an email from the agency inviting therapists to "reward [themselves]" for their dedication by purchasing for them-selves a hot coffee or tea and submitting the receipt to the agency for reimbursement. Upon receiving the email, a normally even-tempered coworker commented to me: "This is insulting. I would almost prefer that they didn't give us anything at all." She went on to explain that she did this job because she cared about the clients, and as such, she didn't require an external reward for her efforts. However, she continued, if she *was* going to receive a thank-you from the agency—and driving in the ice and snow had indeed been quite treacherous, she noted—it ought to be something more substantial than a coffee. For this therapist, a woefully inadequate treat from the agency underscored and rendered problematic—rather than offset—the tacit norm that she remain disin-terested in compensation.

Enacting Agency (and Disavowing Structure) in Accounts of Post-Agency Work: Case Studies in Professional Life Course Narrative Self-Management

Nearly every therapist that I met while conducting my research began their clinical career by working in an agency setting. Among those who had been out of graduate training for a few years and obtained their clinical licenses, the majority had either already departed from agency work or were actively forming plans to do so in the near future. When I did encounter therapists who worked at community mental health agen-cies for significantly longer than the norm, they had usually ascended to supervisory positions that came with small-scale but non-negligible privileges such as a modest pay raise, reduced client caseload (to offset clinical supervisory duties), reduced billable productivity requirements, greater scheduling flexibility, or "dibs" on treating the most interest-ing, cooperative, or otherwise desirable clients. Even given these perks of promotion, agency work appeared to take a toll on its more senior clinicians as much as it did on its entry-level therapists. Across WBH and CRC, I watched two experienced clinical supervisors in addition to Abigail try (with varying degrees of success) to break away from agency work over the course of my twenty months of fieldwork.

The following discussion presents three case studies of therapists who had already transitioned (or partially transitioned) from agency work to private practice at the time of my interview with them. My aim in examining these cases is to foreground a phenomenon that I term *professional narrative self-management* wherein therapists attempt to work out—through the act of crafting a personal career trajectory narrative—the ambivalence, frustration, and guilt that stems from the structural contradictions that pervade their everyday work lives. For each case, I name and characterize what seems to me to be the primary strategy deployed by that therapist for smoothing out, imposing order upon, or otherwise making sense of a set of fundamentally inadequate yet inescapable options. I conclude with a meditation on the second-order effect—namely a sort of structural alienation—that is actualized in the moment of agentive individual self-narration.

Case 1: Claire (Strategy of Sublimation)

When I met Claire—a thirty-year-old Caucasian woman and Licensed Clinical Social Worker (LCSW) from what she describes as an educated, middle-class, Midwestern family—she was working full time at Wellness Behavioral Health as an outpatient therapist and supervisor of social work interns. Though she would mention regularly that her professional specialization (honed through dozens of hours of continuing education) and area of greatest interest was the treatment of trauma across the lifespan, much of Claire's clinical work at WBH consisted in running twelve-week-long cycles of a discipline-based "support group" for parents of children diagnosed with Attention Deficit Hyperactivity Disorder. At Claire's request, I co-facilitated two cycles of the parent group, which ran on Wednesday evenings concurrently with a children's counterpart group that met with another supervisor and intern one floor below. Each week, the children were sent home with worksheets bearing titles such as "You Can Know What to Do Without Being Reminded" and "You Can Learn to Sit Still," to be completed before the next group meeting and subsequently returned to the agency in the client's homework folder. Without fail, Claire seemed to devote at least half of the parent group's meeting time to the extraction of sheepish explanations of incomplete or lost assignments from the children's tired and hungry caretakers. Week after week, the parents would stare down at their phones and occasionally nod off as Claire perfunctorily chided them—her own boredom palpable—on the need to set better examples of organization and time management for their inattentive children. For the twelfth and final session, the two groups would reunite in a half-hearted "graduation" ceremony, after which Claire would promptly—if reluctantly—commence recruitment of the next cycle's clients.

I reconnected with Claire two years after completing my therapy internship. In the time since I had worked with her, Claire had resigned from her staff position at WBH, earned a certificate in Health and Wellness Coaching, and enrolled in a costly online PhD program in Integrative Medicine. She had also become a commission-based independent distributor of nutritional supplements for a multilevel marketing company. For the time being, Claire explained, she maintained part-time employment at another community mental health agency, where she primarily provided clinical supervision to service providers. But since leaving WBH, she went on, Claire had "establish[ed] [herself] as an entrepreneur," creating a "holistic wellness"-focused LLC through which she assisted clients around the world in "reaching [their] full potential" by offering them nutritional, weight management, and skin care products as well as integrative life coaching sessions via phone and Skype. It was into this business that Claire narratively projected herself and her professional future as a therapist, with agency work quietly receding from the horizon.

In our interview, Claire recounted a career trajectory driven, at first, by an increasing awareness of—and desire to actively intervene in—social and structural problems impacting the lives of school-aged children. Though she initially planned to major in early childhood development and elementary math and science education, the college courses that Claire undertook in those areas made her unexpectedly "receptive to a theme of non-school-related hardships which impeded children's learning." As a result of her exposure to this area of interest, Claire decided to switch her undergraduate major to social work with the goal of becoming a school social worker. Upon learning that she needed a master's degree in social work to obtain the job she wanted, she borrowed approximately $60,000 in student loans to attend a graduate program at an Ivy League university. "I was very focused on being located in the school in order to reduce barriers to services," she explained, "and did not want to engage in private practice."

At this point in the interview, Claire's narrative voice became more passive, as she described a series of contingent turns and disjointed opportunities that carried her along from one social service organization to another between 2008 (when she graduated with her MSW) and 2014 (when she enrolled in the doctoral program and began to move away from agency work):

My first job . . . was as an OB Social Worker. I provided case management and therapy to pregnant patients in the health center. I was paid well—25 dollars an hour—and enjoyed the work. I engaged in weekly supervision with my licensed supervisor, who pushed an understanding and application of systems theory and how it impacted my clients. I left after a year due to moving out of the area. My second job was a supervisor and individual and family therapist at a residential treatment facility for teens. I was not paid well, at fifteen an hour. It was not good working conditions, and I received sporadic supervision from an unqualified coworker. Some of the work was fulfilling, but mostly it was long, draining, thankless hours of endless work. One aspect which made this situation a poor fit for me was that I was bringing a trauma-informed, strengths-based perspective to treatment, while my coworkers were focused on a punishment-based approach. After earning my license I moved to another area and took a position as an outpatient therapist. I was surprised to learn that having a full license was not a requirement of the job and thought that I could have transitioned away from my previous position sooner. As an outpatient therapist I met individuals and families in the office to provide psychotherapy. After a few years I moved to the Chicago area where I continued to be an outpatient therapist [at WBH].

Absent from this portion of the narrative is any explanation of Claire's deviation—intentional or otherwise—from her career goal of becoming a school social worker. She offers no account of a shift in her clinical interests or of institutional factors that might have motivated her to abandon her single-minded focus on "being located in the school," in spite of having made a point of emphasizing this focus to me earlier in the interview. Instead, she matter-of-factly recounts an aimless trajectory in which pay rate does not correspond to level of experience, and qualifications associated with licensure are rendered unclear if not nonexistent. Claire makes mention once of her preferred therapeutic modality (trauma-informed, strengths-based), but gives no particular indication that her career moves afford her progressively better opportunities to work in this way (and indeed, my observations of her job responsibilities at WBH would suggest otherwise). At the same time, she stops short of naming or critiquing a system that repeatedly derails her efforts to follow through on the social mission for which she sought training. Even when she is able to articulate the complaint that her second job amounted to "long, draining, thankless hours of endless work," Claire immediately retreats from a structural analysis of her frustration and turns to an interpersonal one, citing incompatibilities between her own clinical orientation and that of her coworkers as the reason that the position was "a poor fit."

If Claire's style of narrating these four successive jobs performs and indexes an experience of floundering within a profession that inexplicably denies her the opportunity to carry out the very sorts of work to which it socializes her to feel a commitment, her description of the next phase in her career marks a reclaiming of Claire's sense of her own agency. In contrast with the passivity and aimlessness of her sentences noted above, Claire's account of returning to graduate school and establishing a private life coaching practice is couched in a language of choice, progress, and intentionality:

> While at WBH I was treating a few clients with Binge Eating Disorder (BED). I did my personal research for resources and attended conferences in order to obtain further training. When I attended the ANAD [National Association of Anorexia Nervosa and Associated Disorders] conference, I was surprised to see that they were presenting the same information I had already found on my own and deemed insufficient. I decided to return to school for the PhD program in order to add to the field specifically in creating more informed and holistic approaches to treating BED . . . I am now focused on expanding the research base related to how mind-body

practices support the change process . . . As I move forward in my career I will continue to focus on coaching and holistic wellness. Since establishing myself as an entrepreneur, I have become more mindful of financial considerations such as time for money compensation and the use of leveraged income . . . I've also changed my mindset away from accepting the expectation that I need to work 60 hours a week for a low salary which only compensated me for 40 hours and never have savings. I am now focused on working fewer hours, making more money, and utilizing technology . . . to grow my business. My goal is to work part-time from now on, without compromising my health, economic responsibilities, or family obligations.

Without directly acknowledging her rejection of the impossibilities of agency work, Claire nonetheless performs a turn away from grappling with structural issues—whether those impeding children's learning or those within the profession of social work—through her discursive mobilization of an entrepreneurial ethic of autonomy and self-determination. Thus, as she talks about making the transition from WBH to research and private practice, Claire agentively *deems* existing information insufficient, *decides* to add to her field, *establishes* herself, *changes* her mindset away from low expectations, *move[s] forward*, and *focuses* on her chosen values and goals. One may compare two parallel sentences in Claire's agency work and post-agency work narratives, each beginning with the phrase "I was surprised," to further illustrate Claire's discursive alignment of her own agency and authority with her retreat from social services: Whereas Claire's first narrative registers unactionable surprise over discovering, in hindsight, that her claim to authority was obscured by structural ambiguity ("I was surprised to learn that having a full license was not a requirement of the job and thought that I could have transitioned away from my previous position sooner"), her surprise "to see that [purported experts] were presenting the same information I had already found on my own and deemed insufficient" in the second passage indicates a recognition of her own authority that Claire is able to act upon.

Claire's social media presence in the persona of "Coach Claire"—a central element of her private practice business model—echoes and often visualizes the embrace of the tropes of agency, self-direction, and

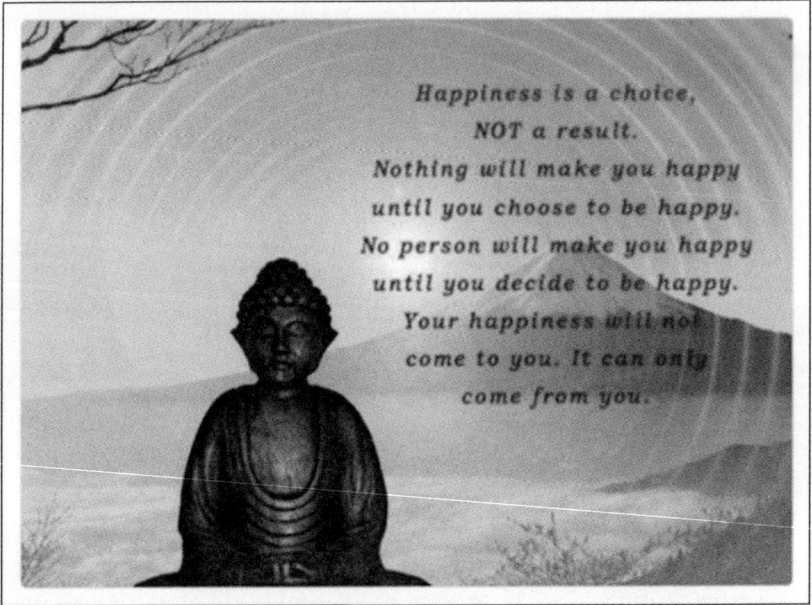

Figure 3.1. A meme posted by Coach Claire with a reminder to readers to manifest the life outcomes that they desire by choosing to be happy.

individual accountability that emerge in her professional life course narrative. Distinctly anti-structural in their framing of the origins of—and remedies for—psychological distress, Coach Claire's Facebook, Twitter, and Instagram posts both model and market to clients a life organized around the principles of choosing and "manifesting" happiness, creating inner peace, and exercising power through self-control (see figures 3.1–3.4). With short messages such as "Going thru a crisis? Look for the opportunity. Not sure how to move forward? Msg me and use coaching to get moving!" Claire positions herself as clearing for her clients a pathway to success that is impervious to social context.

Claire states on various social media outlets that she is passionate about "supporting young professionals in gaining work/life balance." More specifically, she writes that her coaching practice

specializes in supporting psychotherapists with carrying out the wellness and health practices needed to support a life in service to others. Without support, burnout is a near-certainty in this field—but it doesn't have to be that way! I can help you to identify your goals, core values, and self-care action steps, and then bring them to life. Start living a fulfilled life today!

When I asked about this specialization, Claire explained that in teaching other helping professionals to feel empowered and satisfied in their ongoing work "in service to others" at mental health agencies, she is able to maintain continuity with "the mission of social work":

I do feel an obligation to the mission of social work. This is one of my driving forces for gearing my coaching practice toward supporting providers . . . [A] therapist who feels powerless and exhausted is less effective at properly supporting clients to take control of their environments . . . I have found that there are many factors which create an environment that can lead to burnout, as well as many mitigating factors. One of these factors is locus of control. For example, especially when

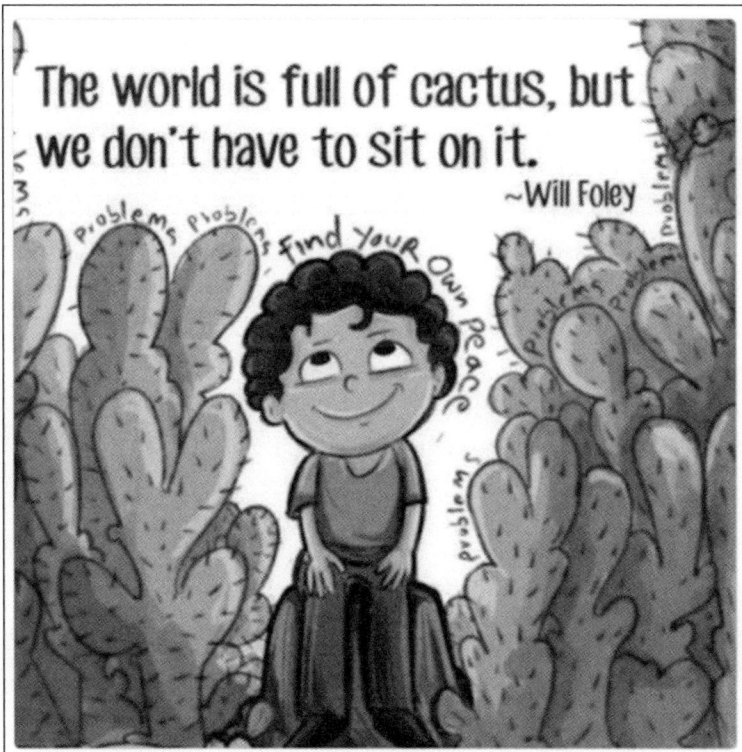

Figure 3.2. Agency, choice, and autonomy override social context.

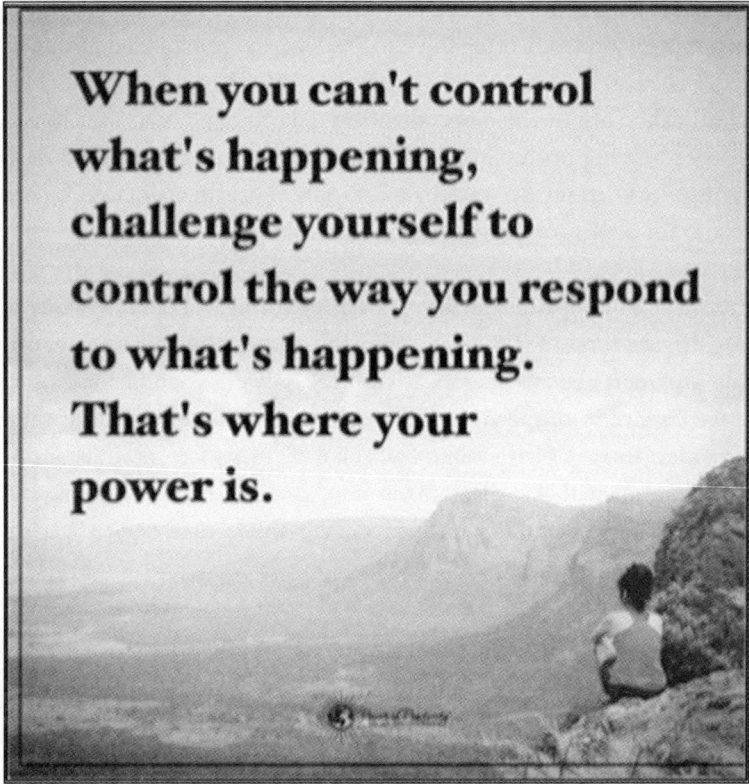

Figure 3.3. Coach Claire urges readers to use the power of individual self-control.

working in an agency, providers can begin to experience a lack of control. This sense can either be reduced or increased based on leadership in the organization. At WBH, the lack of control and micromanaging of providers was quite pervasive and stifling . . . Personally and as a coach, I identify my areas of control and exercise choice and power in those areas rather than allowing the sense of lack of control to spread to personal life.

Here, Claire once again approaches the articulation of a structural tension within agency work—namely the sort of hierarchical organization of power that may have required Claire to lead therapy groups at WBH that were far outside of her area of clinical interest—only to propose an alteration of personal mindset as the appropriate response to such tensions. She transforms the concept of burnout from a structural symptom that is "a near certainty" for early career therapists into a preventable state of mind; having thus reframed the problem, Claire is able to view her coaching project—teaching providers to adapt themselves to the structural contradictions that she herself escaped—as a form of social work.

By her own account, Claire enters the field of social work because she appreciates the profession's propensity to theorize problems in broad social and structural terms. Ironically, however, she is ultimately unable or unwilling to apply this sort of analysis to the forces that guide and constrain her own career trajectory, working discursively instead to expand the definition of "social work" to encompass the more individualistic and entrepreneurial coaching practices to which she is attracted. Claire's strategy of narrating and navigating her career path, then, seems to be characterized by a sort of *sublimation*: She redirects

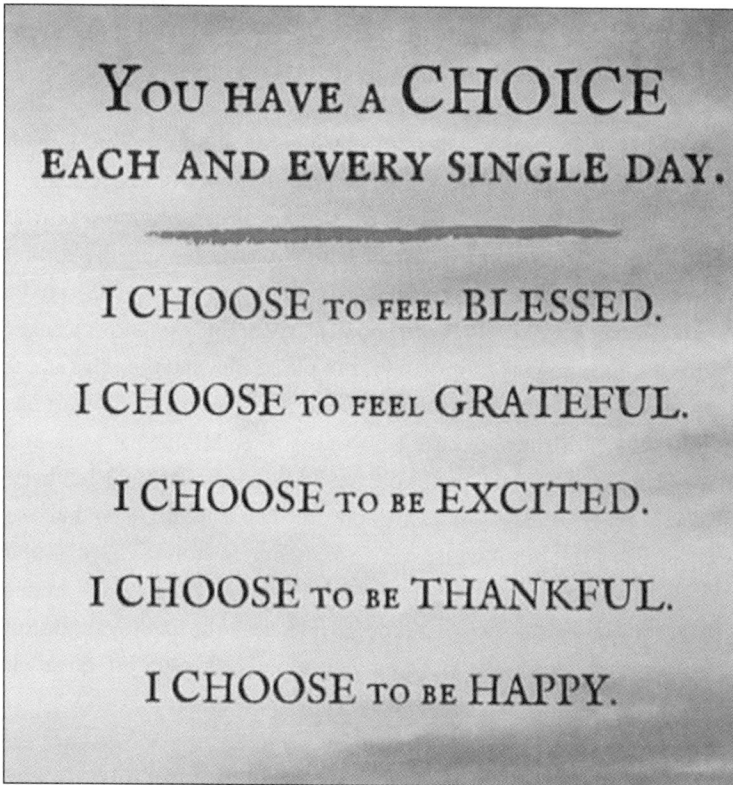

Figure 3.4. One of Coach Claire's many shared memes privileging choice and positive attitude as central to wellness.

her ambivalence around agency work and its structural problems into an embrace of inward-directed ideologies of empowerment and self-care. Furthermore, by helping other helping professionals to similarly minimize the impact of *their* structural conditions so that they may continue working in agency settings, Claire is able to avoid encountering the anxiety-producing possibility that she *has*, in fact, abandoned the social mission of her field—a possibility that Claire, having dispensed with her belief in the deterministic role of social context, would perhaps not be well-equipped to tolerate.

Case 2: Emily (Strategy of Class Dis-Identification)

I come from a very Protestant, very ultra-conservative family. My dad was a radiologist and my mom was a Lutheran schoolteacher. Yeah, definitely ultra, ultra, conservative. And my dad—it's interesting—he's very Western medicine and, you know, [believes] that there are specific illnesses and here are the treatments. So when I got into therapy, they were like "what?" They thought it was all silly and my mom was like "are you going to do aroma therapy?" It was like that to them. And my dad's understanding of psychiatrists, out of the pecking order, you know of who has the highest IQ in the medical field, from his take, they are the bottom of the barrel. Those are the ones who are not the sharpest. And then to be a social worker is like the—the dirt on the shoe of the, you know. 'Cause I started out pre-med my freshman year to please him and then that didn't happen. It wasn't a good fit. Then I shifted. And they're like: "What? Social work?" And I have a niece who wants to go into social work and they're like: "Tell her how poor you are! Did she see your car? Tell her!" He wants her to be an engineer, so—but she lives close by . . . and he's so worried that I might influence her. "She's going to work as hard as you do!" Because, just to supplement my income, I clean a friend of mine's apartment. Her family owns a building and I clean the hallways and stuff and so my dad will say "is that what you want [your niece] to do at 45? She's going to be cleaning apartments?!"

The above quotation, which came near the end of my interview with Emily, encapsulates a form of class dis-identification and attachment to downward mobility that was at the center of Emily's strategy of professional narrative self-management. A Doctor of Clinical Social Work with a PhD from a prestigious program, a teaching appointment at the Chicago School for Psychoanalytic Psychotherapy, and a home and private therapy practice in an affluent suburb, Emily appeared superficially to have attained many of the normative markers of success in her chosen field. Yet throughout her narrative, with a curious mixture of self-deprecation and pride, Emily repeatedly made sure I understood that her business practices, values, lifestyle, and identity were not those of a middle-class psychotherapist.

Emily's account of her career trajectory begins with a depiction of several of her experiences of deeply fulfilling—almost idealized— therapeutic work with the poor in social service settings, unencumbered by bureaucratic obstacles or financial worries. In particular, this portion of Emily's narrative focuses on two female role models, both of whom achieve high status as clinicians and intellectuals while remaining seemingly indifferent to matters of income and dedicated to what Emily understands to be the meaning of social work—that is, "working with more vulnerable populations that don't necessarily have the resources to get their basic needs met." In contrast to the received wisdom that Emily struggles against in her educational institutions—which present the treatment of structural and psychological issues as almost incommensurable projects—she finds examples, in these mentors, of clinicians who seamlessly integrate case management tasks with interpretive interventions in their work with the poor. By extracting a set of guiding principles and practices from her impressions of the mentors and foregrounding her own implementation of these in each stage of her professional trajectory, Emily is able to fashion an account of her career path that erases some of the potential distinctions between agency work and private practice. Specifically, as we will see, Emily attempts to narratively reconcile her commitment to providing psychoanalytic psychotherapy to the poor and vulnerable with her transition into private practice by embracing the trope of self-sacrifice, and by aligning herself with the working class. In so doing, Emily preserves integrity and consistency, but undermines the very need for a higher income that motivates her turn to private practice and obfuscates the structural conditions that prevent her from earning a viable living doing the work she enjoys as an agency social worker.

Emily explained to me that while earning her master's degree in social work and completing her assigned field placement "at a hospital in
an in-patient unit in a fancy schmancy suburb," she arranged a second,
simultaneous therapy internship under the supervision of an unconven-
tional psychiatrist who taught at the medical school of the university
that Emily was attending. "I was working 24/7 and it was all sort of nuts,
but I somehow had a hunch that [this psychiatrist] was absolutely somebody I wanted to spend as much time [with] as I could."

> What [the psychiatrist] was doing was providing psychiatric services pre-
> dominantly to homeless people. She would move around into different
> shelters or establishments in the area and people would kind of drop in
> or some would have standing appointments. She was cool as shit. She
> would show up in her jeans and her ragged T-shirts and just sit there. So
> she had two interns, and I was one of them. She wanted to do more of
> the medication management and then have, you know, the internships
> be more of the deeper talk therapy. So I would just kind of drive around
> with her to the different places and built up a small caseload. I was so
> impressed with her.

Emily admitted that she had never tried to understand the psychiatrist's institutional status, and that she had no recollection of whether or
how the psychiatrist earned an income. What impressed upon Emily's
memory—and what she worked to communicate to me—was the image
of a selfless clinician who was not motivated by professional success, and
who appeared completely comfortable in working-class surrounds. Only
as an afterthought, and in response to my specifically probing the topic,
did Emily acknowledge that her mentor might have been wealthy and
even a bit famous; even then, such information was narratively mini-
mized and never integrated into the character of the psychiatrist with
which Emily identified:

> I have such a bad memory. I think [the psychiatrist] had been on Dona-
> hue or something? She's not somebody who was trying to make—to get
> any publicity for herself, but I think she wrote a book if I remember
> correctly . . . Yeah, you know, I'm sure because she was faculty at the
> medical school, so I'm sure she was doing some publishing at the time . . .

It's all kind of fuzzy . . . I know she was teaching at the hospital, but I don't know if she was full faculty or what. But just her clothes, her car—that doesn't mean she didn't have a ton and maybe part of it was intentional to not drive people—you know, to not drive up to places . . . But there wasn't a lot of discussion at all with her about [money]. People kind of paid what they had. In fact it was such a non-issue, I can't remember. Yeah, I don't know how it transpired . . . She had one [office] space, but it was right in the park where she would go to the different shelters. I think I went there for the interview initially. You know, a total dive.

In her final year of the MSW program, Emily continued to intern under the psychiatrist. She somewhat proudly noted that by then, to her parents' dismay, she would sometimes put her own physical safety at risk by driving alone to meet with clients in the homeless shelters: "I remember my family being scared, like, 'what are you doing?' . . . Or I'd worry because I've always [driven] clunkers that would die and so as I'm leaving at ten o'clock at night I'd think 'how do I get home?'"

Emily got to know several of the staff therapists at one of the shelters, and admired their approach—conspicuously absent from her formal training at school—to bringing clinical techniques into the social service context:

It was a homeless shelter for street kids that some would spend the night there and some would just drop in. What that looked like was [the therapists] would just hang out, and kids would come. Sometimes it would be a set appointment. Sometimes it would just be, you know, it'd be shooting pool with one of them and we'd say, "can we go talk?" And we'd go off and talk. But there was a structured way of understanding what we were doing, that the intention was that we would engage them in a therapeutic process, you know. The administration saw that. You know, they were hoping they weren't just shooting pool; that eventually we were sitting down . . . Whereas, in my coursework, [the professors] were giving really concrete suggestions. Cognitive behavioral [therapy] and family systems were really big, but [social context] wasn't talked about, even though it was an MSW program. It wasn't talked about in terms of—the context wasn't thought about in terms of what that means clinically. It's weird, that there were courses on social issues and dynamics and then clinical [courses], but somehow there wasn't a course that blended those let alone—or talked about techniques that take both of those [into account] . . . But I think I learned [at the shelter], and I remember having this realization that there were a couple therapists that worked there full-time that I just really respected. One guy, his name was Pete, and I just remember following him and listening to how he thought about stuff and it ended up being pretty helpful to draw from his experiences . . . What drew me to him was that he could be practical and really think about the practical side—the needs of the kids—the immediate needs in terms of safety and food and shelter. A lot of them had legal issues and whatnot. So he had a very practical approach but then also thought about issues psychologically. He would talk about their behaviors in ways where he seemed to unpack it, and wonder about it and different dynamics. I don't remember any particular theory or school of thought necessarily, but there was something where I could tell he was really engaged and thoughtful.

After earning her master's degree, Emily moved to Chicago and began working as a therapist at a community-based recreation center and social services agency in what she described as "this very posh neighborhood" in the suburbs. There, Emily found her second role model in the figure of the agency's queer, socially conscious, politically progressive director, Beth. Like Emily, Beth placed an emphasis on providing poor clients with therapeutic services that were attentive to both social context and psychological processes. For Beth, the key to accomplishing this lay in establishing a strict policy of no "third party interference," and particularly in refusing to join the panels of any non–PPO managed care plans. With obvious respect, Emily described the agency's stance under Beth:

Beth was *so* against any third party . . . she was *all* about it in the training, the philosophy was no third party, you know, it was based on the client's needs and you don't need people intruding in the treatment . . . so [the agency] had a sliding fee . . . The highest fee patient was eighty [dollars], and then it slid down to five. I think the caseload—even though it was in this neighborhood that you would assume that everyone within a ten-mile radius has transportation and things sustaining them—there were quite a few people coming in that were paying five or ten. And down the way there was government-assisted housing and stuff.

Inspired by Beth's example, Emily decided to pursue her PhD in clinical social work at the same psychoanalytically oriented program Beth had attended—an elite school with a socially progressive reputation. The program allowed Emily to continue working at Beth's agency for nine months out of the year and travel to the campus during the summers for intensive coursework. But even in this school, Emily was disappointed to discover, the faculty wielded a shared taxonomy that classified patients struggling with poverty or structural problems as incompatible with psychoanalysis. Emily recalled the frustration of presenting a case from the agency in Chicago to her professors:

> The faculty and the people I had to present cases to, for them everything would line up along Oedipal/pre-Oedipal. And if somebody's pre-Oedipal then you can't really do anything. You can't do any analyzing. You just have to hold their hand and give them practical resources. But if they're Oedipal, then you analyze and don't worry about the practical. So I'd present cases—and I failed my first orals and I—part of it was I was talking about a case and I was analyzing her psychologically and they kept saying "Rome is Burning! What do you mean? She has this, this, and this and you're talking to her about the meaning?" . . . She was losing jobs, getting electricity shut off. Engaging in some self-destructive behaviors. So they were wanting me to hospitalize her. And at the time I was still working in [the agency] and Beth's angle was, "What? We're not going to line her up on some continuum and, you know. Yes, we have to worry about some of the practical, but what is all of this leading to?" She kind of held both, so I had that on one end and then my supervisor from the school was like, you know, "this is ridiculous! You're missing the point." . . . You know, there shouldn't be any unpacking of what's going on because "Rome is burning!" That just runs through my head. They were like "Roooome!" And I'm like, "I know but I'm trying to *understand* Rome!"

Once again, it was the unlikely space of the agency—and not the progressive classroom—that represented, to Emily, the ideal synthesis of practical problem solving and deep interpretive work with vulnerable clients.

The beginning of a period of eight years while working on her doctorate, in which Emily resigns from agency work and takes a job at a profit-driven group psychotherapy practice, marks a significant turn in Emily's professional life course narrative. Here, for the first time, Emily speaks in negative terms about her employment situation:

EMILY: I got pregnant and felt like, "ok, gotta go make some more money," because my partner is in his own business and didn't make a ton. And at the time he had just insurance for himself and I'm thinking "okay, I'm going to have a baby, how are we gonna do this?" So then I signed up with this private practice which I felt like I really sold my soul to do. It was a hellish experience. [The boss] was all insurance panels, very bottom line. "How much money are you bringing in?" Just very—not clinical at all. He was very concrete in his understandings of the patient and he just wanted everybody to get on as many insurance panels as possible, no matter how intrusive. Like some panels are more intrusive than others and it doesn't matter if you're having to say everything about the patient as long as you get reimbursed. So in the beginning I only agreed to sign up on some because I read through them; they have these huge applications. After a while, though, I realized they all stink, and so I jumped from there to just break from that whole process. 'Cause it was just hell. 'Cause with managed care, it's—you have to ask how many sessions you can give and somebody on the line is filing their nails, and they'll tell ya "oh, I'll give you five sessions."

TALIA: And it wasn't one of those things where you could just play the game and tell them the diagnosis—or tell them the words they need to hear—but actually not really share anything personal about the patient?

EMILY: And I did that and I could sleep at night because I would tell myself that's what I was doing. But after a while, he started running into trouble because I brought a group of people with me from my caseload at [the agency] that was sliding scale. So he was like, let's see, what's his standard fee? It was $125 and then you could slide to $60, and I had people coming in that were paying me $15. So he agreed to hire me with the idea that I would, you know, eventually phase those folks out and build up . . . So when that wasn't happening there was some tension there, and I felt pressured to then change the nature of my caseload but it didn't seem right so it was just always

this source of tension. And I remember doing it and actually feeling, like, a sense of shame or something when I would talk to other
colleagues. To admit that oh my goodness I was on a managed care
plan . . . Because Beth was so against third party . . . so I went from
that to "get on these panels!" and "how much money are you bringing in?" And it was tough because my daughter at the time got really
really sick and was in the hospital the first two years of her life on
and off. So the bills were piling up so then part of me was like, "okay
I need to make more money" but it was just this, like, what am I doing? I'm submitting referral forms for a managed care panel! This is
everything I didn't want to do.

In spite of the claim that Emily had "sold [her] soul" in order to support her family financially, according to her narrative, Emily continued
to make major economic sacrifices at the group practice to avoid compromising her professional standards. Because working with managed
care panels, in Emily's view, required "feeding a database" with invasive
information, privileging short-term and superficial treatment modalities,
and using pathologizing diagnostic labels to ensure approval of services,
Emily opted over time to "find a way to do out-of-pocket" instead with
nearly all of her clients at the practice. She would factor in the cost to her
clients of taking the train out to the suburbs for their therapy sessions,
often leaving herself with hourly fees as low as $7.50 after handing over to
her boss his 50% cut of all session earnings.

At the time of our interview, one year had passed since Emily had left
the group and opened a private practice of her own. "Now I hang my own
shingle and just do my own thing, and it's nice not to have the pressure
from [the boss] and from the whole group. So I very much prefer that,"
she told me. When I asked whether the new business was more lucra-
tive than Emily's previous job, she said that it was hard to tell. As her
own boss, Emily chose to do self-pay with most of her clients, charging
$10, $30, $35, or $60 per hour depending on the client's resources. She
had yet to find out whether not having to split her earnings would offset
the overhead costs of owning her own business, but anticipated that she
would "get somewhere around the same, maybe a little less" than she
had earned before. As we gazed out the window of the downtown Chicago coffee shop in which we were sitting, I inquired: "Do you ever think

about getting an office around here and charging $200 an hour?" Emily
smiled.

> It's funny, I envision doing the opposite. I would like to get out of [the
> suburbs] because it's such a hike for some of my clients. I just have a lot of
> guilt with people trying to come from the city out to see me. So I picture
> myself one day setting up shop [in Chicago], maybe not right around
> here. And I go back and forth because I think "oh, why don't I just do it?"
> And then I think "oh, my family" and, you know, to do that I would have
> to spend less time . . . with my family. And my income with [my husband]
> is such that he makes enough to cover our living expenses but not over
> that. So like I'm the safety valve for savings . . . So then I'll think, "well,
> should we figure out how to just live on his and save on his?" And then
> I can do more of what I envision? Like, how I picked my internships was
> based on what I expected myself doing for years to come once upon a
> time, so I feel like I do some of that [now] but it's not enough.

Emily's fantasy of abandoning her efforts to save money and opening a private practice in the city so that she can better serve the poor is
telling in several ways: It acknowledges, in one sense, that Emily's career
path from agency to private practice has taken her far away from what
she envisioned herself doing "once upon a time." But in the same ges-
ture, it continues Emily's narrative project of flattening the typical distinctions between the two endpoints of the normative career trajectory
by transforming the icon of material success for a psychotherapist—the
downtown private practice—into an envisioned opportunity for deeper
self-sacrifice and greater precarity.

Like many therapists, Emily is funneled along the normative career
path by forces largely outside of her control. Her transition from agency
work to private practice is, perhaps, made all the more painful because
Emily identifies so fully with her agency clinician role models (notwith-
standing the facts that the psychiatrist's credentials afford her different
opportunities from those available to Emily, or that Beth eventually decides to resign from her position as agency director) and is shielded from
the sorts of experiences that often generate ambivalence about agency
work for many therapists. Since Emily cannot resist movement along the
trajectory itself, she instead tries intensely to narrate and enact resistance

to any concomitant changes in her clinical practices, client population, and class status. Emily grounds this resistance to change in a consistent rejection of managed care insurance panels. While such a rejection is not unusual in itself—indeed, many therapists resent the intrusions of managed care on their clinical work, and there are innumerable books and websites available to private practitioners specifically instructing them on how to disentangle themselves from the managed care system—Emily equates managed care with shameful clinician profit where other private practice therapists might complain about the panels' low reimbursement rates (Henneberger 1994). In Emily's career path inversion, eschewing managed care in favor of only self-pay and PPO is no longer tantamount to selecting a wealthier client pool; instead, it facilitates (or at least does not hinder) the maintenance of a working-class caseload.

Emily's selflessness and steadfast commitment to her values are remarkable and, in my view, quite admirable. But to understand the significance of the rigorous claims to downward mobility and attachment to working-class identification that anchor Emily's narrative—as well as her carefully managed, self-undermining declarations of both needing to earn more and preventing herself from earning more—one must recognize that Emily is attempting discursively to stretch herself into a professional arrangement that is structurally impossible for her to attain. Despite her best efforts, Emily cannot beat the system and remain a psychoanalytic social worker in a homeless shelter. But rather than find fault in the system that obstructs her, she takes on the burden individually—to the point of holding a side job as a janitor—and class dis-identification emerges as a symptom in her narrative.

Case 3: Abigail (Strategy of Bargaining)

I interviewed Abigail—my clinical supervisor at Wellness Behavioral Health who resigned from her position in the middle of my internship year—a little over two years after her switch to full-time private psychotherapy practice. We had not been in contact during the intervening time; indeed, I was only able to track her down by sending her an appointment request via the form on her private practice's website.

In many ways, Abigail and I re-entered our former relationship of supervisor/trainee for the duration of the interview, with Abigail positioned as the experienced mentor guiding me through the steps of opening a therapy business in the event that I should decide to do so one day. In contrast to Claire or Emily, Abigail did not devote much of our conversation to a description of the early stages of her clinical training and career, other than to remind me that she had been at WBH from the moment that she obtained her master's degree in counseling until she resigned from agency work ten years later; that prior to her resignation, she had already transitioned from full-time to part-time status at WBH; and that from day one of her career, she had "always had a little private practice" near her home in the suburbs north of Chicago. Explaining that while unusual, it is in fact legal for unlicensed therapists to see patients privately as long as they arrange to do so under a supervising therapist's license, Abigail launched her version of a career trajectory narrative by remarking that the specter of full-time private practice had always been there for her due to her having established one on the side. What varied over the years of her employment at WBH, according to Abigail's hindsight account, was the degree to which the miseries of agency work were present and exerted their pull on Abigail in the direction of her private practice:

> [F]rom the time I left my graduate school, I always had a few [private practice] clients and I did that through the entire ten years. So in terms of how you make that leap, I think part of it for me was that I always had some little structure. I always had office space and, you know, my cards and voicemail numbers. It's just basically a little structure so I knew that I could do that. So then when I went down to part-time [at WBH], I think what I realized is *my god, I'm making more money in less time.* You know, than I'm making at the agency. And that started to really, like, weigh on me. And I think it wouldn't have been so much of a motivation to leave if it just hadn't gotten worse and worse. Just, I mean, in terms of the amount of expectations on us without any kind of, you know, whether it's financial remuneration or even just—even thinking about our self-care. Unfortunately, it seemed like nobody was able to take the time to wonder how we're doing. So it was terrible, depressing. The staff meetings were depressing and people were really unhappy but . . . it was already so overwhelming with what [my supervisor] was doing that she didn't even feel compassion. It was just skipped right over, right? Like, "well, I know you

guys are working really hard, we really, really appreciate you, and here's some more things you have to do."

Recalling the overwhelming impression of ambivalence and contradiction with which I had been flooded upon hearing Abigail's comments on her resignation from WBH two years prior, I inquired about the status of feelings such as guilt in Abigail's understanding of her career trajectory today. This time, she appeared to possess no shortage of surety, readily endorsing an experience of guilt while squarely locating that experience in the fully resolved past:

> Yeah, I'm glad you said that, because . . . I *did* feel guilty! And I think that being able to structure things the way that I did has really, you know, taken care of that . . . I really grappled with leaving for a few reasons. One, I do appreciate the social justice aspect of having agencies, which to me mean you can provide services to the disenfranchised, you know, people who don't have other options. And to me, I've always considered private practice to be somewhat elite. I mean, there's other analogies in other areas, you know, not just the mental health field but there's public aid, public defenders, right? And then there's people who have money to pay real lawyers. Like in so many areas, there's this, you know, people who just don't get the same quality typically because of not having the means. And so that's always bothered me.

Having named the sources of her potential guilt, Abigail quickly assured me that she had absolutely no regrets about her decision; she was "done, definitely done" with agency work, and had "not looked back for even a second." She then enumerated, at some length, a series of bases for her present lack of ambivalence. First, she reiterated her growing awareness over the course of ten years of the insufficient remuneration—either monetary or in the form of care or compassion—offered by WBH: "I started to feel like, wow, I'm just working my ass off and I'm just thinking—I mean, at the end of ten years, I was making $25 an hour and that's just not cool!" In spite of her own "incredible dedication," Abigail explained, she simply could no longer endure a workplace environment that showed such little regard for her wellbeing. Here, Abigail emphasized—as she had two years earlier—how unusually long she had lasted in community mental health compared to other clinicians. No longer speculating about the psychopathological roots of her devotion, however, Abigail simply credited herself for having done more than her share of agency time, and expressed a wish for a greater number of her colleagues to take on more of this burden: "For me it was like, come on—ten years is enough. If everybody could put in a few years in this area, it would be great."

Next, and central to her narrative, Abigail detailed the decisions she had made about how to structure her private practice that "allowed [her] to leave in good conscience." She had instituted a "significant sliding scale," inviting some of her Medicaid-funded clients at WBH to continue working with her privately for $25 per session:

> One of the things that I agreed to do in my own mind, in order to leave, was that I agreed to take clients if they receive monthly disability benefits. You know, they can't work, they receive mental health disability and they have Medicaid, which means that they can't pay for anybody outside an agency, which you may know. These days, it's changing a little and I think Medicaid is now being privatized . . . in some areas like through some insurance companies. So that's really recent and I'm kind of looking into that, but just all this time . . . you couldn't see anybody privately with Medicaid. So I basically said to some people that I was seeing at the agency, "if you want to follow me, then I will charge you $25 an hour."

Abigail had also accommodated a set of clients who wanted to follow her from the agency to private practice by getting in network with their Blue Cross HMO plan, which, she explained, "took an *enormous* amount of effort." Furthermore, true to her word from two years prior, Abigail had rented out a second office in a middle-class suburb that was near WBH and far from her primary practice. She commuted to this office one day a week to see her former WBH clients who, Abigail noted, "are really clear that I did that for them."

Abigail acknowledged that for the sake of her own quality of life and material comfort, there were limits to the sacrifices she was willing to make "to be able to honor and continue to have some social justice" in her work. For what she termed "diversification" purposes, Abigail balanced out her Medicaid and HMO clients with PPO clients whose insurance

would reimburse her $128 per hour, as well as with clients who could af-
ford to pay an out-of-pocket fee ranging from $100 (which, Abigail com-
mented, was still low compared to her colleagues) to $135. Moreover, she
had decided not to accept any additional Medicaid clients, and made a
point of explaining to existing ones that the tradeoff for her discounted
fee was a lower priority status in her schedule:

> Basically how I contract with people—especially $25 an hour people, and
> I have a handful of them—is that's what you're paying me and I under-
> stand that's what you can afford and that means you can't have prime time
> spots. You can't come in at prime time hours, where I have people who
> can't come in any other time, like private insurance people. And I may
> need to bump you. You know, I mean we kind of say, "hey, I can't do this
> time but can I move you around to this time," and they're fine with that.
> That's how we work it out.

Abigail stressed that the compromises she had made in order to retain a number of her clients from WBH were particularly important to
her sense of professional integrity because they enabled her to provide
therapeutic continuity to individuals who especially needed it, because
of their "significant trauma histories and attachment disorders." Such
individuals—the kind that Abigail specialized in treating—were fundamentally, in Abigail's view, "agency clients":

> These are what I call "agency clients." They have long-term trauma his-
> tory. They don't function well. The healing or improvement work that
> you see is very small and it's never going to look like, you know, big leaps
> and bounds of recovery. It's just: are they able to have a little more peace
> in their life, little less symptoms of post-traumatic stress disorder, which
> most of them have? So that's what I got, this creates *my* version of a pri-
> vate practice, which allows for both, you know, that population as well as
> people who can afford to pay or have insurance to pay.

While seeing these agency clients in her private practice was meaningful
for Abigail, she conceded that there were other individuals with similar
trauma issues whom she had seen at WBH but was not comfortable taking with her because "they're not outpatient people, in terms of they

need a crisis line, right? They need more support than I could really offer in private practice without too much anxiety for me. So, that was very hard for me and I still think about that."

Abigail concluded her narrative by mentioning two ways in which she felt that her trajectory from agency work to private practice was distinct from that of other therapists she knew. First, building on her statements about the nature of agency clients, Abigail declared that unlike many private practitioners, she had not decided to make the switch in order to escape the sorts of lower-functioning individuals that she associated with trauma and poverty:

> I'm not a private practitioner who's going for the elite North Shore . . . I think oftentimes, people in private practice are looking for the worried well, because they pay. They have, you know, they can pay out-of-pocket or they've got the insurance and there's a . . . link here between people who are lower functioning and the degree of trauma that they have and if we did the research, we'd find it. In my ten years, you're not necessarily going to find as much of those much more complex issues in private practice. Because oftentimes, those are the people that have been so wounded that they don't function very well and that's why they come to an agency! So yeah, I think there's a link here to being less functional and not being able to maintain an income that allows you to have the resources to go to somebody in private practice.

Here, Abigail distinguished her willingness (or even preference) to engage with the complexities of so-called agency clients from a willingness to do case management, to which she said she had never been well suited:

> Case management is not therapy and I don't want to do it . . . And I think at one point this would have sounded arrogant but it doesn't feel like arrogance anymore, just an observation: I have some real skills to be able to do some real work with people, so I don't want to waste that on doing case management. There are people who do that really well, and I think we should all do what we are drawn to do. I mean, I had a colleague [at WBH] who was hired at the same time I was to do the

same project—homeless shelter case management—and she's a great case manager and that's what she wanted to do. She didn't want to go deeper. She didn't want to help people go deeper. She really liked making sure that they got resources and she was great at it. I sent people to her, and she sent the people to me that wanted to do the deeper work, and that worked.

Abigail's second point of career path distinction pertained to her status as a single woman. In contrast with her earlier critiques of agencies as unsupportive environments, at this point in her narrative Abigail drew attention to the relative safety and stability of an agency paycheck and benefits compared to the risk inherent in embarking on a business venture on one's own. Borrowing the psychoanalytic notion of a "container"—meaning a maternal person or setting that protects the patient by receiving their unwanted or overwhelming thoughts and feelings and returning them in a less destructive form (Bion 2013; Winnicott 1953, 1971)—to characterize the reasons that some therapists might depend on the structure of agency work, Abigail went on to observe that most (woman) therapists besides herself who *did* leave the safe container of the agency did so with the financial support of a spouse:

> Most of the people I know—I don't know if this has come up in your research—but the women I know who've gone into private practice from agencies, they *all* had other income and support. I'm the *only* person in my group that did it without any other income or support . . . To go from agency to a private practice, there's no way to do that and have a whole practice. So you are taking a financial risk, right? There's no way because you can't physically have a full practice before you leave the agency to go onto your own practice, does that make sense? There's not enough hours in the week, right? So if you did what I did, which is start part-time, you still don't have enough people part-time to make a full living. So there is a piece of, like, how are you going to make that work?

In the midst of saying this to me, Abigail discovered and disclosed (in a manner consistent with her discursive style as a therapist and clinical supervisor) a sense of pride in her own independence. She neatly wrapped up her narrative by formulating her current-day success in private practice—as opposed, perhaps, to the successes of her married colleagues—as a sort of karmic return on her longtime commitment to agency work and agency clients, exclaiming: "You know, as I'm speaking that aloud, I feel kind of proud! Like, I feel kind of great around that, and maybe that's part of what I feel—that those of us who want to be a part of social justice, that the universe takes care of us!"

When Abigail initially left WBH, her comments evinced an intense ambivalence around pursuing a professional status shift that seemed to feel to her simultaneously inevitable, well deserved, and shamefully self-indulgent. Two years later, much of this ambivalence has dissipated, and Abigail is able to articulate some of the structural circumstances that led to her decision. She does, however, work narratively to reconcile within her own trajectory the conflicting norms that structured her initial ambivalence. Abigail's principle strategy for accomplishing this reconciliation is through enactments of *bargaining*: She makes an agreement with herself "in [her] own mind" to create ways to continue seeing some of her clients from WBH in return for allowing herself to focus on a pool of new, higher-paying clients; she "contract[s] with" her "twenty-five an hour people" about the exchange of a low priority in Abigail's schedule for a discounted fee, thereby acquiring (and narratively indexing) an externalized form of validation of her internal strategy. Ultimately, these narrative moves permit Abigail to frame her career trajectory as a special bargain with the universe, in which her unique demonstration of commitment to social justice in the past—and her concessions to the same causes in her present practice—is rewarded with well-deserved pride and the alleviation of guilt.

Notably, Abigail's narrative strategy relies on a frequent invocation of her own exceptionality—first in her preference for lower-functioning, complex trauma cases over the North Shore worried well, and later in the distinct symbolic significance of opening her private practice as an unmarried woman. In her insistence on such (legitimate) points of distinction, Abigail may help to reify the dichotomous categories of "agency client" and "outpatient client," even as she asserts her own willingness to muddle them. After all, Abigail's descriptions of "[her] version of a private practice" rely on an a priori separation of the types of clients who generally *belong* in agencies—because of their complex and traumatic histories, which in turn predispose them to be poor and lower functioning—from those clients who would never be found outside of a private practice. It is only by virtue of Abigail's idiosyncratic skill set and ethical commitments that certain Medicaid-carrying "agency clients" are allowed to do "real [long-term, introspective] work"—the sort of therapeutic work not often available in agencies—with Abigail, first at WBH and then in the even more unlikely setting of a private practice. In other words, Abigail's narrative effectively demonstrates her extraordinary initiative, resourcefulness, and professional integrity precisely by *not* opening up a more *generally* fluid conceptualization of the types of clients and services appropriate to community mental health versus private practice settings. In fact, Abigail's division of *her* WBH clients into two types—those that could receive an invitation to follow her to private practice, and those that she was not comfortable removing from the agency—functions as a process of fractal recursivity (Gal and Irvine 1995), entailing the production of "ever more distinctions applying the same axis of differentiation within itself" (Gal 2016). Moreover, Abigail's narrative reliance on exceptionality resists a ready extension of her indictment of agency work to the general plight of other therapists, whose career trajectories are tacitly interpreted as either defined by dependence or exemplifying privilege and greed.

Conclusion: Professional Narrative Self-Management and Structural Alienation

We have seen in this chapter that therapists are socialized into a set of mutually undercutting and incompatible narratives about their professional identities and aspirations. They are encouraged in training to learn to equate their credentials with a desire to help the disenfranchised and a disinterest in profit or prestige, while they are simultaneously immersed in pedagogy that sets them up for professional dissatisfaction when working with the poor. Upon embarking on clinical careers in agency settings, therapists manage everyday contradictions and frustrations at different moments by suppressing, temporalizing, or identifying with their exploited roles. They do not necessarily encounter their own structurally generated ambivalence regularly; moreover, that ambivalence may be tempered or offset by the fulfilling aspects of doing work that feels consonant with the social justice mission of the profession. For these reasons, in spite of the availability of a narrative arc into which therapists may insert themselves that demands a shift from agency work to private practice—and despite the existence of institutional and material barriers that at times indisputably obstruct therapists from sustaining their careers in agency settings—therapists often experience an intense degree of guilt or ambivalence around following the normative career path. A common response to these affective experiences is for therapists to attempt to reclaim their own moral agency and professional integrity through *emplotment* (Mattingly 1994)—the crafting of a career trajectory narrative that internally resolves (within the therapist's individual narrative) and temporally organizes the structural impasses in which the therapists are caught. For Claire, this narrative resolution takes the form of a rejection of structure and social context, and a redefinition of social work through an elevation of ideologies of choice and entrepreneurship. In Emily's narrative, demonstrations of intense self-sacrifice enable her to performatively flatten the distinctions between agency work and private practice. Even Abigail—whose narrative comes closest among the three cases to naming the sociological and material conditions motivating her career shift—individually takes on the burden of reconciling structural oppositions through the bargains she makes with herself, her clients, and the universe.

In using such strategies as sublimation, class dis-identification, and bargaining to locate themselves within narrative frameworks that resolve structural tensions, therapists' professional trajectory narratives constitute a form of self-management in the expanded or metaphorical sense of this term that is being traced throughout the book. As we have seen, discourses on self-management as a universally empowering clinical treatment modality for mood disorders turn on an erasure of social or structural context, and a privileging of sovereign individual agency. A similar logic appears to be at work here: Structural tensions and differences—and the impact of these on therapists' desires, dispositions, and actions—necessarily recede from the storyline when therapists aim to recuperate agency through the autonomous management of their own professional trajectories. Thus, professional life course self-management may facilitate *structural alienation*, even as it is entwined with therapists' efforts to *decrease* certain forms of structural inequality within their individual practices. As illustrated in the case studies, therapists' reliance on narrations of their life decisions and strategies as acts of free will and social-aesthetic choice can help to obscure—and thereby naturalize and reproduce—the very constraints and disparities (e.g., in their professional socialization process, and in the distinction between agency and private practice) that drive the therapists to seek self-recuperation through narrative emplotment in the first place.[16] As we will see in the next chapter, such alienation from—and disavowal of—political economic structures can have far-reaching consequences for mental health treatment delivery, as this disavowal animates a number of powerful discourses rationalizing particular kinds of therapeutic relationships and temporalities as appropriate or inappropriate to disparate classes of clients.

Billable Services and the "Therapeutic Fee"

*On the Work of Disavowal of Political Economy
and Its Re-Emergence in Clinical Practice*

"There May Be an Awkwardness That They Need You to Sit With"

Huddled in the corner of an expansive, featureless classroom on the top floor of a chain university building in downtown Chicago, my small cohort of clinical counselors-in-training at the Chicago School for Psychoanalytic Psychotherapy (CSPP) listens as our instructor, Emily,[1] tries to define what it is to establish a "therapeutic alliance" with a patient.[2] We meet on Saturday mornings, earlier than any of us would prefer to be awake. The hours reflect our adjunct instructors' employment first and foremost as clinicians, occupied during the business day with well-established private psychotherapy practices. The entire center in which we receive our training often feels like a strange apparition: a collection of psychoanalytic murmurs springing up during off-hours in makeshift classrooms amid the half-completed creations of culinary school students and the model spines of an orthopedic school, leaving no trace of itself when these other inhabitants return.

Emily's voice is small, and her hands shake when she teaches. She explains that today we will only be talking about conscious-level components of the therapeutic alliance, including various forms of explicit agreements that are made between the therapist and the patient. Of utmost importance, we learn, is that the therapist create safety and stability by maintaining a consistent approach to "those aspects of the helping relationship that are not necessarily congruent with how we would handle ordinary social relationships"—things like gently but unfailingly resisting the patient's efforts to engage in small talk on the way to the therapist's office, holding firmly to the agreed-upon session length, or explaining to a patient why you recognize, but will not fulfill, her wish for a hug. So, too, with the practice of charging a fee. "The patient needs to know that we have clear expectations about the fee," Emily tells us.

> It is important to convey how stable we are, even in chaotic moments in the patient's life, by staying consistent with this issue. I charge a fixed consultation fee, and during the consultation sessions, we will talk about money and what a fair fee would be. If [managing] money seems to be an issue for my patient, I won't go too low, to avoid colluding with them . . . Our patients need to know that we are present, consistent, and reliable— they will push for more, but when you cave, it actually hurts them . . . If we are too quick to reassure patients or to act on their longings, we are suggesting that the patient's pain can't be survived or managed, or that we can't bear to hear it or muddle through it. So when a patient says they can't pay, instead of jumping to "no worries, you'll pay next week," there may be an awkwardness that they need you to sit with.

Emily's message was met with considerable resistance from my classmates and me, all of us interning at the time at mental health agencies serving low-income clients. How could we talk about such a thing as a "fair fee" for psychotherapy, we asked, when there was nothing particularly equitable about the system of healthcare delivery in the United States? And how were we to distinguish between those patients whose financial struggles were legitimate and the ones for whom avoidance of the fee was a psychological symptom? Emily was not unsympathetic to such concerns—passionately committed to social justice, she had devoted most of her clinical career to treating underprivileged individuals in agency settings. As mentioned previously, she currently offered therapeutic services to working-class patients in her private practice for as little as $10 per session, supplementing her own modest income with occasional janitorial work. Yet in response to our queries, Emily advised: "Make your decision about what's fair based not just on your political or social views. When deciding what to charge, think about stability, safety, patient-centeredness, and the alliance."

The following week, Emily raised the issue of the fee again, conceding that she had thought it over and come to the realization that a better term than "fair" for what our stance toward setting and maintaining a fee should be was "therapeutic." This time, Emily had brought along textual expertise to bolster her pedagogy: She handed to each of us a copy of pages 13 through 24 of a typewritten paper that looked to have been Xeroxed dozens of times, onto which the words "Spring Conference, 1989" had at one point been scribbled. The paper was written by an eminent psychodynamic psychotherapist and contained a section that was widely regarded, according to Emily, as the authoritative word on fees for psychotherapy.

The paper's section on fees begins with a brief acknowledgment of the practical and material functions of remuneration. However, its focus lies in an articulation of the fee's critical role in facilitating a strong, effective, and intimate relationship between the therapist and patient. To that end, the paper describes at some length two aspects of the fee's therapeutic function. First, it explains that the fee can "serve as an important safeguard for the therapist." Because the fee "may take on meanings related to self esteem for the therapist, and to feeling valued professionally by one's patients as well as by one's self," its collection "make[s] it less likely that the therapist will require other gratifications from the patient." This monetarily mediated elevation of the therapist's self-esteem is theorized as ultimately serving the patient's clinical interests by affording the patient access to an experience of *unmediated* empathic attunement during the therapeutic encounter: Psychotherapy, the paper argues, is "a subtle process which requires that the therapist feel free of preoccupations so that he can allow himself to attend to the experience of being with the patient in an empathic mode . . . Feeling deprived of appropriate professionally derived gratification . . . produces a situation which is bound to be a disservice to the patient, because the therapist cannot function optimally under these conditions." To this point, Emily shared that in her experience, she had come to realize that her fee was too low—that it was not a "therapeutic fee"—when she found herself distracted from the therapeutic alliance by resentful ruminations about the cost of her patient's clothing: "It's not that there's a set dollar amount that is necessarily too low to be therapeutic. But I know that there's a problem with the fee if I'm talking to a patient and thinking to myself: '*If she can't afford to pay me more than x dollars per week for therapy, how did she buy those expensive shoes?*'"

While the conference paper's first point is focused on the therapeutic qualities that the fee effects in the *clinician*, its second point about the significance of the fee foregrounds the liberty and equality that the *patient* accrues by paying an amount that does not feel discounted or too easy:

> The patient is more likely to feel free to expect something from the thera-
> pist, to demand the therapist's skill, attention, tolerance, and understand-
> ing of disruptive feeling states if he feels that he is paying a fair fee. It is
> likely that the patient will allow himself more freely to express disap-
> pointment or anger at the therapist if he feels he is paying a fair fee. It
> may be difficult to express such negative feelings if the patient feels the
> therapist is doing him a favor by seeing him at a fee which seems too
> little. In this sense, the reparative meaning of the fee—the sense that pay-
> ing money to the therapist may help to repair the fantasied damage done
> via the patient's anger or retaliatory feelings—may get lost if the fee seems
> too low.

As in the paper's first, therapist-oriented point, the argument here suggests that the fee, when properly set to a therapeutic rate, works in the
service of the therapeutic relationship while rendering its own media-
tion invisible: The patient is theorized as requiring a support person who
can hold (Winnicott 1960; Slochower 1996) and endure (or, in Emily's
earlier words, "sit with" or "muddle through") the patient's "disruptive" affects. Indeed, it is the drama (or at least the patient's fantasy of a
drama) of damaging and then repairing the therapeutic relationship—
and the experience of participating in a relationship that can survive this
process—that is understood in contemporary psychodynamic theory to
heal the patient (Bowlby 1979, 1988; Winnicott 1971). The therapeutic or
fair fee, according to the above quotation, plays an integral role in the
unfolding of this drama both because it affords the patient the emotional
"freedom" to damage the relationship and because it functions as a
repair to that damage. In other words, the fee—provided it is appropriately high—becomes a meaningful component of the therapeutic process
rather than merely the medium of exchange for the service of psychotherapy. Only when the fee is set too low, according to the paper, does its
therapeutic function "get lost," forcing the therapist and patient into an

uncomfortable recognition of their economically mediated transaction. Explaining that "[a] patient may wonder what you want from him, if he is not paying a fee which he regards as fair," the paper offers the example of a patient of the author's who, the night after having had his fee lowered, dreamed about a barber demanding sexual favors in exchange for a haircut. Emily seconded this point as well, stating that "a low fee can make boundaries feel fuzzy when they need to feel fixed," and recalling a patient of hers who had felt himself more Emily's equal, and had experienced greater therapeutic benefit, after voluntarily raising his own fee from what he had termed "the village idiot rate."

In the months of my fieldwork that followed these classroom discussions, I repeatedly encountered this striking compulsion on the part of psychotherapists to produce elaborate discourses that semiotically transformed the labor relations in which the therapists participated into something continuous with—and at times even constitutive of—therapeutic care. This work of alignment was not limited, as I might have expected, to private practice therapists who—at least in many instances—received large cash fees directly from their patients. Rather, it was just as prevalent in therapists' talk about billing in agency settings, in spite of the facts that agency clients seldom paid out-of-pocket for therapy and agency clinicians' (fixed) salaries were not directly impacted by the amount of money reimbursed to the agency in exchange for client services. This chapter examines the production of such discourses among private practitioners at CSPP and workers at Wellness Behavioral Health (WBH) and Community Recovery Center (CRC). Building from the arguments already laid out, I propose that, bound within a structurally contradictory profession that prescribes upward mobility on the one hand and a selfless commitment to helping the underprivileged on the other, therapists at each stage of their career path—a path whose normative trajectory begins at an agency and culminates in private practice—attempt to manage the ambivalence that these divergent imperatives invoke by working discursively to disavow the role of political economy in shaping their professional activities. This strategy of disavowal, while differently instantiated based on the therapist's institutional status and the styles of reasoning that are intelligible in particular kinds of clinical settings, often crystallizes around the rationalization of clinical decisions pertaining to billing procedures in terms of moral principles concerning therapeutic appropriateness. In the process of this reframing of economic considerations, therapists articulate and legitimate a class-differentiated *moral economy of mental healthcare* that reasserts precisely the market-based logics that they seek to transcend. Specifically, the ways in which therapists make moral sense of the economic constraints around their professional practices with working-class clients in agency settings leads to a figuration of those clients as autonomous actors who are clinically best suited to participation in a time-limited series of present-moment exchanges. In contrast, therapists' moral discourses around fees for middle-class patients in private practice settings bring the patient and clinician together in something akin to a gift economy (Bourdieu 1977) that entails an ongoing social relationship and the transmutation of economic into symbolic capital.[3] A consequence of therapists' disavowal of political economy—and particularly of their mobilization of the category of therapeutic appropriateness in exporting the economic to the moral domain—is a naturalization of class disparities in therapeutic temporalities and relationships.[4] These seemingly appropriate disparities index, and transmit to the recipients of mental health services, broader "variegated" (Brenner et al. 2010) neoliberal ideologies regarding entitlement to care, self-responsibility, and political belonging.

Moral Economy as a Register of Disavowal

Historian E. P. Thompson introduced the term "moral economy" in his seminal work, *The Making of the English Working Class* (1963), and subsequently developed the concept in his 1971 paper, "The Moral Economy of the English Crowd in the Eighteenth Century." Writing against what he viewed as the tendency of his contemporaries toward "a crass economic reductionism . . . [that obliterates] complexities of motive, behaviour, and function," Thompson argued, in his analysis of the eighteenth century "food riots," that the actions of the English crowds were not driven merely by hunger or by "elementary economic stimuli" (1971, 78). Rather, he contended, the grievances of the peasants and laborers emerged from a "moral economy of the poor"—a popular consensus regarding the legitimacy or illegitimacy of certain practices that was, in turn, "grounded upon a consistent traditional view of social norms and obligations, of the proper economic functions of several parties within the community" (1971, 79).

Because the aim of Thompson's intervention was to ascribe agency and self-consciousness to the rioting masses and thereby complicate the presumed causal link between the crowd's material realities and their actions (Fassin 2009), his analysis needed to foreground the ways in which moral economy functioned as a nuanced, internally coherent system that operated outside of—and prior to—capitalist political and market economy. To accomplish this, Thompson repeatedly cited notions of tradition and paternalism as undergirding moral economy, positioning these modes of valuation in opposition to the new *laissez-faire* model that "entailed a de-moralizing of the theory of trade and consumption" (Thompson 1971, 89). Thus, Thompson claimed that the English crowd acted according to "a selective reconstruction of the paternalist [model]" (1971, 98), and described acts of looting in the wake of rising bread prices as "legitimized by assumptions of an older moral economy, which taught the immorality of any unfair method of forcing up the price of provisions by profiteering from the necessities of the people" (1963, 63). Though Thompson would later write that he had never meant to imply such a sharp dichotomy between morality and market economics (Thompson 1991), his work has often been read this way in the social sciences, leading to a proliferation of studies that treat moral economy as inhering in poor or dominated populations or situated only within developing, precapitalist societies (e.g., Scott 1976).

Alongside these stricter appropriations of Thompson's category, hundreds of studies have taken up and expanded the concept of "moral economy" in nearly every conceivable direction (Fassin 2009). Among these expansions is a corpus that argues for a reintegration of the purportedly dichotomous domains of moral and market economy, pointing out the ways in which the two are in actuality complementary and even interdependent. Martin Kohli, for instance, writing on retirement as an element of moral economy in contemporary Germany, endorses Thompson's call to trace the "social logic of reciprocity," but asserts that

[a]nother part of [Thompson's] argument is less convincing: that the moral economy is valid only in the pre-industrial economy, and after a prolonged agony is giving way to the newly emerging market economy. It

is more plausible instead to consider the latter as a new form of economic organization giving rise to its own moral economy on which it depends for its functioning. (Kohli 1987, 127)

For Kohli, an understanding of the "taken-for-granted beliefs of fairness in the relation of efforts and rewards" is integral to an analysis of the lifelong engagements of workers and management in a wage labor market (127). Minkler and Cole (1992) argue, similarly, that political and moral economy are "not such strange bedfellows" and that limiting the application of moral economy solely to analyses of premarket economies robs the concept of its potential for larger relevance. Didier Fassin (2005, 365) makes the case for a reading of moral economy as "the economy of the moral values and norms of a given group in a given moment" and, from this point of departure, uses the concept to provide an analysis of immigration policies and biopolitics in contemporary Europe. Michele Rivkin-Fish, in an ethnographic examination of dental education in the contemporary United States, treats the country's system of commodified healthcare as a type of moral economy into which dental students are socialized as they "learn sets of assumptions regarding participants' rights, responsibilities, and entitlements, notions that define the kinds of claims they can make on each other and society at large" (2011, 187).

In this chapter, I follow Rivkin-Fish, Kohli, Fassin, and others in thinking about the ways in which moral economies articulate with—rather than stand outside of—political economy and free market logics. Departing in focus somewhat from these scholars, however, my central aim is not to demonstrate the presence of moral values and norms embedded within contemporary economic systems and public policies; instead, I trace a process through which a moral economy of psychotherapeutic care is structured by—but comes to appear as though it is disconnected from—market logics and ideologies, even as it enforces and reproduces them. My use of the term "moral economy" here serves to underscore the idea that under conditions in which actors are driven to disavow their relationship to political economy, one strategy they may deploy is to shift discursively to a moral register, exploiting the presumed immunity of the moral order to baser economic considerations.[5] The resulting moral discourses, I contend, are pernicious inasmuch as they efface their own economic bases, thereby stabilizing and rendering natural unequal practices that might be better served by a recognition and interrogation of their underlying economic logics.

Therapeutic Fee as Gift: The Transmutation of Capital in Private Practice Billing Discourses

Given the contradictory ways in which psychotherapists are professionally conditioned to both disregard and pursue capital, it is not surprising that matters pertaining to fee collection should comprise a site of ambivalence that therapists attempt to manage through a shift to a more agreeable moral register. Indeed, among academic and practicing psychotherapists there exists a robust literature lamenting the "resistance among us to exploring [the issue of money and fees for treatment]" (Shields 1996, 233; see also Herron and Welt 1992; Monger 1998; McWilliams 2004) and offering various ethical or psychoanalytic explanations for this "money taboo" (Trachtman 1999; Wolfson 1999). Financial planners have even developed their own local idiom to write about the phenomenon, diagnosing mental health professionals as "money avoidant" and publishing studies that suggest that "when compared to other occupations, mental health professionals report significantly lower levels of financial health" (Britt et al. 2015).

Expanding on the opening vignette of the chapter, we will examine the manner in which a disavowal of money matters takes shape among psychotherapists in private practice, as well as the consequences of the strategies that therapists in such settings deploy. I argue that therapists' moral discourses on the therapeutic function of the fee in private practice figure the clinician and patient as socially connected in a kind of gift exchange relationship characterized by ongoing relational support and the shared perception of unmediated intimacy. This figuration draws from national ideologies regarding class and entitlement to care, and it naturalizes notions of the middle class as more deserving of, and better suited to, enduring forms of social support.

A close reading of the messaging found on a private practitioner's website is instructive to our understanding of the ways that matters pertaining to payment and fees are enfolded into the construction of an unmediated therapeutic relationship: Matthew Brown worked for many years in social service agencies—first as clinical staff and later as a supervisor and director—before earning his doctorate and shifting focus to academic administration at CSPP and private practice. Today, Matthew's psychotherapy office is on the highest floor of a beautiful art deco building with a prestigious street address in downtown Chicago.

A section of Matthew's business website devoted to questions and answers about his fee opens with a statement that is reminiscent of the sentiment that many therapists aspired to express in the professional life course narratives analyzed earlier—that is, that by leaving community mental health for private practice, the therapist has not abandoned their commitment to helping the poor. Matthew asserts that psychotherapists like himself, who have trained as clinical social workers, are deeply invested in the mission of making therapeutic services "available to all, regardless of income." He goes on to explain that for this reason, he strives to "maintain a balance" between seeing patients who are able to pay his fee of $175 per session and reserving "a certain number of appointments" for those who are unable to pay the full amount.

In the next sections of his website, Matthew elaborates several aspects of his billing policies. First, he promises not to raise a patient's fee once it has been set: If the initial, agreed-upon session fee was $90, for example, then it will never increase over the course of the treatment. Next, Matthew explains that any negotiation around the fee must occur in the context of a larger discussion about the patient's financial obligations as well as what Matthew terms "the required commitment to the work of psychotherapy," emphasizing his belief that the latter "must be a real commitment." Finally, Matthew requests that patients pay him directly, no less frequently than once per month.

The website section goes on to justify a billing policy that would seem incompatible with Matthew's stated desire to make his services available to all—that being the fact that he is not on any insurance panels. It explains that the reason for this policy is that psychotherapeutic work is "intense, highly personal, and absolutely must be confidential." Accepting private insurance, it reasons, would mean that Matthew "promised to follow the dictates of a corporation" instead of focusing "solely on the needs of a unique, one-to-one psychotherapeutic relationship" between himself and each of his patients. As such, it would amount to including an unwelcome "third party in the room."

For Matthew and Emily, who had instructed my classmates and me on the fair or therapeutic fee, the fee both symbolizes and helps constitute the therapeutic relationship, which lies at the heart of the therapeutic process. As a representation of the relationship, the fee is reliable and consistent: Like the relationship, the fee's stable dollar amount withstands the passage of time and survives chaotic turns of events in the patient's material or emotional life. Indeed, by foregrounding his policy of never raising a patient's fee once set, Matthew marks the therapeutic relationship as one that is insulated from market logics such as inflation, thereby decoupling psychotherapy from other examples of fee-for-service arrangements with which it could potentially be associated. In a sense, Matthew's statement about the stability of his fee is paradoxical in that it at once announces the financial relationship of therapy and renounces certain pecuniary interests on the part of the therapist. This duality, again, helps to set therapy apart as a special kind of relationship that operates outside of typical market logics and temporalities. Through a logic that collapses economic and psychological investment, the fee also stands for, as Matthew phrases it, a promise of loyalty on the part of the therapist—and it reflects, in turn, the patient's "real commitment" to the potentially long, arduous, and expensive work of psychotherapeutic treatment. Even the *form* of the fee—the surety of its repetition, and the fact that (for Matthew and many private practice therapists) it applies retroactively to the previous month's therapy sessions—seems symbolic of a relationship characterized by trust and continuity.[6] Finally, the very existence of an elaborated discourse on the meaning of the fee—both on Matthew's website and in the academic paper that Emily draws from—indexes a therapeutic process in which every aspect of the encounter is thoughtful, deliberate, and not compromised by third-party interests or bureaucratic considerations.[7]

As an instantiation of the therapeutic relationship, the fee is presented by Emily and Matthew as *that which renders possible* the intersubjective processes that constitute the work of psychotherapy, such as empathic understanding and the containment of "disruptive feeling states." Rather than understanding the fee as something that mediates in an economic transaction, or that externalizes and objectifies the value of the therapist's labor, in this formulation the fee potentiates a unique, financially *unmediated* relationship between therapist and patient characterized by collaboration, mutual respect, and intimacy.

It is, in one sense, ironic that in private practice therapists' moral discourses, it is the fee that is identified as allowing for the possibility of "intense, highly personal," and unmediated empathic work—after all, unlike at the agency where a therapist's salary is fixed and only indirectly dependent on client fees, in private practice the therapist's income is determined by what the patient pays. In a rather literal fashion, then, the private practice therapist and the patient engage in what would appear to be an undeniably transactional exchange of cash—ideally (as Matthew requires) from the patient's own bank account, sent via personal check to the therapist—for a service, leaving no question as to whether their ensuing relationship was a mediated one. But instead, as the meaning of the fee is folded into a moral framework of therapeutic value, the fee undergoes a conversion from money into symbolic capital. It ceases to mediate, and instead seals and strengthens the bond between the two parties that jointly disavow its exchange function.

But in another sense, one could argue that the economic structure undergirding clinicians' moral discourses of the "therapeutic fee" recalls that of a gift exchange and that, as such, it is unsurprising that only in the predominantly middle-class setting could there be a shared "misrecognition . . . of the reality of the objective 'mechanism' of the exchange" (Bourdieu 1977, 5–6). By this reading, it is *because* private practice patients possess sufficient capital that they are able to give the therapist a "gift" and thereby enter into a horizontal social relationship that appears to operate outside of the logic of market exchange. Such relationships, as Pierre Bourdieu, Georg Simmel (1950), and Jacques Derrida (1992) remind us, are sustained, and accomplish their misrecognition, by incorporating into them intervals of time between gift and counter-gift. Here, similarly, fee discourses and policies facilitate a figuration of therapist and patient as collaborators in an enduring social relationship—rather than as participants in a series of economic transactions—both by theorizing the fee as an index of mutual, long-term commitment and formally by building a temporal delay into the exchange of fee for service. Accordingly, as private practice therapists rationalize the fee as therapeutic, they naturalize as appropriate only to middle-class patients a supportive therapeutic relationship with an ongoing, open-ended temporality.

Billable Services and Appropriate Care: The Production of Moral Discourses in Agency Settings

In contrast to the "therapeutic fee" discourses deployed by psychotherapists in private practice, which invoke a politics of immediation (Mazzarella 2006) in order to refigure a potentially anxiogenic form of economic exchange as a morally positive enactment of mutual trust and intimacy, agency therapists generate moral talk regarding therapeutic appropriateness in order to achieve an alignment between the constrained set of services for which they are able to bill and the clinical needs of their clients. Consider the understandings around fee and therapeutic services elicited in the case of Jamal, an uninsured ex-convict with no employment history who came through my office for an intake at WBH: Following the agency's protocol for uninsured clients, I administered a document called the "Financial Interview," and determined that with his nonexistent income, schizophrenia diagnosis, and history of psychiatric treatment in prison, Jamal readily met the criteria for the Illinois Department of Human Services/Division of Mental Health Eligibility Group 2: The "Non-Medicaid Target Population." As "a DMH-2," Jamal was entitled to a very limited set of mental health services—including a few sessions of case management, but no psychotherapy—paid for by the state. If he wanted a long-term therapist, he would need to come up with $15 per session in cash to see a student, or $60 per session to see a licensed clinician.

In supervision, I learned that occasionally, a therapist would conduct a total of four off-the-record psychotherapy sessions with a DMH-2 client by billing for the therapy under the "Case Management" code. However, I was advised that in Jamal's case—given his psychotic symptoms and tendency to miss his appointments, psychotherapy was not appropriate at any rate. "In community mental health," my supervisor explained, "it's more of a revolving door. We get clients who are ambivalent, less motivated, or not ready for change." The best care I could provide for Jamal would be to meet with him a couple of times to help him apply for health insurance and persuade him to follow through with his scheduled psychiatric evaluation.

But the next time I saw Jamal, he arrived in a lucid and upbeat state, announcing that he had just seen the psychiatrist and had already submitted the CountyCare insurance application on his own. To my surprise, Jamal then asked: "Can I tell you about a dream I had last night? It's the first one I've remembered in years." Jamal recounted a dream of trying to ride an elevator up to his birthday party while avoiding other passengers who wanted to harm him. Grinning for the first time since I had met him, Jamal declared that his dream was about needing to find some peace from his intrusive, paranoid thoughts "so I can make it up to that party at the top of the building!" At the end of the hour, Jamal thanked me several times and promised to call and schedule his next session soon.

I returned to my supervisor, excited to tell her about Jamal's unexpected capacity for relational, insight-oriented therapeutic work. "It's nice that he opened up that way," my supervisor said, "but I wouldn't spend too much time on that kind of work with him, going forward. It's not really appropriate or relevant to his treatment. What he needs is to be empowered to better manage his appointments and begin to get his life in order without the support of a therapist." Thus chastened and feeling slightly defeated, I went back to my desk and wrote a note about Jamal's progress toward enrolling in a Medicaid managed care program. Later, in my biweekly clinical consult session with a psychoanalyst from CSPP, I would recount the story and receive instruction on how I could have proceeded with dream interpretation "if this were a patient you were seeing in long-term analysis." My internship ended before I had the chance to talk to Jamal again in person.

The case of Jamal is illustrative of the fact that, as in private psychotherapy settings, agency clinicians would prefer to understand their practices as arising directly out of the client's therapeutic needs rather than as dictated by economic factors. Thus, when faced with a billing protocol that is incompatible with an individualized, long-term, relational style of treatment, therapists may naturalize the service limits imposed on the client by viewing them as conveniently coinciding with what is most clinically appropriate—even when they are presented with evidence to the contrary.

Everyday Alignments in Agency Therapists' Usage of Billing Codes

Jamal's case was somewhat unusual owing to his lack of any insurance coverage. However, even in the treatment of Medicaid-funded clients at the two agencies, I regularly encountered similar instances of discursive work aimed at resolving clinicians' ambivalence through an alignment of billing-related decisions with assessments of therapeutic appropriateness. Unlike private practice patients, for whom therapists' disavowal of political economy helped to produce a sustained social connection, agency clients were subject to moral rationales that inserted them directly into (rather than freeing them from) a logic of present-moment economic exchange, and that were oriented toward a horizon in which the client would not receive therapeutic support.

One way in which billing constraints at agencies were translated into moral principles that naturalized, as therapeutically appropriate, interventions that denied clients access to ongoing relational intimacy was the standard practice of providing services coded as "Community Support." This convention was introduced to new clinicians almost immediately upon hire, as the following vignette from a New Staff Orientation illustrates:

> Four days into the weeklong New Staff Orientation at RecoveryNet's main office, I file into a darkened room lined with computer monitors for a training on how to write service notes. Going through the orientation with me are about 25 other newly minted social workers and counselors (as well as a peer recovery specialist and a few other miscellaneous clinical staff), all of us soon to be scattered across RecoveryNet's 100-plus Chicago-area programs for adults with severe and persistent mental illnesses.
>
> The goal of the afternoon's training is to teach us how to choose the billable service code that best describes the interaction we had with a client, and to train us in the art of producing a written narrative of that interaction that will satisfy criteria for Medicaid reimbursement. We begin with a straightforward distinction: "Client-Centered Consult," or "CCC," is the code that one uses to bill for interactions that the clinician has *about* a client *with* another professional—such as a phone call with the client's physician. The client is usually not there when we perform a

service that is coded as CCC. "Case Management" can also be conducted in the client's absence and is, we are told by the training presenter, "something that you're basically doing *for* the client, that they couldn't do for themselves."

After covering these services quickly, the presenter moves into the heart of the training: a discussion of when and how to use a service code called "Community Support" versus one called "Therapy/Counseling." "We want to lean towards Community Support whenever possible," the presenter explains. Unlike instances of case management, she elaborates, Community Support "is really an opportunity to teach [the client] something rather than create a dependence on you to do it for them." This sort of teaching toward independence, we learn, is of great clinical value to our client population, and is oftentimes more appropriate than Therapy/Counseling, which the presenter describes as a clinical interaction that would tend to "look a lot more backwards" into the client's past.

Having established that in the majority of instances, the kinds of sessions that we will be having with our clients will fall under the "Community Support" heading, our presenter asks the group to participate in an exercise wherein we collectively write a Community Support service note based on a description that she provides about a meeting with one of her former clients. The client is a man diagnosed with bipolar disorder who used to cut himself and who, the presenter adds, "is employed, but that's always been shaky." We are told that the client's treatment goals are to "learn better coping skills to deal with changes in his moods," and to "strengthen his natural supports," namely by improving his currently tumultuous relationships with family members.

"I come in to see the client at his job," the presenter narrates. "He hasn't shaved, and looks upset. He describes a whole bunch of difficulties he's having at work, mainly due to his feeling that his boss hates him. He says he's been thinking about cutting, but has managed to stop himself. He then describes recent positive interactions with his sister."

Our presenter stops there and asks: "Ok, so how do we break this down into a note?" We practice writing the opening sentence of the note, which, we are told, should "give a nice, tight definition of the mental health reason for the visit—of 'this is why we're here.'" The presenter explains that instead of naming the client's diagnosis in this sentence, we want to choose actionable symptoms that can then be linked to specific, tangible interventions. We settle on: "Due to client's history of self-harm and low self-esteem, staff met with client to review progress using independent coping skills."

Next, our attention is directed to a handout—which I later re-encounter posted above my desk at CRC—listing suitable examples of "intervention verbs" according to the type of billable service used with the client. The longest list on the handout is the one for "Community Support" services. Defined as "[s]ervices consisting of therapeutic interventions that facilitate illness self-management, skill building, use of natural supports, and use of community resources," the "Community Support" list contains verbs such as "Coached," "Directed," "Modeled," "Planned," "Practiced," and "Taught." One column over on the handout is a list of intervention verbs for "Therapy/Counseling" services. Defined as "[f]ormal and ongoing counseling/therapy sessions with a [client] with the goal of ending or reducing symptoms related to his/her emotional, cognitive, and behavioral problems," this list includes the more contemplative "Analyzed," "Explored," "Reassured," "Shared," and "Understood."[8]

The presenter then imparts to us a straightforward guideline to be followed when writing service notes: For every 15 minutes of billable time spent with a client, a service note should contain a sentence with one intervention verb. To practice implementing this rule, we are asked to draft three sentences describing what we did in our hypothetical 45-minute visit with the bipolar man. The presenter takes suggestions from our group and gently re-works them as she writes the service note on a white board at the front of the room.

"So what did we do with our client?" she asks.

"Maybe we can ask the client why he believes his boss hates him?" someone offers.

"Sure, we want to help the client identify his triggers," the presenter responds, scribbling "*Identified triggers at work*" onto the board. "What else?"

A trainee volunteers: "Talk about how he thinks about cutting when he feels bad?"

The presenter prompts: "That's like what he *does*, that he feels bad. So the *development* is around . . . ?" As she speaks, the presenter writes the intervention that she is looking for on the board: "*Reviewed alternative coping mechanisms with client.*"

Turning back to our group, the presenter then asks: "And what do we do about the sister?"

"*Listed ways to continue to receive positive support from his sister*" rounds out this section of our imaginary service note.

Note that although there is certainly some overlap in the lists of intervention verbs, the verbs that are designated as "Community Support"—exemplified by those selected by the presenter in the group-written note—generally describe interactions that position the clinician as a temporary support whose role is to be instrumental in the client's movement toward independence or "recovery" (Myers 2015). Distinctly non-intimate or relational, these verbs—and the types of meetings with clients to which they refer—are ones that reflect and aim to facilitate the client's ability to autonomously "self-manage" a mental illness or to seek support from outside of a formal therapy context if needed (i.e., through "natural supports" and "community resources").

When I began working at RecoveryNet/CRC, I initially believed that the content of trainings such as this one would bear little resemblance to what would occur during actual clinical encounters with clients. I suspected that a vast, easily discernible, and openly acknowledged divide existed between the sorts of relationships and interactions that clinicians had with clients "on the ground," and the ways in which those relationships and interactions had to get translated so as to become exchangeable for dollars of Medicaid reimbursement.[9] These expectations were *partially* correct, in that my therapist informants would certainly agree that the interminable documentation they were made to produce did not capture the depth or complexity of their experiences with clients. But what surprised me was the frequent *lack* of disjuncture between the ways that clinicians evaluated and described clients for the purpose of satisfying billing-related regimes, and their *clinical* assessments of clients' capabilities and treatment needs. I soon came to understand that at CRC, therapists not only learned to label their client sessions with the "Community Support" billing code; they also tended to subscribe to the belief that the code genuinely reflected the kinds of support best suited to their clients, and they interacted with clients accordingly. Thus, when I asked my coworkers why we generally billed sessions as "Community Support" rather than "Therapy/Counseling," their responses emphasized the dual convictions that the "Community Support" code most accurately reflected their clinical interactions (e.g., "It's primarily because ['Community Support'] is the best way to describe the service"), and that such interactions were the most appropriate form of care for the agency's clients (e.g., "[Our clients] don't tend to [have] regularly scheduled appointment[s], working on therapeutic concerns"). Only one clinician cited as a secondary reason for the billing preference (after first mentioning the greater appropriateness of Community Support services to the client population) that she had gotten a vague "vibe" that "Medicaid would be more likely to reimburse unlimited coaching versus therapy." It was not until I posed the question to an employee in the agency's quality assurance department that I received confirmation that the guideline was indeed motivated by managed care billing constraints: Therapy/Counseling services, I learned, required a time-consuming reauthorization procedure after twenty hours per year. No such limitations were imposed on Community Support services, which were reimbursed at the same rate.[10] The billing protocol thus both encoded and structured notions of the kinds of services agency clients needed or deserved, but the economic origins of these notions went largely inaccessible to clinicians, who had translated them into moral principles of therapeutic appropriateness.

The Figuration of Agency Clients as Market Actors

While technically there was no annual limit on the number of hours of Community Support services that a clinician could bill to Medicaid, and many clients did indeed receive this service for multiple years or longer, therapists—who themselves often were oriented toward a horizon of departure from agency work—talked in ways that aligned the objectives and implicit temporality of Community Support services with notions of how best to work with their clients. Specifically, therapists' talk conveyed to the clients—and to one another—moral principles that were focused on equitable exchanges of effort in present-moment interactions, and that envisioned the client's future autonomy from therapeutic support. For example, therapists frequently reminded each other in team meetings that it was clinically detrimental to "work harder than your client" or to expend effort toward the client's improvement if the client was not willing to do the same. Similarly, one supervisor described the goal of clinical work to me as "making yourself unnecessary," and encouraged therapists to support clients in learning how to navigate their worlds without the help of the agency. Even the pervasive talk within agency settings about service "reimbursement"—a term that I never heard used among therapists in private practice, but which arguably calls attention to a temporal delay between the moment of care and the moment of payment not unlike that which is set up in the private practice relationship—becomes a language for continually recalling the client's indebtedness and obligations to reciprocity. In such ways, clients were continually constituted as market actors who could only participate in a futureless logic of immediate exchange. Lacking the forms of social and economic capital that paradoxically allowed private practice patients to transcend this logic and acquire social ties with their therapists built on mutuality and open-ended time, agency clients were repeatedly reinserted into economic paradigms as therapists disavowed the role of billing protocols in their clinical thinking.

Conclusion: Moral Economies of Mental Healthcare

Private practice and agency clinicians both deploy a moral register in order to negotiate structural contradictions and reframe problematic economic imperatives in terms of therapeutically appropriate practices. In so doing, they unwittingly reproduce and naturalize a class-differentiated *moral economy of mental healthcare* that ascribes to middle- and working-class clients radically unequal therapeutic needs and entitlements. Private practice clinicians' discourses on the "therapeutic fee" construct psychotherapy as something that is collaborative, long-term, individualized, and, above all, based on a close interpersonal relationship. These discourses suggest that patients' problems are not to be resolved autonomously, but rather in and through a relational matrix. As such, private practice patients receive a message that validates and normalizes their need for ongoing social support.[11] Agency clients, in contrast, are figured through therapists' moral discourses as somehow constitutionally unfit for a healing process based on interpersonal support, and better suited to interventions that focus on building the client's own motivation and self-sufficiency.

Although therapists shift to a moral register as a strategy for reframing and disavowing the political economic tensions that structure their professional lives, their resultant discourses, ironically, end up reasserting the very market logics that the therapists seek to overcome. Specifically, they set up in microcosm the same uneven or "variegated" (Brenner et al. 2010) expectations about neoliberal governmentality, self-responsibility, and entitlement to care that pervade contemporary US social policy and the public imagination—namely, that those individuals with the fewest economic resources are the ones who are most required to minimize "dependency" and behave as market actors (Peck 2001), while those who have the resources to do so may convert their money into social capital and thereby participate in social relationships that ostensibly operate outside of a logic of exchange.

Put another way, classic anthropological analyses of gifts have demonstrated that one does not ever truly give or receive a gift for "free": In every instance, the gift is actually "part of a system of reciprocity" that has to be returned in some specific way so as to "[set] up a perpetual cycle of exchanges" (Douglas in Mauss 1990, xi). What sets gift exchange apart from adjacent practices such as loaning or swapping, for example, is the norm that its return must be "*deferred* and *different*" (Bourdieu 1977, 5, emphasis in original) so that the parties involved may sustain solidarity by disavowing their joint participation in a form of market exchange. As this chapter has shown, even though the provision of psychotherapy in *both* agency and private practice settings usually consists of a time-deferred exchange of a fee for a service—and, furthermore, even though the cash fee in the private practice case passes more directly from the patient's hands to the therapist's—the ways that private practice therapists theorize and talk about fees promote their reinterpretation as gifts, while billing talk at agencies foregrounds the relationship of immediate exchange with the client-as-market-actor. The difference is productive of meaningful consequences for the kinds of therapeutic services considered appropriate to each setting's respective population, subtly suggesting and shaping what recovery, self-responsibility, and support might entail for one class of citizen versus another. At the same time, of course, the treatment disparities that therapists' billing discourses help to produce are not created in a vacuum—instead, they are continuous with broader, yet often invisible, ideologies and practices that apply the ideals of neoliberalism in differential ways. Inasmuch as this chapter traces a mechanism for the relief of structurally induced therapist ambivalence that leads to the fortification of problematic, class-differentiated notions of governance and moral responsibility, it tries to heed Gershon's (2011) call to mobilize the anthropological imagination in an effort to "delineat[e] where and how neoliberal perspectives fail to provide adequate and equitable ways of living" (546).

In emphasizing the potential for unintended harm caused by therapists' efforts to effect a felicitous alignment of economic and therapeutic imperatives, I do not mean to assert the analytic priority of market relations or the superficiality of psychotherapeutic care (i.e., care as merely a rhetorical claim produced in moments of misrecognition). Nor do I wish to suggest that the two domains of economy and care are mutually exclusive; that "authentic care" can or must operate outside of spheres of economic exchange. Rather, the point that I aim to make is that problems arise when therapists are systematically asked *both* to perform care labor within uncomfortable political economic regimes *and* to participate in a collective professional disavowal of the constraints that such regimes may produce. I remain open to the possibility, in other words, that under certain conditions a private practitioner's higher fee may indeed serve a therapeutic function—or that for some agency clients, the types of mental health services most easily reimbursable by Medicaid may in fact be entirely congruent with the forms of care most therapeutically appropriate to them. My concern is with a professional reluctance to acknowledge economy and therapeutic care as distinct—albeit deeply intertwined—domains whose logics and ends are not always in full alignment. When the continuity of market relations and care is presumed and institutionally demanded rather than interrogated, we run the risk of naturalizing structural inequalities that could instead be named and problematized.

To return to the broader concerns of this book, what we may take away from the ethnographic data provided in this and the previous chapter is a strange symbiosis between a sort of discursive/narrative self-management *mobilized* and *enacted* by therapists as a strategy for disavowing structurally produced ambivalence, and an aspiration or need for clinical self-management *attributed to* those clients who are immersed in the very structural contradictions that therapists seek to overcome. Self-management—at least in symbolic or performative gestures—at once affords therapists the means to assert a degree of choice and autonomy over a compromised and structurally overdetermined professional trajectory, and paradoxically helps to solidify and naturalize the treatment disparities that exist at distinct nodes along this career path. It leads, specifically, to an erasure of the role of structural constraints on the therapist's designation of appropriate care for clients in agency settings, and consequent figuration of the agency client as a self-managing market actor. In contrast, the self-managing discourses that therapists produce to make sense of their private practice work open up a space of possibility for social solidarity and intimacy, if not for structural recognition.

5

"If You Close My Clinic, I Will Die"

*Structural Subordination and "Unwilling" Radicalism in a
Grassroots Mental Health Consumer Protest Movement*

Early one morning in August 2014, on a desolate corner of a depopulated
neighborhood on the South Side of Chicago, I lined up with some seventy members of the Mental Health Coalition (MHC) to board a yellow
school bus bound for downtown Chicago's City Hall. This was, as leaders of the coalition kept reminding the crowd, a historic day. As noted
earlier, around three years prior, the City Council of Chicago—under
the governance of its newly elected mayor, Rahm Emanuel—had unanimously approved a budget that closed six of Chicago's twelve public
mental health clinics. The six clinics that were closed had been located
in low-income neighborhoods throughout the city, with four of the six
situated on Chicago's predominantly Black South Side.[1] All six clinics
had provided free, long-term psychiatric and therapeutic services, sometimes for decades, to economically marginalized and often uninsured
adults diagnosed with severe and chronic mental illnesses. Rooted in
the "clubhouse" or community drop-in center model that emerged with
deinstitutionalization and the JFK-era Community Mental Health Act
of 1963, the neighborhood clinics were beloved by their consumers as
spaces that offered mental healthcare as well as social activities, leadership opportunities, or just a local place to go and spend time with
culturally similar peers and staff.

Since the time of the closures, the MHC—a grassroots activist coalition led by former consumers of the shuttered South Side clinics—had
organized dozens of protests, letter-writing campaigns, an "occupation"
in which they barricaded themselves inside of the Woodlawn Mental
Health Center, and even a sit-in at the mayor's office—all with the goal
of compelling the city to restore and maintain its public mental healthcare system. A major step in this pursuit, the coalition believed, was to

be granted a City Hall hearing to address the issue of the clinic closures. This would finally provide consumers with an opportunity to testify and set the record straight about what had transpired in the wake of the closings—namely, that many consumers had not been successfully "transitioned," as the city had claimed, either to the remaining public clinics or to private community mental health providers; that instead, as the coalition's press release that August morning stated, consumers "fell into severe depression, addiction, psychosis, incarceration and general crisis due to losing their clinics and/or therapists" (Dardick 2014). The Mental Health Coalition also hoped that the hearing would function as a forum in which it could present to city officials its painstakingly researched public mental health policy and budget recommendations.

After years of setbacks, the hearing day had finally arrived. To ensure as wide a consumer presence as possible, the MHC had chartered a bus, arranged for carpools throughout the city, and combed the South Side of Chicago looking for consumers who were out on the street. Boxes full of SUBWAY® sandwiches and potato chips had been procured. Three hours had been set aside at City Hall for the hearing, during which time, we had been told, anyone who wished to testify would be given three minutes each to do so.

By looking closely at several moments from the MHC's long-anticipated City Hall hearing, as well as at other dynamics and conflicts related to consumer-led public mental health activisms in Chicago during the time of my research, we can gain insight into the practices and experiences surrounding the coalition as a kind of perverse endpoint to the logic of self-management that we have been tracing. We have already encountered a group of "professional bipolars" who embraced the clinical self-management paradigm in hopes of achieving some degree of agency, self-responsibility, and control over their own disordered brains, as well as explored the realm of *therapists'* discursive self-managerial practices, examining how the mobilization of particular narratives enables clinicians to lay claim to moral agency and professional integrity at the expense of disavowing structural forces. We have seen the ways in which therapists' "self-management" of political economic constraints—both those constraints guiding the therapists' own professional trajectories and those influencing the therapeutic services they are able to provide to clients—work to naturalize class-based disparities in the forms of clinical self-management and concomitant styles of subjectivity and agency (i.e., as more or less socially distributive) offered to different patient populations. In each of the above instances, self-management was a mode that was in some sense "chosen" or claimed by its user as a means—though not necessarily a successful one—to achieving and indexing a desired form of self-determination. At the same time, each of those examples of self-management gestured toward the reality that in the contemporary United States, the duty to perform full and autonomous self-direction—and to individually take on and attempt to resolve structural constraints—falls most heavily on the shoulders of those who are structurally vulnerable and who are therefore especially *limited* in their ability to achieve such autonomy. As we look deeper at the ways in which disenfranchised individuals are forced to self-manage in a literal sense[2]—not principally out of a desire for greater autonomy, but as a survival strategy in response to the disappearance of the institutional structures on which they depend for essential mental healthcare—we will see the ironic and unjust forms that self-management can take when its ideology is pushed to the extreme. If the self-management paradigm began to appeal to psychiatric (ex-)patient activists in part because it resonated with some activists' desire to be more independent from the state apparatus, then the Mental Health Coalition's *unwilling* radical self-management—necessitated by, and aimed at remediating, insufficient state support—brings the paradigm full circle.

The Rise and Fall of the Woodlawn Clinic

Before we turn to the meanings and uptakes of self-management in the context of poor and racially marked consumers' responses to public abandonment, it is helpful to review the history of those institutions that the consumer activists we are discussing sought to preserve. In 1959, the Chicago Health Department (now the Chicago Department of Public Health [CDPH]) opened its first Community Mental Health Center—the Mid-South Mental Health Center on the South Side of Chicago. Within three years, Mid-South was one of a robust network of more than fifteen community-based mental health centers that operated under the auspices of the newly established Mental Health Division of the city's Health Department. By the 1970s, Chicago had twenty-two public mental health centers that provided care to thousands of low-income residents of the city.

Even in their heyday, Chicago's public mental health centers were not without shortcomings and complexities: Consistent with what was occurring in other Chicago city departments, the clinics were "infected with patronage" (Bogira 2009, 670); city clinic psychiatrists worked only on a part-time basis; case management and psychotherapy were generally handled by lower-status (i.e., master's-level) clinicians (Bogira 2009). Nonetheless, the centers served vital functions, both for their consumers and for the local economies of the communities in which they were situated. The patronage-based hiring system, though corrupt, offered an important source of stable employment to residents of the clinics' working-class, minority neighborhoods (Lydersen 2013). Moreover, the clinics—which were early to adopt the holistic, collaborative, and flexible therapeutic model of the "clubhouse" developed in New York in the late 1940s (Spitzmueller 2016)—provided compassion, a welcoming environment, and at times even a sense of family to many individuals whose lives would otherwise have been relegated to the revolving door of hospitalization, imprisonment, and homelessness.

Chicago's innovative system of public mental health clinics rapidly became an exemplary model of the federal government's emerging community mental health vision: In 1955, the US Congress had passed the Mental Health Study Act, a landmark policy document that represented the first federal initiative to implement a national mental health program (Spitzmueller 2014). In the final report that came out of this study six years later, the Joint Commission on Mental Health and Illness (which comprised the newly established National Institute for Mental Health and the American Medical Association) identified the key clinical goal of reducing mental hospital populations and re-assimilating patients back into their communities. These recommendations culminated in the Community Mental Health Centers Act of 1963, which earmarked $150 million in federal grants between 1965 and 1967 for the construction, across the nation, of community mental health centers similar to those recently created in Chicago (Spitzmueller 2014).

Announcing the Act to Congress, President John F. Kennedy stated:

I am proposing a new approach to mental illness and to mental retardation. This approach is designed, in large measure, to use Federal resources to stimulate State, local, and private action. When carried out, reliance on the cold mercy of custodial isolation will be supplanted by the open warmth of community concern and capability. Emphasis on prevention, treatment, and rehabilitation will be substituted for a desultory interest in confining patients in an institution to wither away. (Prioleau 2013)

A defining feature of this early community mental health movement was its social theory of mental health, and specifically its conviction that social rejection was a key obstacle for individuals with severe mental illnesses. Indeed, its emphasis on "community" was meant to shift the subject of care and reform from the isolated individual to the broader social environment: Through an initial influx of federal grant support, *communities* were to be nurtured so that they, in turn, could accommodate their mentally ill (Spitzmueller 2014). Relatedly, the mission of community mental health centers, according to the Act's vision, was to foster environments that would proactively *prevent*—rather than merely treat—developmental and psychiatric problems.

Among the Chicago city clinics, the Woodlawn Mental Health Center particularly anticipated and embodied the ideals of JFK's community mental health movement. Founded in 1962 by three Yale psychiatrists as a joint project between the city and the University of Chicago, the Woodlawn clinic was described by its co-directors as a service facility as well as a "laboratory in social and community psychiatry" (Kellam and Schiff 1966, 255). As a social experiment, the clinic was designed to see whether it was possible to create

a public-health-oriented psychiatric treatment context for a circumscribed community. Such a treatment center would allow longitudinal studies of the relationship between psychiatric illness and the social processes of the community. In [the founders'] judgment, such a scientific interest could be pursued only in the context of a basic psychiatric service commitment to the mental health of the community, a commitment that could not be satisfied by duplicating traditional psychiatric treatment services. The commitment to the mental health of a total population required longitudinal methods of assessing mental health need in the community and the development of ways of intervening on a broad scale. (Kellam and Schiff 1966, 256)

The clinic's founders had evaluated sites in twelve different states before settling on the Woodlawn region of Chicago for its community mental health experiment. Criteria guiding the selection had included the existence of a community that was "geographically bounded, identifiable both to its citizens and to the larger governmental context in which it existed as a distinct community"; a "local, specific sanction from the citizens of the community" for the development of a community mental health center; available funding for basic operations through the county, city, or state; and proximity to a university (Kellam and Schiff 1966, 257). Woodlawn, with its marked sociological contrast with the affluent University of Chicago neighborhood of Hyde Park bordering it to the north, satisfied these criteria given the city's interest at the time in supporting the development of its cutting-edge system of neighborhood mental health centers. At a one-day "Conference on Community Psychiatry" marking the dedication of the University of Chicago's new Social Service Administration building in 1965 (Community Psychiatry and Social Work Introduction Statement 1966), Dr. Sheppard Kellam—a director of the Woodlawn Mental Health Center who would soon become a University of Chicago faculty member in the Department of Psychiatry—read to an audience of seven hundred social workers the following description (subsequently published) of the Woodlawn neighborhood:

> [The Woodlawn Mental Health Center] is located in an urban, Negro community of 82,000 people on the South Side of Chicago. Woodlawn is defined as a community both by natural boundaries and by historical tradition. It has been described as a transitional community. It has at times served many ethnic groups as the area through which populations have passed on their way out of the inner city toward eventual middle-class status. In recent years, this ecological function has been hampered by the increasing age of its buildings, by severe overcrowding, low income, and the specific problems of its Negro citizens in acquiring acceptance in the middle-class areas of the larger city. (Kellam and Schiff 1966, 255)

While the Woodlawn clinic founders were initially focused on the provision of comprehensive community care and outreach for the severely mentally ill, they were persuaded by local community leaders to also develop programs aimed at interrupting and preventing cycles of social and developmental disorder. In spite of their lack of prior training in prevention-based programming, the founders expanded the work of the Woodlawn Mental Health Center to include a successful early intervention program that collaborated with neighborhood children, families, and teachers to improve child behavior and school performance (Bogira 2009). Ample funding from federal and state grants was available in the early years of the clinic's existence to support these broad and forward-looking initiatives that aligned with Kennedy's vision of community mental health. Over time, however, federal funding for the Woodlawn clinic and other community mental health centers decreased in accordance with JFK's proposed timeline, while the gradual concomitant increase in the proportion of state support envisioned in the Community Mental Health Centers Act failed to materialize. In 1981, President Ronald Reagan dramatically slashed federal funding for these initiatives and delegated to the states the responsibility for community mental health services through meager block grants (Bogira 2009). Limited resources led prevention programs at the Woodlawn Mental Health Center and elsewhere to fall to the wayside, as clinics had to narrowly focus their priorities on the severely and chronically ill.

In the ensuing decades, as federal Community Mental Health Act funding and then state funding (see figure 5.1) for the Chicago Mental Health Centers declined, Woodlawn and some of the other city clinics managed to survive in large part because of the City of Chicago's unusually central role in the direct management and provision of mental health services. To compensate for budget losses, some public mental health clinics were gradually closed, while the CDPH increased its support of those that remained open through its Corporate and Community Development Block Grants. But even with this added support, the city seemed to be moving decidedly in a direction away from the maintenance of its public clinics. Mental health services at the centers, particularly psychiatry, grew sparser. By 2008, only twelve of the twenty-two city clinics were still in operation and publicly

**IDHS Mental Health Funding to Chicago
Department of Public Health, 2005-2015**

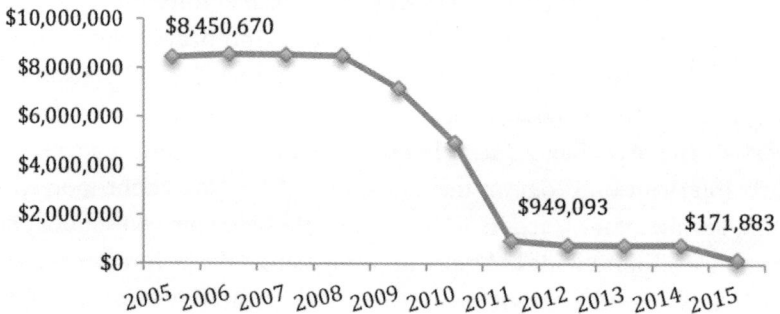

Figure 5.1. Illinois' spending on Chicago's mental health centers decreased from more than $8 million in 2005 to less than $200,000 in 2015—a total reduction of 98% over the course of a decade (Health & Disability Advocates 2015, 2). Reprinted with permission from Barbara Otto.

managed—three on the North Side, one on the near Southwest Side, and eight (including the Woodlawn clinic) on the South and Southwest Sides of Chicago.

In 2009, after the Chicago Department of Public Health failed to adequately implement its new electronic billing system and subsequently was facing a $1.2 million budget shortage, the Daley administration announced that up to five clinics would have to be closed.[3] Four of the five clinics slated for closure, including the Woodlawn Mental Health Center, were located on the South Side of Chicago. In collaboration with its umbrella organization and a local youth activist group, the Mental Health Coalition staged a sit-in followed by a confrontation with Mayor Daley in order to demand that clinic consumers not be punished for the city's administrative errors. In what was described by an NBC Chicago blogger as a "remarkable scene in which a citizen confronted the city's powerful leader and made him look like a weak, weaselly child" (Lydersen 2013), the MHC reduced the mayor to silence and then secured his assurance that the clinics would stay open, albeit with reduced staffing levels (see figure 5.2).[4]

In 2011, in his proposed budget for the following year, newly elected Mayor of Chicago Rahm Emanuel wasted no time renewing the city's efforts to close Woodlawn and five other mental health centers—all but two in predominantly African American communities on the South Side. Emanuel's plan was referred to as one of clinic "consolidation" rather than closure because consumers would in theory be transferred to the remaining clinics or to one of a number of private community mental health agencies. These private agencies, in turn, would receive a total of $500,000 from the city to supplement their federal funding. Through such "community partnerships," Emanuel argued, the city would save between $2 million and $3 million annually while offering better quality and more efficient mental health services to poor and uninsured consumers.

In response to the proposed closures, the Mental Health Coalition—with support from the labor union representing city clinic staff—prepared a report entitled "Dumping Responsibility: The Case Against Closing CDPH Mental Health Clinics." The report argued that the CDPH had failed to consider the high monetary and social costs of its clinic consolidation plan, relative to the small (around 1% of the total CDPH budget) amount of savings that it would derive. It pointed out that even the 1% savings estimate "does not anticipate the increase in costs of crisis services, law enforcement and jails resulting from the disruption of

Number of FTE Psychiatrists at CDPH Mental Health Centers, 2006-2015

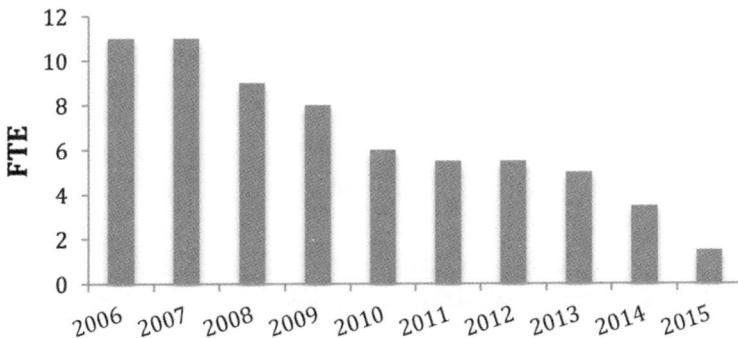

Figure 5.2. Bar graph depicting the decline in full-time equivalent (FTE) psychiatrists employed by CDPH between 2006 and 2015 (Health & Disability Advocates 2015, 3). Reprinted with permission from Barbara Otto.

treatment" (Mental Health Coalition 2012, 5). Furthermore, it contended, clearly the Department of Public Health had not worked out the details of its consolidation plan carefully or collected any data on "the prevalence of mental health disorders, current service capacity or any benchmarks for tracking changes in residents' mental health or access to services" (5). In its hurried enthusiasm over privatization, the report argued, the city had overlooked the many channels through which its plan would add to health disparities in Chicago and disrupt the lives of its most vulnerable citizens, disproportionally harming people of color. In short, the MHC declared the CDPH's proposed clinic closures to be a "disaster in the making"—one that demonstrated the city's cruel, "skewed priorities" as well as its incompetence (2012, 12). Interspersed among the report's pragmatic arguments and figures—including a chart visualizing the racial and ethnic makeup of the consumers at each city clinic and a list of suggested alternative budget line items that the CDPH could cut to achieve its desired savings—were photographs of consumers with descriptions in the consumers' own words of the vital impact of the city clinics. These quotes attempted to convey the gravity of the CDPH's proposed closures by emphasizing that consumers' very survival was at stake: "For me, my therapist is a matter of life or death because I have no one and I am alone," one photo caption read. Another issued the dire forecast that "[w]ithout the clinics some people will commit suicide" (MHC 2012, 12).

On November 15, 2011, the MHC held a ten-hour sit-in outside Mayor Rahm Emanuel's office in City Hall to protest the proposed clinic closures. Donning hospital gowns and holding up a sign that read "Rahm's Psych Ward," twelve consumers sat on the floor by the mayor's door from noon until 10:30 pm, at which time the need for access to a bathroom and drinking water led them to conclude the action (Terry 2011). In spite of these efforts, the very next day, the fifty aldermen comprising the City Council of Chicago unanimously passed Emanuel's proposed budget, including the "consolidation" of the twelve public mental health centers down to six (Lydersen 2013).

On April 12, 2012, just two weeks before the scheduled closing of the Woodlawn clinic, the Mental Health Coalition planned what it euphemistically termed a "party" in celebration of the clinic and its consumers. Hidden within the large barrels of refreshments that consumers wheeled into the building at 63rd Street and Woodlawn Avenue were bags of

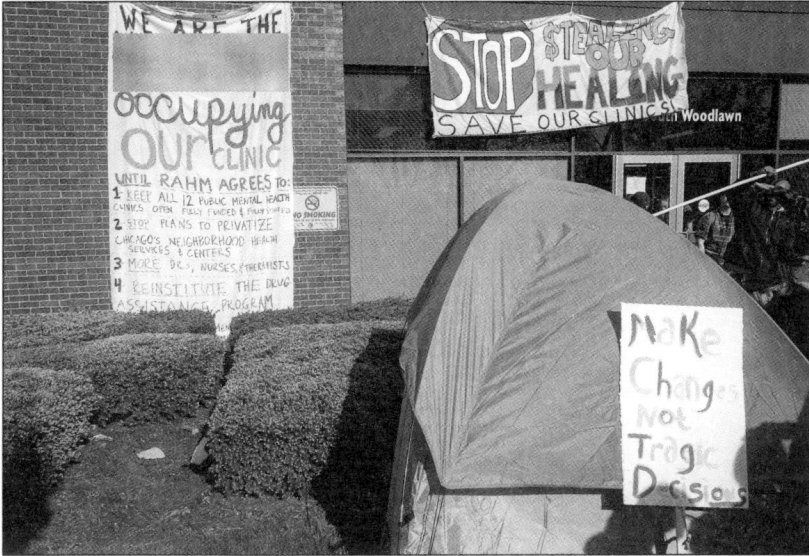

Figure 5.3. The Mental Health Coalition's occupation of the Woodlawn clinic on April 22, 2012. Photograph courtesy of Brett Jelinek used with permission.

quick-dry cement, and enough supplies for twenty people to survive inside the clinic for a month. Two hours into the celebration, the coalition announced its plan to "occupy" the clinic, warning revelers that they should leave if they did not wish to get arrested.[5] Two large banners, positioned earlier in the day on the clinic's roof, were then unfurled. The first banner stated that the Mental Health Coalition would occupy its clinic until Rahm Emanuel agreed to the organization's five demands: "Keep all 12 city mental health clinics public, open, fully funded and fully staffed; stop plans to privatize Chicago's 7 neighborhood health centers; hire more doctors, therapists, nurses, social workers and other clinic staff; reinstate the drug assistance program; and expand the public mental health safety net to cover unmet community needs." The second banner read "Stop Stealing Our Healing—Save Our Clinics" (figure 5.3).

Using metal chains and the concrete-filled barrels fortified with office chairs and vending machines, the Mental Health Coalition members erected a makeshift barricade (figure 5.4) and settled in for what they hoped would be a lengthy occupation. When the police arrived soon after, Caryn Jones—an outspoken, working-class African American

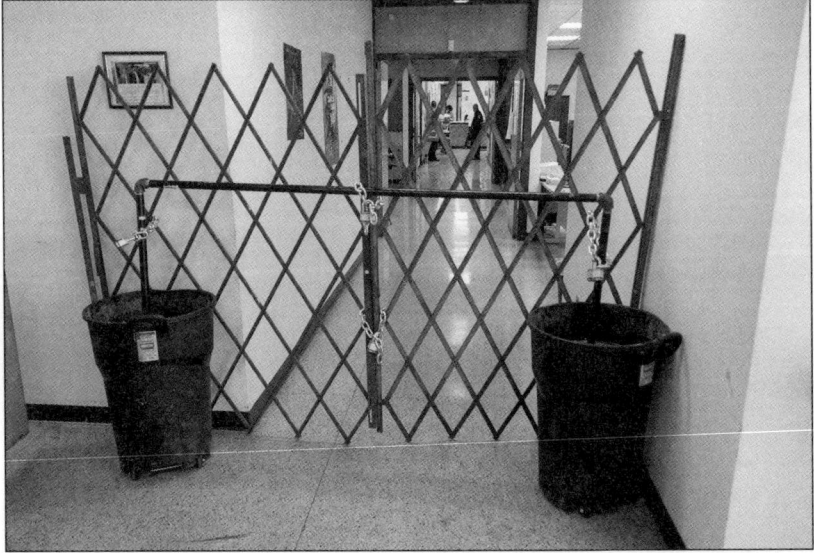

Figure 5.4. Barricade erected on April 12, 2012, for the occupation of the Woodlawn Mental Health Center. Photograph courtesy of Brett Jelinek used with permission.

public clinic consumer and an unofficial leader of the coalition—spoke with an officer through an opening in the barrier. Jones explained that the MHC's aim was to "get the mayor here to negotiate in good faith and stop being a bully" (Lydersen 2013, 119). She added that keeping Chicago's public mental health centers open was in the police department's interest as well as consumers' interest, since it would free up time for the officers to perform their intended job of stopping criminals: "We're not just fighting for us. We think it's unfair the police are forced to be babysitters for the mentally ill. . . . You are being shot at by people who are struggling with mental health issues," Jones said (Lydersen 2013, 120).[6] Ultimately, the MHC's occupation of the interior of their Woodlawn clinic only lasted about nine hours. The night culminated in the arrival of a SWAT team that used chain saws and bolt cutters to break down the barricade and arrest twenty-three people (Lydersen 2013).

Though brief, the occupation was a radicalizing event for many members of the Mental Health Coalition, who during my fieldwork would still occasionally recount how they stood their ground and stuck together, singing songs and chanting throughout the cold night that they spent in the police station lockup. Even after the arrests, for more than a month, at least a few members of the Mental Health Coalition occupied the vacant lot outside of the Woodlawn clinic on a daily basis. One consumer continued his own one-man, round-the-clock occupation, sleeping in the umbrella organization's beat-up van for several weeks after the others had moved on.

The City Hall Hearing on the Closing of the Chicago Mental Health Centers: Unwilling Self-Management and the Politics of Recognition in the Mental Health Coalition

As our yellow school bus made its way through the South Side of Chicago and into downtown, Mike, a young white community organizer who had been working with the MHC since its inception, kneeled backwards on his vinyl seat to address the other passengers. I looked up from the conversation I was having with a consumer who had asked me to help him rehearse his speech for the hearing during the bus ride. Prior to the hearing, Mike announced, we would hold a press conference at City Hall:

> The point of the press conference is twofold: One is to claim this as a victory, that the voices of the people affected by the clinic closures are finally gonna be heard! And the second is to make clear what we want, which is three demands we have today: Reopen the clinics; increase [clinic] funding and staffing in the next budget; and the third thing is join a provider network for Medicaid so that everybody can be served!

This third demand, in particular, had been discussed at length in MHC meetings leading up to the hearing day. The public mental health clinics in Chicago had originally been created to provide services to the uninsured only. At one time a much-needed safety net, in the wake of Medicaid expansion and the Affordable Care Act this qualification had arguably been transformed into a barrier to services for many consumers. It now functioned as a rationale for the city to turn consumers away, and then to justify closures by claiming that clinics were being underutilized. By demanding that the city clinics accept Medicaid payments, some members of the MHC reasoned, the city's not-so-secret plan to starve the clinics would be revealed and thwarted. Moreover, since joining a provider network would bring in revenue for the city, the coalition's demand would divest the city of its excuse that it could not afford to keep the clinics open. Countering these arguments, some MHC members maintained that the city clinics ought to continue to operate separately from any managed care arrangements.

Caryn Jones was to present these demands at the press conference and hearing, together with a budget that the Coalition had created showing that a mere $2 million a year—easily obtainable with a few simple cuts to nonessential city expenditures—was all it would take to reopen the six clinics. Addressing the passengers on our bus, Jones reminded everyone to conclude their testimonials by speaking about their experiences in the city's own fiscal language:

> Every time you see the news, there's people being arrested. Oftentimes they are dealing with frustration and anger and depression. Being put in jail is *not* helping anyone—it is costing the city and the taxpayers a lot of money! So what we want [at the press conference and hearing] is to end *always* by saying: "If the city needs money, they should join the referral networks." 'Cause that will bring in money for the clinics!

As the bus neared its destination, several MHC members slipped on matching, oversized T-shirts bearing the face of one of the Coalition's heroes, Eileen Morgan. A longtime consumer of a now-shuttered South Side clinic, Morgan had earned the respect of the MHC with her willingness to fearlessly confront the mayor of Chicago and her knack, as Mike had put it once, for delivering "a perfectly timed outburst." Morgan's voice itself—loud, sometimes belligerent, and often teetering on the edge of panic—was regarded by the Coalition as an effective tool, so much so that one member credited Morgan with saving the clinics in 2009 when Mayor Daley had first attempted to close them: "I believe," the member stated, "that the reason we got the clinics open was Mayor Daley was afraid that he would have to hear Eileen's voice every time he went to his office!" Printed below the photo of Morgan's face on the MHC's T-shirt was the warning that she had famously shouted to Mayor Rahm Emanuel just weeks before she was found deceased in her home: "If you close my clinic, I will die."

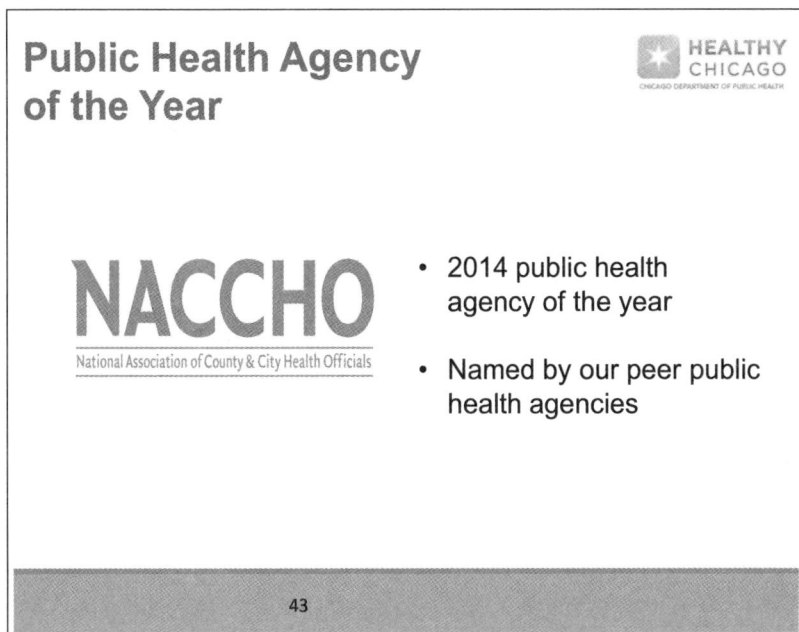

Figure 5.5. A slide from CDPH Commissioner Bechara Choucair's PowerPoint presentation at the City Hall hearing boasting of the department's recent accolades (Chicago Department of Public Health 2014, 43).

The MHC had been informed in advance that the first person to speak at the hearing would be Bechara Choucair, the Commissioner of the Chicago Department of Public Health. "He is a bad person," Jones had advised. "But just let him be bad on his own. Don't boo him." Yet even with this forewarning, consumers could not contain their frustration as the Commissioner delivered a self-congratulatory, nearly hour-long PowerPoint presentation, entitled "Ensuring Access to Mental Health Services For All Chicagoans," reiterating the very mistruths and denials about the consequences of the clinic closures that the consumers had come prepared to debunk (see figures 5.5 and 5.6). Disgusted murmurs rippled through the room as the Commissioner informed his audience that clinics had not been closed, just "consolidated"; that the city had tracked every "transitioned" consumer to ensure that no one had slipped through the cracks; that through its "targeted investments" and "strategic partnerships with private providers," CDPH had actually *expanded*

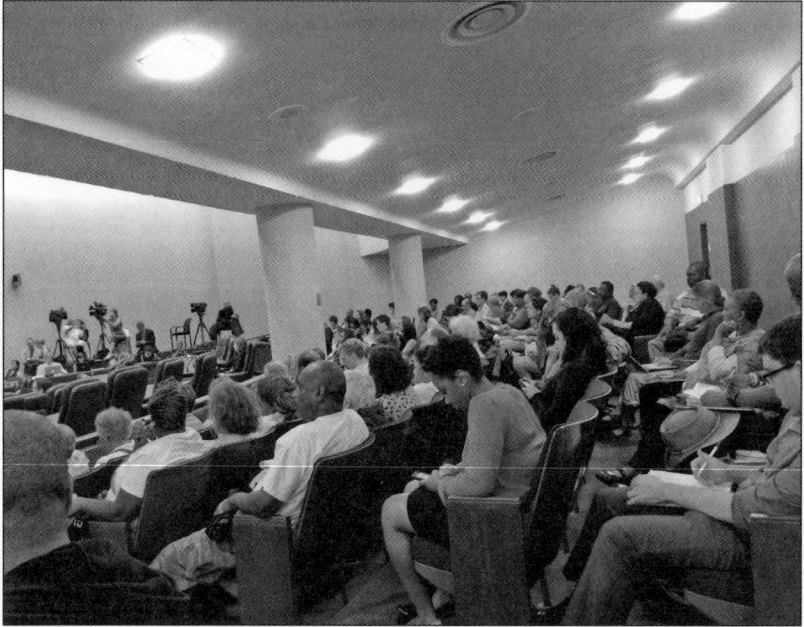

Figure 5.6. City clinic consumers from throughout Chicago wait for their promised opportunity to testify at the hearing on the closing of the clinics that the MHC had fought for years to arrange. Photograph by author.

services at the sites of the former clinics and now boasted award-winning "enhanced specialized care, increased service delivery, and improved patient hours." In a breathless finale, Choucair proclaimed: "Our city is moving in the right direction. . . . Two years after starting our reforms, Chicago's mental health system today is stronger than it was" (Dardick 2014). "Do we have a perfect mental health system in Chicago today? Absolutely not," the Commissioner conceded. "But is our mental health system today better than it was two years ago?" Over a resounding chorus of "*noooo*," Choucair announced his verdict: "Absolutely yes."

Commissioner Choucair's presentation was followed by ninety minutes of testimony from private providers that arguably had benefitted from funding and increased business after the public clinic closures. Most of these speakers, including representatives from Recovery-Net, endorsed the Commissioner's assessment that mental healthcare in Chicago was improving. During this portion of the hearing, which took up most of what remained of the three hours that had been allotted for consumer testimonials, the only MHC member who was called up to speak was Caryn Jones. As planned, Jones did not provide a narrative of her personal experience of losing mental health services, but rather attempted to speak in the bureaucratic register of the city officials. Ironically referencing what Commissioner Choucair had termed in his presentation the city's "three prong strategy" for public mental health reform, Jones enumerated the Mental Health Coalition's own "three prong demands," and then asked pointedly whether or not the city planned to join a provider network. Without acknowledging—much less responding directly to—any of Jones's points or her question, the Chair of the hearing thanked her and moved on.

As the scheduled end of the hearing drew near, and no other consumers had been called up to testify, a young Black activist sitting in the back of the room shouted out in anger: "Commissioner, you are creating genocide! How can you close half of the clinics and say that you have increased services? You're a liar!" "There seems to be some commotion," the Chair remarked. "Can everybody please settle down?" "There is commotion in the back of the room," Jones interjected dryly, "because you have *stacked the deck* with city workers! This is *the people's* hearing—*not* theirs!"

The expression on the Chair's face softened as he faced what remained of the room full of consumers (many had given up and gone home by this point). In a tone of voice that one might use when speaking to impatient children, the Chair reassured them: "Don't worry. We won't leave until *everyone* has a chance to get heard. I've cleared my schedule for the rest of the afternoon, so if everyone can just *calm down*, we can continue with the testimonies. The young lady in the back of the room: Why don't you come up here and tell us your name?"

Next to testify after the "young lady" was Nancy, an experienced Latina consumer activist speaker who delivered a powerful testimonial about her son, who had been shot and died in the arms of his now severely depressed and traumatized brother. Receiving therapy in their neighborhood clinic had been the only thing that had helped Nancy's son make progress toward recovery. Since that clinic had closed, Nancy explained, her son's situation had become hopeless: His mental health services had been "transitioned" to a clinic ninety minutes away via a bus that drove past two cemeteries and rival gang territory, which gave her son traumatic flashbacks. He refused to leave the house anymore. "At one point," Nancy confessed tearfully, "I put a gun in my mouth because I felt like a failure. . . . We want our clinics open. Stop lying to us, and open the clinics back up. Stop killing me. Stop killing my son and stop killing me."

"Nancy," the Chair responded gently. "There are a lot of people here in the room today who would like to help you. We have therapists from RecoveryNet here, we have Wellness Health, we have MetroCare,"[7] he added, naming some of the private providers that had just finished endorsing the city's strategy of closing Nancy's neighborhood clinic.

What becomes evident from these moments in the hearing is that the registers of speech made available to MHC members were only those that facilitated a reinforcement of members' structurally subordinate status. Although MHC members had prepared for the hearing by teaching each other to adopt a more politically effective language—a kind of rhetorical and discursive self-management—when they deployed such language, their interlocutors at City Hall refused to recognize them as the sorts of subjects whose positions the MHC members were attempting to linguistically inhabit. Indeed, even when, in temporal terms, Caryn Jones was permitted to participate in the portion of the hearing characterized by professional and expert discourses (i.e., quantified data, financial logics, use of corporate jargon such as "strategic partnerships" and "targeted investments," absence of personal narratives), Jones's contribution in kind was not viewed as such by the city officials. Instead, Jones and other MHC members were only granted a voice, so to speak, at the hearing when they performed disruptiveness, anger, or emotional volatility. These performances, while somewhat effective, simultaneously enabled the members' powerful audience to depoliticize and delegitimize the Mental Health Coalition by repositioning its members as children or as emotionally out-of-control patients in need of pity and placation. Thus, the shouting activist received no engagement with the *content* of her outburst, including her reasonable question about how the Public Health Commissioner could close six clinics while maintaining that he increased services. Rather, her rational critiques were refigured by the Chair as impatience with waiting for a turn to speak—a problem that the Chair ostensibly resolved as he invited the "young lady" up to the podium. Similarly, Nancy's forceful political message about the critical need for public, neighborhood-based clinics was not only left unaddressed but indeed undermined by the Chair, who patronizingly offered consolation in the form of assistance from the very providers that she had stated were inadequate to her family's circumstances.

As these interactions at the hearing as well as the MHC's valorization of Eileen Morgan's outbursts demonstrate, there appeared to be a recognition by the Coalition of the fact that when acquiring equal footing with one's powerful political opponent was out of the question, the most rhetorically effective strategy might be the performance of instability or anger. While such tactics are not unprecedented within social movements (e.g., Jasper 1998, 2011; Duncombe 2016), in the specific case that I have described, the interactions must be analyzed in the context of a growing body of literature on the intersections of race/racism, gender, class, affect, and emotion work. Building on Hochschild's (1979) theorization of the junctures "between consciousness of feeling and consciousness of feeling rules, between feeling rules and emotion work, [and] between feeling rules and social structure" (560), contemporary work in sociology and critical race theory has begun to trace the nuanced ways in which African American subjects engage with and manage affect. Such work has foregrounded phenomena including the racialization of feeling rules in professional workspaces and effects of this racialization on experiences and performance of emotion work by minority employees (Wingfield 2010); the modulation and bifurcation of emotional display strategies by Black men according to class-dependent social norms and expectations (Jackson 2018); the pressure experienced by nonwhite professionals in institutional spaces around emotion management in the interest of avoiding the reinforcement of negative racial stereotypes (Harlow 2003; Evans and Moore 2015); and the existence of "a particular set of 'binds' and 'freedoms,'" with respect to emotional labor, distinct to those who occupy "unprototypical or 'off-diagonal' social locations"— for example, "those whose race and gender identities convey conflicting, rather than overlapping, stereotype content" (Ispa-Landa and Thomas 2019, 392; see also Ridgeway and Kricheli-Katz 2013; Wilkins 2012; Collins 1998). As in the above examples, MHC members managed their public displays of anger with apparent mindfulness of both the affordances and the limitations of mobilizing the stereotypes through which they knew they were apprehended by those in positions of power.[8] Their semicalculated moments of volatility, like Tricia's act of self-harm discussed earlier, entailed a paradoxical form of self-management that both indexed and undermined the rationality of its enactors.

Given the multiply marginalized status of MHC members (i.e., as working-class persons of color and psychiatric service users), the emotion work that members undertook—in response to the condition of unwilling self-management to which they were subjected—was simultaneously effective, necessary, and self-negating. It thus attests to the extent to which analytic categories such as "free will" and "choice" are poorly suited to the task of understanding the phenomenology of self-management, especially as it pertains to experiences of the structurally subordinated. As we will see, micro-level sociological positioning, in the context of a city wrought with racism and historic segregation, played a decisive role in determining the distinct affective and political self-management tactics available to two structurally subordinated—but unequally so—groups of psychiatric consumer activists in Chicago.

Crowd-Funding Community Mental Health: Public Abandonment and Self-Management via the Migrating Logic of Competition

A few months after the City Hall hearing, I received an invitation to participate in a protest at the offices of the Department of Public Health in downtown Chicago. The protest had been organized by consumers of North Side Mental Health Center (NSMHC)—a public clinic located in a whiter and wealthier region of Chicago that had been spared in the most recent round of closures. Although it remained open, NSMHC had been operating without a staff psychiatrist for several months, ever since the one psychiatrist who had worked there for many years had retired. By this point, many of its consumers were either very low on their psychiatric medications or had run out completely. Some had been stable for years and were now in crisis, too depressed to get out of bed or slipping into psychosis. The city had been stalling for months, I was told, promising that it was actively working on hiring a new full-time psychiatrist but in the meantime doing nothing as the position remained unfilled and the number of people being deprived of basic medication management services rose. North Side's Consumer Council had already sent letters to the Chicago Department of Public Health describing their dire situation, but those letters had gone unanswered. The time had come, the Council had concluded, to ask for help in a way that the CDPH could not so easily ignore—by showing up at the department's door unannounced and not leaving until someone paid attention. The plan was for around fifty NSMHC consumers to meet at their clinic early in the morning, board a bus that the Consumer Council had chartered, and drive downtown to South State Street, whereupon the group would calmly demand that a CDPH official refill, on the spot, their expired psychiatric medication prescriptions. In the likely event that this demand was denied, the group was prepared to get back on the bus and take their message a half-mile away to Mayor Emanuel's office.

That the NSMHC consumers would stage a protest of this sort did not, in itself, come as a great surprise to me: In spite of the fact that they were relatively fortunate to still have a city clinic in their neighborhood, a clinic without even a single psychiatrist was hardly more helpful than no clinic at all. Moreover, given what consumers across the city recognized as the CDPH's plan to starve the remaining clinics of resources and then close them down on the grounds of declining usage, NSMHC consumers had every reason to feel threatened, and to be invested in the struggle to preserve this public service. What was more unexpected to me was an offhand request made at the time of my invitation to the protest: "By the way, it would be best if you don't mention this event to any of the other Mental Health Coalition members. Some North Side consumers don't agree with the Mental Health Coalition's approach— they find it overly confrontational—and they would prefer to keep this event within their group."

Given the plan for the North Side consumers' protest—and, indeed, given what I saw when I attended the action—the notion that these activists would find their own approach incompatible with the Mental Health Coalition's initially struck me as odd: It seemed to me that the two groups' styles of political agitation were rather similar—nonviolent, generally respectful, but insistent and "confrontational" inasmuch as they involved demanding recognition by Chicago city officials. Yet, true to the report I had heard, on the day of the protest at the Chicago Department of Public Health, I noticed that NSMHC consumers seemed to

take every opportunity they could find to distinguish themselves from—
and to announce to themselves and to the general public that they were
not allied with—the Mental Health Coalition. When, for instance, a staff
person at the CDPH made reference to a letter that the department had
received from a leader of the Mental Health Coalition regarding the
same psychiatry crisis that the North Side consumers wished to address,
the NSMHC protesters were quick to insist: "*That's* the Mental Health
Coalition. That letter has *nothing* to do with us!" And later on in the day,
after getting turned away by the CDPH, the NSMHC activists recounted
to each other the morning's events and planned their next step in ways
that brought out and crystallized the group's perception of its own community's identity in (unnamed) comparison with the Mental Health Coalition: Addressing the disappointed group back on the chartered bus, a
NSMHC consumer leader reminded everyone:

> The significance [of today]—it was the numbers of us there. Not the result
> of what we got of them treating us so hostile and so abusive, 'cause that's
> what treatment we received. We stayed polite, we stayed respectful, and
> they just told us, "shoot us an email," like that's gonna solve the problem.
> But I want you guys to feel proud of yourself because this is a big issue
> that you're taking on, on behalf of all of our fellow peers that come to our
> clinic, who couldn't be with us today. . . . Now we're gonna go to City Hall,
> the mayor's office, and we're just gonna let the mayor know what's going
> on and how we were treated. . . . Be prepared for the same scenario we
> saw here. We just kind of, we'll stay together, and if they start treating us
> not in a very respectful way we're gonna maintain our posture. We're not
> gonna yell back. Because we're gonna show them, you know, we're here
> and we're human beings and we are treating you with respect and we need
> that respect back.

The NSMHC leader's words communicated a twofold message: First,
it reminded the protesters that they had advocated that day on behalf
of their "fellow peers," a group that was immediately defined as consumers of the North Side clinic only—*not* the broader population of
struggling city clinic consumers throughout Chicago. Second, the message reaffirmed—and performatively constituted—the NSMHC group's

"posture" as polite, respectful, and quiet, arguably in opposition to the unruliness with which they characterized the Mental Health Coalition.

I left the protest still somewhat puzzled as to why the North Side group felt so strongly about distinguishing themselves from the Mental Health Coalition that they would pass up the opportunity to show greater strength in numbers or to benefit from the attention and momentum that the MHC had already accrued. As we have seen, only a few months earlier, the Mental Health Coalition had managed after prolonged effort to secure an informational council hearing on mental health services at Chicago's City Hall. Ahead of the hearing, a group of Progressive Reform Caucus aldermen who had initially supported the clinic closures vowed to get increased funding for the city's mental health clinics written into the next year's budget, and promised to support the Mental Health Coalition in their continued fight to reopen the six shuttered clinics. In a widely covered press conference on the day of the hearing, Alderman Fioretti—who would later run for mayor of Chicago—stated publicly: "We made that vote [to close the city clinics], and it was probably the worst vote I ever made."[9] A second alderman, Roderick Sawyer, also apologized to the Mental Health Coalition in front of the cameras, lamenting that "[w]e were told no one was going to get lost [and] everyone was going to get served . . . We relied on that when we made a decision. I'm sorry if people were not being served because of that. I am deeply sorry, but I want to make that right" (Fortino 2014). The Mental Health Coalition had been all over the news, and was being painted in a rather positive and sympathetic light. The story that the MHC had tried to tell at the City Hall hearing—that the city had allowed thousands of its consumers to slip through the cracks during the clinic closures, and that mental health services for the poor in Chicago were deteriorating, not expanding or improving as the city claimed—seemed to resonate with the Chicago public. By December 2014, prompted in part by the Mental Health Coalition's activism, Chicago's Public Health Commissioner Bechara Choucair would resign. From a strategic standpoint, it hardly seemed disadvantageous for the NSMHC consumers to voice their concerns collectively with the Mental Health Coalition.

But as I learned more about the two groups' political strategies and goals, I came to understand that the Mental Health Coalition and NSMHC

Consumer Council had entered into an antagonistic structure guided by a neoliberal logic of self-management and competition—a logic that migrated from the city to the community level, calling into question the very definition of "community" in the process. This logic drew on and exacerbated long-standing racialized geographies and sociopolitical tensions in Chicago. As such, it worked to magnify and render irreconcilable the relatively small differences in class status and material resources between two disenfranchised consumer activist groups. Ultimately, in its move to privatize what had historically been the public provision of mental health care, the City of Chicago helped to effect a radical shift in the meaning of "community mental health" to one in which communities were refigured as self-interested entrepreneurs that had to compete with one another for scarce resources.[10] This shift played into the city's interests by encouraging consumers themselves to carry out the project of privatization at the local level. As they embraced a new notion of community that redefined empowerment as the community's ability to create and manage its own mental health services without relying on a broader public infrastructure, NSMHC consumers ruptured the potential for grassroots solidarity and unwittingly participated in a micro-level reproduction of the very structural inequalities to which they had been victim.

Salvation, Legislation, and Privatization on the North Side of Chicago

In 1991, Chicago announced its first major round of budget cuts to public community mental health, scaling back its renowned system of nineteen city clinics down to twelve. Faced with these imminent closures, a group of mental health professionals, consumers, and local advocates around the North Side Mental Health Center (NSMHC) created an organization called the Coalition to Save Our Mental Health Centers (CTSOMHC), whose stated mission—like that of the Mental Health Coalition that succeeded it—was to "maintain services and prevent closures and budget cuts." The CTSOMHC, by its own account, worked for thirteen years "in communities throughout Chicago to unite residents, empower mental health consumers, and ensure that anyone struggling with a mental illness was able to get the help they needed" (Coalition to Save Our Mental Health Centers 2017a).

The CTSOMHC's strategy began to shift in 2004, when, it notes, "over a decade of budget cuts, center closures, and privatization resulted in a fragmented mental health system where those in need were left unserved" (2017a).[11] Even as it critiqued the consequences of privatization, the CTSOMHC, beginning in 2004, decided to pursue a new strategy that would look to sources outside of the city—essentially, that would carry out a kind of crowd-funding—to gather resources that would help "save" NSMHC alone. No longer preoccupied with the goal of saving or reopening *all* of the remaining city clinics, the CTSOMHC began to focus its attention exclusively on NSMHC, whose staff had been reduced by the city from fourteen to six in 2004, and thus no longer offered services such as couples counseling, substance abuse treatment, or crisis intervention.

To address these service shortages, the CTSOMHC and NSMHC community placed an advisory referendum on their neighborhood's ballot in the 2004 and 2008 elections, asking voters to approve a new "Expanded Mental Health Services Program." The program would be funded by a nominal increase in neighborhood residents' property taxes, and would supplement the reduced city clinic services for the NSMHC community. When the two referenda passed, the coalition worked with state legislators to draft the Community Expanded Mental Health Services Act, a piece of legislation that gives any community in Chicago the authority to create an Expanded Mental Health Services Program that is initiated, funded, and approved by the community (Coalition to Save Our Mental Health Centers 2017a). In March 2011, Illinois Governor Pat Quinn signed the bill into law. And on October 29, 2014—just weeks before I would attend the protest organized by the NSMHC Consumer Council to which the MHC was not welcome—the Kedzie Center, Chicago's pioneer clinic under the Community Expanded Mental Health Services Act, held its ribbon-cutting ceremony and began to offer mental health services to residents of the neighborhood surrounding NSMHC only.

In its own written history of the Community Expanded Mental Health Services Act and the resulting Kedzie Center, the Coalition to Save Our Mental Health Centers repeatedly invokes the notion of community. However, in comparison with the vision of community conjured by President Kennedy in 1963 or by the founders of the Woodlawn

Mental Health Center, the meaning of the term here is no longer suggestive of the state's responsibility to help integrate all consumers into
their local environments. Boasting that "[n]owhere else in the United
States can one find a program and a mental health center tied so directly
to the community it serves," the CTSOMHC frames its achievement as
"plac[ing] communities back at the forefront of mental health by allowing them to initiate, fund, and oversee their own mental health services"
(Coalition to Save Our Mental Health Centers 2017b). According to this
redefinition of community mental health—undoubtedly a felicitous one
from the City of Chicago's perspective— not only are consumers better off with semi-privatized mental health services, but they are further
empowered by taking on the responsibilities of procuring and funding
those services themselves.

In picking up and furthering the logic of privatization and competition that began at the city level, the NSMHC helped to establish and
magnify sociopolitical differences between their consumers and those
of the Mental Health Coalition, protecting their own group's needs via
their marginal class advantage at the cost of solidarity across the two
groups in pursuing their original project of preserving public mental
healthcare in Chicago. Contained within the NSMHC Consumer Council's critique of the MHC as unruly and overly confrontational were a
set of entrenched "racialized assumptions and biases" linking madness,
Blackness, and political activism—assumptions that "are historically
embedded into the very DNA of healthcare delivery systems, and shape
interactions and outcomes long before the participants appear on the
scene" (Metzl 2010, 202). These biases, while always already present,
might have been subdued or sublimated early in the Mental Health Coalition's development when NSMHC consumers—who themselves were
quite poor, predominantly nonwhite (Latinx), and uninsured—saw the
future of their own mental healthcare as dependent upon the successful fight by city clinic consumers across Chicago against the CDPH's
privatization efforts. Once in the neoliberal mode of self-interested
entrepreneurialism, however, NSMHC consumers engaged in a kind
of "narcissism of small differences" (Freud 1930) and focused on the
greater resources available within their community, as it was believed
that residents of Woodlawn could not afford to voluntarily raise their
own property taxes.[12] Through a sort of fractal recursiveness (Gal and

Irvine 1995),[13] NSMHC consumers—themselves victims of structural violence and race- and class-based healthcare inequalities—thus used available forms of ideological, affective, and political distinction to become the dominant portion of the dominated class (cf. Bourdieu 1984; Freire 1970), bolstering a system that (as many MHC members understood it at the time) diverted public resources from a group similar to, but slightly more disadvantaged than they were.

That the Chicago Department of Public Health's agenda of privatizing mental healthcare was taken up and carried out by way of disidentifications and competition between two socioculturally and politically marginalized groups is consonant with the findings of "a growing number of authors [who] have drawn attention to how discourses and policies of multiculturalism [are not antithetical to but in fact] form . . . part of the neoliberal project" (Muehlmann 2009, 469). For example, in an analysis of the enforcement of fishing restrictions and denial of "indigenous rights" by the Mexican federal government to the Cucapá, anthropologist Shaylih Muehlmann demonstrates how Mexican policies and discourses around "authentic" indigenous identity effect "a restructuring of the political arena that drives a wedge between claiming cultural rights and claiming control over the resources necessary for those rights to be realized" (Muehlmann 2009, 476).[14] This "neoliberal incarnation of multiculturalism," Muehlmann argues (476), achieves the dual ends of constraining class-based political organizing and "transfer[ring] . . . state responsibilities for mediating social conflict to civil society" (469). In the Chicago case, similarly, the NSMHC consumer group's access to resources depended upon their disavowal of commonalities with MHC members and amplification of a cultural distinction—articulated in the racist registers that permeate Chicago's sociopolitical geography and history.

Conclusion

While racial differences and in particular anti-Black sentiment were never explicitly named by the NSMHC Consumer Council as a source of tension between their group and the Mental Health Coalition, the North Side group's will to differentiate itself from the MHC by discursively aligning itself with normative (white) middle-class ideals of comportment—and the MHC with stereotypes of African American aggression and unruliness (Wilkins 2012; Wingfield 2007, 2010)—encodes and reproduces pronounced racial tensions that are deeply set in the City of Chicago (Ansell 2011; Moore 2016; Seligman 2005; Hirsch 1983; Pacyga 2009). Taken together with the Public Health Commissioner's patronizing reception of the MHC at the City Hall hearing described earlier, these findings suggest that the MHC was simultaneously compelled by those in power to perform out-of-control-ness in order to be recognized and heard, and marginalized by would-be allies in part for using this available strategy. In spite of the fact that the NSMHC group was neither predominantly white nor middle class—and in spite of similarities in the two groups' fundamental interests and pro-test practices—local and national ideologies about race, violence, and mental illness (Metzl 2010) converged to reinscribe the MHC's struc-tural subordination through the work of self-management.

Analyses of mental health consumer activism in the United States have often been conceptualized according to a binary (or perhaps a telos, e.g., McLean 2000) of radical anti-psychiatry "survivors" on the one hand and neoliberal patient "consumers" on the other (Carr 2021; cf. Sedgwick 1982). These accounts, while attentive to the differences in interests, goals, and demographics of ex-patients ("survivors") ver-sus consumers, have centered around the related struggles for "self-determination" and "choice." Struggles for either self-determination or consumer choice both take for granted access to institutions, categories, and services from which the consumer might want to distance themself or construct a new kind of relationship. In contrast to such projects, the MHC's politics centered on a will to reverse state abandonment and regain inclusion into these very institutions. MHC members had, in a tragic and ironic sense, an *excess* of unwanted independence or "self-determination," in that they *wanted* to depend on the state apparatus for support and could no longer do so. Indeed, for better or worse, the more time passed without MHC members regaining their public services, the more the coalition itself became members' mental healthcare rather than the vehicle for gaining access to formal services. As one member explained to me in an interview, "I am always a conversation away from suicide. This movement has saved my life, because I have been able to not selfishly look at how I want to die, but I have been able to interact with people that want to live, and to help them. And they have helped me. So [the Mental Health Coalition] means . . . it means not wanting to die."

Loosely following the work of Clarke et al., who write about a form of "unwilling selfhood" in which "people are required to act as consumers whether they understand themselves in such terms or not" (Clarke et al. 2007, 138), we can see that theorizing the politics of the MHC requires a concept of *unwanted* self-management, or unwilling radicalism of the structurally subordinated. In such a politics, death seems to always lurk in the background as a polemical anchor (Judith Farquhar, personal communication): Public health policies can only be denounced, as we saw in the case of the MHC's Eileen Morgan T-shirts and Nancy's plea at City Hall, on the basis of whether they will literally kill their subjects. Healthcare itself, under such conditions, may reside—powerfully, even—in the relationships of mutual aid and community that emerge between unwilling self-managers, but its horizons seldom exceed that of sustaining bare life (Agamben 1998). It would take time—years beyond the period in which I was carrying out my research—before Chicago's publicly abandoned, unwilling self-managers were positioned to imagine, articulate, and begin to demand a different moral calculus of care: one that could escape stark life-or-death absolutism and competitive logics of scarcity to seek everyday forms of support and even flourishing.

6

Use of the Self

Boundary Maintenance, Subjectivity,
and Cybernetic Entanglement

The Blurriness Is Completely Normal

At the start of my second and final year of clinical training at the Chicago School for Psychoanalytic Psychotherapy (CSPP), my classmates and I received what felt like a ritually significant email from the head of the school, introducing each of us to the Clinical Consultant with whom we had been selected to work for the duration of the academic year. Because I was receiving supervision from Abigail at my practicum site (WBH), the email explained, I would meet with my CSPP Clinical Consultant only every other week, with the purpose of "augmenting" my work with Abigail and helping me to "start to understand [my] cases in terms of psychodynamic theory and technique." The email concluded with some words of advice:

> I also want you to know that it's common for new psychotherapists to find themselves coping with strong feelings in their work that come not only from their clients and their situations, but also from within the psychotherapists themselves. This is completely normal, and is valuable to talk about with your Clinical Consultants. Part of developing a professional sense of oneself involves working to understand and manage what you as therapists bring to sessions, in addition to what your clients bring to sessions: those histories and present-day feelings will all intersect in each session, so it's your task to try to sort it out. All of that means that you can find yourselves talking about your personal lives with your Clinical Consultants, and that's fine; they want to know who you are. You're not required to share deeply personal information—that's for you and your

therapists to talk about; but sometimes the distinctions between work and personal matters feel blurry in our work, so it makes sense to rely on your Clinical Consultants to help you sort out whether to take something to your personal therapy, or to talk about how the blurriness comes up in your work, which, again, is completely normal.

With some trepidation, I contacted my Clinical Consultant, Andrew, and set up appointments for biweekly morning visits to his spacious and comfortable office in a skyscraper on Michigan Avenue with a view of Chicago's Millennium Park. And so my life began to trace a circuit, week after week, traversing and landing upon some of the nodes of greatest affluence followed by the spaces of poverty and abandonment that comprised the city's psychotherapeutic landscape. It was dizzying, almost— dropping myself into and out of these disparate communities that were both co-constitutive and invisible to one another; shape-shifting to inhabit and disinhabit the role, the practices, the very forms of selfhood and relationship that each of the spaces demanded or allowed; and now learning to talk about the same client/patient on alternating weeks from theoretical perspectives that felt worlds apart. Two mornings per week, I would set out from Hyde Park to the western fringes of Chicago to work a nearly twelve-hour day at WBH, often driving home, exhausted, at ten o'clock at night. On other weeknights, and every Saturday morning, I caught the number 6 express bus that would carry me out of Hyde Park and deliver me downtown to my classes at CSPP, bypassing a view of the gritty neighborhoods in between via Lakeshore Drive. On clinical consultation weeks, I took the Metra train to the Loop to meet with Andrew unless I was running late, in which case I would drive and pay an exorbitant parking fee due to the fact that in 2008 the Chicago City Council had, under then-Mayor Richard M. Daley, sold the city's public street parking meters to a private company for $1.15 billion (Byrnes 2023). Even the days in which I did not have to travel to clinical classes, practicum, or supervision felt fractured, divided as they were between time spent in meetings and actions with MHC members around Woodlawn, and time spent writing and thinking about my research on the University of Chicago's manicured grounds.

In this chapter, I look closely, through the kaleidoscopic lens of my own multi-sited clinical ethnographic experiences, at variations in a dimension of self-management alluded to in the email above from the head of CSPP: that of the ways in which boundaries between personal and professional—between self and other, or sometimes between self and world—are either firmly enforced or permitted to become "blurry" and porous across sociologically disparate therapeutic settings. Throughout this book, I have contended that context-particular mobilizations of self-management—inculcated and reinforced through clinical professional trajectories and other mechanisms—work to naturalize a system of class-stratified patient subjectivities, such that only wealthier individuals in private practice settings are afforded access to what I have described as a *cybernetic* model of selfhood and agency premised on ongoing social support, while poorer individuals are ascribed an unrealizable model of autonomous subjectivity that, at its extreme, borders on social abandonment. Furthermore, I have suggested that injustice inheres in the fact that the cybernetic model of selfhood, in its normalization of the patient's need for enduring relational connection, empathic attunement, and distributed agency, is fundamentally more livable and humane than the autonomous model.[1] While I continue to endorse that position in general, this chapter delves into some of the nuances of the diverse ideologies and practices regarding boundary maintenance and appropriate extensions of the self that I encountered among clinicians in both private practice and agency settings. At the risk of complicating my prior analysis, I argue here that the relational psychoanalytic approaches to the management of mental illness that were made available primarily to middle-class patients entailed *some* aspects of cybernetic being— namely inasmuch as they acknowledged and made therapeutic use of affective flows across individual selves—but often failed to accommodate a cybernetic understanding of the interconnectivity of self and material world. I theorize this distinction as related to the core psychoanalytic concepts of "use of the self" and "enactment," respectively. Moreover, I propose that certain case management practices, while not conceptualized as such in agency settings, could be understood as invoking a "use of the self" in precisely the cybernetic sense of self as continuous with the material world that psychoanalytic avoidance of enactments foreclose. Finally, I examine the distinct ways in which both private practice and agency therapists often stop short, in their interventions, of treating selfhood and agency as cybernetically embedded in a network of historical and structural forces.

"Use of the Self" in Private Practice

In my second to last clinical consultation with Andrew, I brought along a stack of process notes (Bender and Messner 2003) about a client, Lisa, with whom I had been working for several months as a counseling intern at WBH. As Lisa's therapist, I had been feeling completely out of my depth: Our sessions were disorganized, confusing, and vaguely hostile, with Lisa alternating between criticizing me as "meek" and ineffective, and complaining that I did not do a good job of anticipating and meeting her needs. She had taken to calling me by the first name that she had come up with for the imaginary fiancée of one of her grown sons (from whom, I believed, she was estranged), and would make offhand remarks about how she felt certain that my mother-in-law had been disappointed with the size of my wedding.

By this point in the practicum year, Abigail—my initial WBH supervisor who was quite relationally inclined—had resigned, and I had been added to another busy clinician's roster of intern supervisees. As a result, and given the limited time remaining in my internship, Lisa's apparently low level of functioning and financial precarity, and the general ethos of the agency, I was advised to avoid getting sucked into Lisa's drama and to instead focus on two practical treatment goals: connecting Lisa with an attorney who could help her apply for Social Security Disability Insurance (SSDI), and persuading Lisa to enter into WBH's Psychosocial Rehabilitation (PSR) day program, where she would receive what the agency described as a more intensive level of "structure and routine for clients that suffer from severe mental illness."

In contrast, as I reclined on his plush couch, Andrew read my process notes aloud slowly and deliberately, pausing to muse about the nature of Lisa's psychotic disturbances, her transference toward me, and her fantasies of merging with her sons and with her therapist. "There are two options for understanding the significance of Lisa's merge wish," Andrew explained. "Either it is a defense, or it is the expression of a wish for the fulfillment of a primitive need that she never got met." Andrew suggested that I take it as a working hypothesis that the merger was a primitive need, and that I attempt to provide Lisa with "close empathic attunement." If the hypothesis proved correct, the "static" in the session—Lisa's yelling, her disorganized thoughts, and her delusions—would "quiet down" over time, and I would see improvement. In that scenario, I could expect to see Lisa's symptoms resurface in moments of "empathic rupture" between myself and her. On the other hand, Andrew said, if by merging with Lisa I was "colluding with a defense," the therapy would "come to a standstill" and Lisa would not improve.

Andrew's recommended approach to my therapeutic work with Lisa—inactionable as it was given that only three weeks remained in the practicum—calls forth a relational psychoanalytic principle that my private practitioner instructors at CSPP tried to model and explicitly teach in the classroom: the "use of the [therapist's] self." Nearly every course that was offered as part of the master's-level clinical training at CSPP—in topics ranging from "Professional Ethics" to "Counseling Methods" to "Psychodynamic Theory" to "Bio-psycho-social Assessment" to "Substance Abuse Treatment"—devoted considerable attention to the need for the therapist to know, develop, remain true to, and offer their "self" to the patient in the psychotherapeutic encounter. Only through such use of the self and the therapist's courageous and vulnerable embrace of "authenticity" (Miller et al. 1999) could a "real relationship"—which, we were taught, was the cornerstone of psychotherapeutic effectiveness—be attained (Gelso 2011; Gelso et al. 2012). In one course, we read about the necessity of integrating "the personal self with professional and technical self" through the therapist's inculcation of a deep awareness of their own "natural attributes," styles of thinking, preferences and discomforts, and "personal solutions to lifelong dilemmas" (Edwards and Bess 1998, 98):

> The psychotherapist's personality and personal experiences should be the "filter" for all professional knowledge. So often we have been led to believe that it must be the opposite—that we should sublimate our natural tendencies and force them into a professional discipline. No technique . . . should ever be applied to a therapist's own work if it feels in the slightest incompatible with the therapist's sense of self. (1998, 99, emphasis in original)

While we learned about the attempts of clinicians and scholars to operationalize "use of the self" (e.g., Dewane 2006), at its heart the concept was presented to us as both intuitive and ineffable. "Use of the self" was "[t]hat which distinguishes a clinician [who uses technical skills coupled with practice wisdom] from a magician" (Dewane 2006, 544; Baldwin 2013); it was "difficult to describe since we would diminish that which makes us unique by trying to define it" (Dewane 2006, 544; Edwards and Bess 1998); it had to do with inhabiting a state of full presence, and with allowing a kind of openness to the other that follows from a sense of security with oneself. In an essay assigned in my Counseling Methods class, pioneering family therapist Virginia Satir describes her own use of the self this way:

> [W]hen I am fully present with the patient or family, I can move therapeutically with much greater ease. I can simultaneously reach the depths to which I need to go, and at the same time honor the fragility, the power, and the sacredness of life in the other. When I am in touch with myself, my feelings, my thoughts, with what I see and hear, I am growing toward becoming a more integrated self. I am more congruent, I am more "whole," and I am able to make greater contact with the other person. (Satir 2013, 25)

Just as Andrew had done in the clinical consultation session, my instructors at CSPP took every pedagogical opportunity that arose to encourage my classmates and me to use our selves in ways that allowed us to learn about, empathically attune to, and promote change in our patients through the flow of affect across the boundaries of our porous subjectivities in an ongoing relational process (Freedberg 2007). It was not unusual for an instructor to present notes or even formal written case studies about their own patients in class in order to illustrate the ways in which they relied on the self as an instrument for the transmission and receipt of affect and the generation of insight: One instructor described his visceral experience of the pain of his adolescent patient who came to her therapy sessions wearing spiky heels and a black and silver dress—evoking the knife she had been using to engage in physical self-harm. Another shared a detailed account of her decade and a half of clinical work with a patient diagnosed with bipolar disorder with psychotic features, whose symptoms were reduced only when the therapist shifted her orientation from one of service provision to one that focused on the establishment of relational connection. Likewise, in classes, we were encouraged to actively work on "expanding the intersubjective space"—one instructor likened it to a balloon that could become more or less deflated—by using our selves to notice and process affective changes in the room, and by relating to the course material on a personal as well as professional level. Similarly, we were expected and sometimes prompted in our written work to perform openness and boundary blurring by bringing our life histories and emotional responses to bear on the academic topic at hand.

So routine was the invocation of use of the self among everyone I interacted with at CSPP that I sometimes forgot how rarified of a concept it was in settings outside of the middle-class relational psychotherapeutic milieu. Oftentimes, as with my WBH supervisor's advice about Lisa or in the case of Jamal described earlier, time constraints and clients' urgent problems rendered a more contemplative and intersubjectively porous approach to treatment impractical. In those circumstances, use of the self was, almost literally, a luxury that neither the agency therapist nor the client could afford. In other instances—such as the transactional injunction recited in agency settings to "never work harder than your client"—the avoidance of an affective use of the self, or an insistence upon extremely impenetrable emotional boundaries, felt more ideologically rooted. At one point, at CRC, I worked with a client who was particularly demanding and somewhat manipulative toward me. In supervision, I was advised to use my self as an instrument: The ways that the client's psychological makeup seeped into me and colored my personal affective experience were "good data" that would help me to understand how other people in the client's life experienced her. In terms of my interactions with the client, however, the supervisor instructed me to "put up boundaries and don't give at all." If the client had nothing to "push against," the supervisor explained, she would "fall flat on her face."

In their willingness to conceptualize the self as a porous recipient and transmitter of affect (Brennan 2004), and to apprehend the relational "use" of that self as fundamental to therapeutic healing, clinicians at CSPP gave patients access to some vital aspects of what I described earlier as a *cybernetic model of selfhood and agency.* Anthropologist

Gregory Bateson, writing about Alcoholics Anonymous as a cybernetic corrective to Western philosophy's epistemologically unsound theory of selfhood, points out the absurdity of defining the self as localized and bounded within the individual body:

> [C]onsider a blind man with a stick. Where does the blind man's self begin? At the tip of the stick? At the handle of the stick? Or at some point halfway up the stick? These questions are nonsense, because the stick is a pathway along which differences are transmitted under transformation, so that to draw a delimiting line across this pathway is to cut off a part of the systemic circuit which determines the blind man's locomotion . . . The total self-corrective unit which processes information, or, as I say, "thinks" and "acts" and "decides," is a system whose boundaries do not at all coincide with the boundaries either of the body or of what is popularly called the "self" or "consciousness." (Bateson 1972, 324)

Bateson argues—and I would agree—that "when the underlying epistemology is full of error, derivations from it are inevitably either self-contradictory or extremely restricted in scope" (1972, 327): As he describes with the example of "alcoholic pride" and I have demonstrated in the phenomenon of clinical self-management, an epistemological refusal to locate selfhood and agency intersubjectively creates paradoxes and double binds; it places impossible and at times deadly demands on individuals to exhibit autonomous, unilateral self-control. Conversely, a cybernetic understanding of selfhood and its therapeutic "use" as exceeding the bounded individual is the precursor to a vital shift from "symmetrical" to "complementary" relationships (Bateson 1972); from a "logic of choice" to a "logic of care" and social support (Mol 2008).

Cybernetic Limitations: Containment Versus Enactment

The understanding of selfhood as continuous with and available to the other that undergirded "use of the self" at CSPP thus aligns in some significant ways with Bateson's cybernetic epistemology. However, as the quotation above suggests, Bateson's model locates selfhood and action within a system that is far more expansive than only the intersubjective space and affective flow between the therapist and the patient. For

Bateson, self as "total self-corrective unit" must also include a notion of embodied human subjects as coextensive with—and ultimately inextricable from—the material world with which they interact: hence the nonsensicality of trying to draw a line delineating the end of the blind man and the beginning of his stick. We could look at the example of Tricia's cutting and hospitalization in similar terms: The scene that Tricia describes is not intelligible if we try to parse it in terms of a delimited agent—the sovereign individual "self"—who purposively acts on a delimited object; it begins to make sense only when we conceptualize Tricia's self and her agency as distributed across a human and nonhuman network that includes Tricia's razor, her medications, the hospital, her boyfriend, and so forth.

The ways in which therapists at CSPP taught and invoked "the use of the self" often did not extend to a cybernetic understanding of self as inseparable from the material world. In fact, a second term of art that figured prominently into my CSPP training—"enactment"—was regularly referenced to problematize or critique those instances in which the therapist could be seen as failing to adequately enforce the boundaries of the therapeutic frame, such that too much of the surrounding physical world entered into the session.

The origin, meaning, and utility of "enactment" as a distinct category are contested among those in the psychoanalytic community who write about it (Aron 2003; Bettelheim 2022). Related to and preceded by Freud's equally nebulous concept of "acting out"—which first denoted a memory recalled "by action" rather than "by speech"—"enactment" was unintentionally coined in a paper by Theodore Jacobs (1986) about countertransference (Bettelheim 2022). It was "originally seen both as a behavioral breach of therapeutic norms and an obstruction to therapeutic progress. This is particularly vivid in severe mutual boundary violations such as sexual encounters between therapist and patient" (76). In its more mundane forms, such as those that typically arose in discussions at CSPP, "enactment" is used in contemporary psychoanalytic discourse to describe "a collapse in the analytic dialogue in which the analyst is drawn into an interaction where he unwittingly acts, thereby actualizing unconscious wishes of both himself and the patient" (Bohleber et al. 2013, 517, cited in Bettelheim 2022, 76). Enactment is, therefore, what some psychoanalysts would call a "failure of containment"—and the degree to which it either derails the therapeutic process or offers an opportunity for progress depends on "the analyst's recognition of what has happened and his/her role in it, interpretation of what has happened, and restoration of the 'as if' verbally based therapeutic relationship" (Bettelheim 2022, 76).

At CSPP, in a class on "Methods in Psychodynamic Psychotherapy," the instructor drew heavily on a text by British relational psychoanalyst Patrick Casement (1991) to explore the distinction between uses of the therapist's self that helpfully facilitated containment or "analytic holding" (Winnicott 1960) and those that crossed a line into the detrimental territory of enactment. In a discussion in the book about his work with a suicidal patient ("Mrs. F"), Casement describes the dramatic improvement he sees in Mrs. F when he offers to meet with her more frequently during a period of time when she is experiencing great distress:

> It had been a feature of Mrs. F.'s whole life that she had always been seen as the strong and self-reliant person, upon whom everyone else could lean. She felt she must never let anyone know of her frightened and dependent self. Instead, she usually tried to hide this in order to preserve some contact with others, whom she experienced as leaving her whenever she showed signs of being needy. She had relied on medication to help her in this hiding. When suppression still did not obliterate her feelings, she increased the dose to the point of nearly obliterating herself. Her suicide bid, therefore, was an attempt at finally eliminating those feelings which she could no longer manage alone . . . Mrs. F. gradually dared to draw upon my availability openly, rather than secretly, and the effect of this "relationship-holding" was startling. She began to discover that her own most difficult feelings of distress could be contained within a relationship . . . Over a period of several months, Mrs. F. began to develop a different kind of security, now based upon her use of an outside dependability which she could internalize and consolidate within herself. Her new-found strength was different from her life-long self-sufficiency. (Casement 1991, 118)

At the conclusion of the chapter about Mrs. F, Casement summarizes those qualities of containment that make for the most effective use of the therapist's self through analytic holding:

> Analytic holding . . . is always based on a capacity to tolerate being genu-
> inely in touch with what the other person is feeling, even to the extent
> of feeling those feelings oneself . . . Patients have taught me that when I
> allow myself to feel (even to be invaded by) the patient's own unbearable
> feelings, and if I can experience this (paradoxically) as both unbearable
> and yet bearable, so that I am still able to find some way of going on, I can
> begin to "defuse" the dread in a patient's most difficult feelings. (Case-
> ment 1991, 127–128)

From these and similar passages, we learned in the class that our most
important task as therapists would be to open up the boundaries around
our selves so that we were available to receive and feel—and, thereby,
share and diffuse—those affects that our patients could not bear to experience on their own, just as Casement had done for Mrs. F. We worked
on training this empathic capacity like a muscle, reading our instructor's
real or hypothetical therapy session transcripts and practicing responses
that conveyed affective understanding and connection rather than reas-
surance, problem-solving, or pity. Feedback, or interpretations, that we
gave to our patients would ideally then emerge from our recognition of
the feelings induced in us by the patient, and from our relational awareness of why the patient needed us to experience those feelings.

These intimate and highly valorized uses of the self for containment
were contrasted in our class with enactments, which we learned were
bound to occur occasionally and typically required processing and rem-
edy. Enactments, our instructor explained, comprised a class of dilemma
that threatened "the frame"—meaning the therapist's boundary rules
within which the therapeutic process takes place (McWilliams 2004;
Bleger 1967). What constituted an enactment might to some extent depend on the therapist's preferences or on characteristics of the particular
patient, but certain actions—engaging in physical touch, attending social
events or special occasions, and receiving even small gifts, for instance,
as well as the fee deviations described earlier—were nearly always best
to avoid.[2] In a chapter that we were assigned on "analytic holding under
pressure," Casement presents an extended clinical sequence about a patient, "Mrs. B," who needed to "relive" in therapy her traumatic childhood experience of seeing her mother faint while Mrs. B was in surgery

following an accident that had left her severely burned, and requests an enactment from the therapist. "Mrs. B," Casement writes,

> began to stress the importance of physical contact for her. She said she was unable to lie down on the couch again unless she knew that she could if necessary hold my hand, in order to get through this reliving of the operation experience. Would I allow that or would I refuse? If I refused she wasn't sure she could continue with her analysis. (Casement 1991, 131)

Feeling increasing pressure to acquiesce to the patient's wish, Casement makes the "defensively equivocal" reply to Mrs. B that while some analysts would not contemplate allowing her request, he realizes that she might need to have the possibility of holding his hand in order to get through the experience (Casement 1991, 131). Mrs. B feels relief, prompting her to hand-deliver a letter to Casement on a Sunday expressing (in the symbolic terms of a dream) her renewed sense of hope in the treatment. In their next therapy session, Casement determines that his initial response had been a mistake. He tells Mrs. B that

> I had thought very carefully about this, and I had come to the conclusion that this tentative offer of my hand might have appeared to provide a way of her getting through the experience she was so terrified of; but I now realized it would instead become a side-stepping of that experience *as it had been* rather than a living through it. After a pause I continued. I said I knew that, if I seemed to be inviting an avoidance of this central factor of the original experience, I would be failing her as her analyst. I therefore did not think I should leave the possibility of holding my hand still open to her. (1991, 132–133, emphasis in original)

Upon hearing Casement's refusal to go through with the enactment, Mrs. B becomes enraged and delusional. Over the next several sessions, she addresses Casement as her unavailable mother and as a homicidal surgeon. Casement begins to feel that he is in an impossible position, where he is unable to use his self appropriately to sustain an analytic holding environment: "There appeared to be no remaining contact with me as analyst" (136), he laments. Eventually, however, he is able to interpret the feelings that he realizes are engendered in him by Mrs. B in a way that gets through to her:

> Very slowly, and with pauses to check that the patient was following me, I said to her: "You are making me experience in myself the sense of despair, and the impossibility of going on, that you are feeling . . . I am aware of being in what feels to me like a total paradox . . . In one sense I am feeling that it is impossible to reach you just now; and yet, in another sense, I feel that my telling you this may be the only way I can reach you."
>
> She followed what I was saying very carefully, and slightly nodded her head. I therefore continued: "Similarly, I feel as if it could be impossible to go on; and yet, I feel that the only way I can help you through this is by my being prepared to tolerate what you are making me feel, and still going on." After a long silence Mrs. B. began to speak to me again as analyst. She said: "For the first time I can believe you, that you *are* in touch with what I have been feeling; and what is so amazing is that you can bear it."
>
> I was then able to interpret to her, that her desperate wish for me to let her touch me had been her way of letting me know that she needed me to be really *in touch* with what she was going through. This time she could agree. (Casement 1991, 136, emphasis in original)

Ultimately, by using his affective self, Casement is able to open up the "right" kinds of boundaries between himself and the other, while not compromising, through enactment, the integrity of those boundaries between self and material world—including, here, between the therapist and the physical body of the patient—that are deemed vital to the treatment process. In the terms of Batesonian cybernetics, Casement's interventions can be seen as instantiating a model of selfhood that is connected to and continuous with the other in its affective communication, but that must be physically delimited in a manner that coincides with the boundaries of the individual body.

Use of the Self in Agency Settings

On a winter morning, I met my CRC supervisor at her car and drove with her to pick up a client, Anne, at Anne's apartment in the Rogers Park neighborhood on the Far North Side of Chicago. My supervisor had been providing "Community Support Individual" (CSI) services to Anne for more than five years, but was going to be transitioning her to my caseload and had decided to facilitate our introduction. "Anne is one of my favorite clients," my supervisor had laughed, "but I'm not supposed to say that!"

When Anne joined us in the car, she gave my supervisor a list of shops that she wanted to visit that day. This, my supervisor told me, was their weekly routine: "Anne always knows the places that have the best prices for cigarettes and other things that she likes to get." We drove around for an hour or so, my supervisor and I waiting in the car while Anne went into various stores, returning with some groceries, lottery tickets, and the cigarettes. My supervisor explained that I would soon inherit her role of being listed as the payee for Anne's monthly disability checks. To continue the system that Anne and my supervisor had established, I was to request Anne's disability money from the CRC office manager in weekly installments. A check would then be made out to me, which I would need to cash at the bank prior to each meeting with Anne.

As described earlier, activities such as my supervisor and Anne's weekly shopping routine—sometimes glossed (but not necessarily billed) as "case management"—were a central component of clinical work at CRC and, to a somewhat lesser extent, at WBH. Much of the time, agency therapists at CRC interacted with clients by accompanying them to medical appointments, holding their place in line at social services offices, moving their furniture, contacting their landlords, balancing their budgets, planning their diets, helping them apply for jobs, or drinking coffee with them at Starbucks. When a client of mine whose appetite was poor spoke nostalgically about trips to the candy and soda shoppe from his youth and asked if we could visit one, we got in my car and drove to an old-timey place in town to enjoy root beer floats and packs of Bazooka bubble gum. Another client was busy and trying to lose weight, so we conducted our sessions while taking brisk walks together on the city streets around the agency.

These sorts of activities were not always entirely unproblematic: There were certainly moments when agency therapists felt taken for granted, bored, or over-qualified for the client work that we were routinely expected to take on. However, across the agencies, there was a notable lack of any discourse worrying that using the therapist in such ways was inappropriate, or that it would break the frame and impede a therapeutic process. Indeed, it would have seemed an absurd fiction to insist that the world could be neatly bracketed out of the clinical encounter in such a fashion, or that therapeutic work could be conducted entirely in the verbal realm of the "as if," without involving any action. In the context of my training at CSPP, I felt certain, the vast majority of CSI services provided in agencies would potentially qualify as enactments. Yet, of course, the word "enactment" was never uttered at WBH or CRC; it was simply a given that working with a client entailed an openness to the blurring of physical boundaries—it meant, more often than not, stepping into the client's material world and being an active participant in it.

When we drove clients around Chicago in our cars or cashed their disability checks, we did not talk about what we were doing as a "use of the self."[3] But perhaps we might do well to start reconceptualizing the work in this way, toward the dual ends of expanding our models of selfhood toward greater cybernetic connectivity and envisioning a more sociologically diverse range of patient populations as entitled to, and able to benefit from, a distribution of the self.

Conclusion

Understanding the ways in which a given therapeutic framework espouses a more or less cybernetic philosophy of self and agency is not only, as Bateson has it, a matter of epistemological correctness. It is also a matter of epistemic justice (Fricker 2007; Chapman and Carel 2022) for, as we have seen, context-specific differences in the ideological ways that boundaries around personhood are opened up or fortified have real implications for patients' access to livable models of subjectivity and self-management that promote flourishing—implications that tend to fall inequitably along race- and class-stratified lines.

In this chapter, I have proposed that even as these systemic inequalities persist and require urgent remediation, there might be something of value to learn about the cybernetics of selfhood from both private practice *and* agencies' settings: Relational therapeutic approaches taught and used by private providers at CSPP are rooted in a conceptualization of humans as intersubjectively connected through the push and pull of affect across porous boundaries. As such, these approaches offer patients a model of subjectivity that normalizes the human need for ongoing relationship and mutual support. At the same time, in its intense privileging of affective entanglements of selfhood that are contained within the analytic frame, and its assiduous avoidance of an extension of the use of the therapist's self into the patient's broader material world, relational psychoanalysis of this sort may miss opportunities to think about and intervene in crucial sociopolitical aspects of patients' lived experiences. Indeed, contemporary scholarship within the psychoanalytic community is increasingly concerned with the need within the field to think intersectionally, engage in social critique, and better attend to society's complex structural and political problems if psychoanalysis is to remain viable and relevant into the twenty-first century (Tolleson 2009; Auestad 2012; Lapping 2011; Layton et al. 2006; Vaughans and Harris 2016; Altman 2020; Brickman 2018; Grand 2014).

The therapeutic activities of agency workers, on the other hand, make use of the therapist's self in some important material ways that private practitioners are unable or unwilling to explore. In so doing, agency settings seem to implicitly acknowledge greater interconnectedness between person and material world, which could potentially open up liberatory possibilities for rethinking selfhood and agency. As we have seen, however, these possibilities do not obtain for agency clients; the sorts of cybernetic entanglements of person and world that I have argued are modeled by case management and community support interventions fail to afford agency clients full recognition as distributed, relational beings with concomitant entitlement to affective porosity and ongoing support. Instead, agency clients are constantly pointed toward a horizon, however unachievable, of self-sufficiency and independence. Perhaps we would do well, across clinical training and practice settings, to more intentionally theorize the work that agency therapists do with their clients as a different kind of intimate use of the self rather than its opposite, and to appreciate the cybernetic entwinement of selves and material supports as a valid form of human subjectivity rather than always as an aspirational means to an autonomous end. Indeed, there may be many underutilized, positive ways to enact a use of the self that is cybernetically embedded in a material world in ways that are compatible with a frame that also emphasizes relationship and affective porosity, even in case work with the poor (Segal 2012; Berzoff 2012).

Furthermore, as with private practitioners, therapists in agency settings must go even further than our current practices allow to see our clients' selves as produced in and through a web of historical, political, and structural forces. This includes, of course, our conscious reckoning with the structural influences on—and effects of—our own psychotherapeutic institutions in the production and unmaking of client subjectivities.

Conclusion

What do YOU think Chicago's mental health care system should be like—from now until 2025?

At once beautifully open-ended and impossibly ambitious, the above invitation to re-imagine the future of public mental health services in the City of Chicago—disseminated on paper fliers and circulated via a social media event page—drew a crowd of approximately sixty consumers, clinicians, and allies to a South Side church for an all-Saturday community meeting in the fall of 2014. The meeting—one of a series of "Town Hall" gatherings organized by the Mental Health Coalition—had been conceived in the wake of the Chicago Department of Public Health's disappointing handling of mental health consumers' hard-won City Hall hearing on the clinic closures several months earlier. Its aims were both practical and performative: In an effort to counteract a potential loss of organizational momentum or the collective slippage into despair that seemed all too plausible after the anticlimax of the hearing, leaders of the MHC had decided to adopt a longer-range perspective on the project of improving public mental health services by drafting a "Ten Year Plan for Mental Health Care in Chicago." This shift in temporal strategy was framed by the MHC, rather self-consciously, as a reclamation by city clinic consumers of the ability and authority to make decisions about their own mental health services. Appealing to the power and legitimacy of concerned citizenship, the community meeting announcement positioned consumers as effective—rather than defeated—actors more capable than the City of Chicago of producing sound healthcare policy: "The Chicago Department of Public Health refuses to look seriously at the needs of our mental health system, listen to those who use it, or make a plan to support and strengthen mental health services for all Chicagoans," the event flier asserted. "So we, Chicagoans who care deeply about our city, will take on this task."

Upon arriving at the church, meeting attendees were welcomed effusively by Caryn Jones and invited to sit down and enjoy a hot catered lunch from a local Caribbean restaurant. They were offered small pads of blank notebook paper—the three sections of which Jones had labeled with the titles of the meeting's breakout sessions—and provided with a brief primer by Jones on how to make use of these pads. ("You write notes if there's anything that you want to say when someone else is talking but you don't want to lose your train of thought. If there's any ideas that you want to share, write them here. If people have said things that you think are important, write them in here.")

Jones also directed each participant's attention to a basket full of ceramic butterflies that she had painstakingly adorned with paint, glitter, stickers, and rhinestones at her home the previous evening. The butterflies, Jones explained, were to serve as mementos of the day that attendees could keep and cherish. Attached to each butterfly with a ribbon was a small card, onto which was typed the following message:

> Butterflies are a symbol of resurrection, hope, joy, and new beginnings. It is a symbol of rebirth and a transformation of change: meaning out with the old and in with the new. We must go through several growth experiences in life before we experience our true purpose and get to a place of inner peace in life. WINNING THE BATTLE FOR THE RIGHT TO BE WELL IS INEVITABLE—YOU MUST BELIEVE—THE VICTORY IS OURS!

This tone of generativity and optimism was invoked by Jones throughout the town hall event in her role as the meeting's emcee. "We have moved mountains; now it's time to put *property* on our mountains," Jones declared in her welcome address. The City Hall hearing, she reminded attendees, was but a minor setback—even perhaps an opportunity for growth and learning—in the Mental Health Coalition's grand telos. The fundamental and self-evident *rightness* of the MHC's cause would ultimately ensure justice and victory; it was only a matter of patience and persistence before a better future would arrive for city clinic consumers.

Before splitting up into the breakout groups, Jones asked all of the community meeting participants, in the spirit of the butterfly, to free their imaginations and share their dreams of what an *ideal*—rather than a simply adequate—public mental health center would look like. Mike, who had been standing at one corner of the room translating Jones's words into Spanish for an attendee, chimed in to emphasize to the group that the brainstorming exercise would be something of a paradigm shift for the Mental Health Coalition:

> I want to encourage everyone to really be creative today. Usually, we're reactive to what the city's doing to us. Usually, if the city's gonna close our clinic, we need to stop them from doing that. Or the city's letting psychiatrists retire? We need to stop them from doing that. But we never take the time to really think about what *we* are doing and where we are going. So instead of us reacting to the city, let's force the city to react to us and *our* plans. And so today, don't limit yourselves by what you think is impossible, right? That's why we said ten years—maybe it takes us more, maybe it takes us less to get there, but the idea is not a specific time period; the idea is *our* dream; what our community needs to survive; what services we need.

If only for a few hours of one exceptional day, MHC members were to give themselves permission to operate outside of the stark politics of bare life (Agamben 1998) and death that so often take hold of individuals who find themselves caught in a "zone of social abandonment" (Biehl 2005) and that had determined much of the Coalition's discursive self-management strategy; they were to inhabit the very relational world from which they had been systematically excluded—a world in which forms of state care existed not to stave off the threat of death, but to ensure continued wellbeing and create the conditions for flourishing.

Attendees' fantasies, long stifled by the struggle for mere survival, started out modestly with a reconstitution of the six recently closed city clinics. Then, gradually, the original preventative and community-engaged features of Chicago's community mental health system that had been budgeted out of existence years earlier began to reappear in the collective imagination. Excitement swelled as meeting participants voiced visions of a public mental health system that conducted outreach to reduce the stigma of psychiatric illness, offered resources for consumers with criminal records, developed programming for youth,

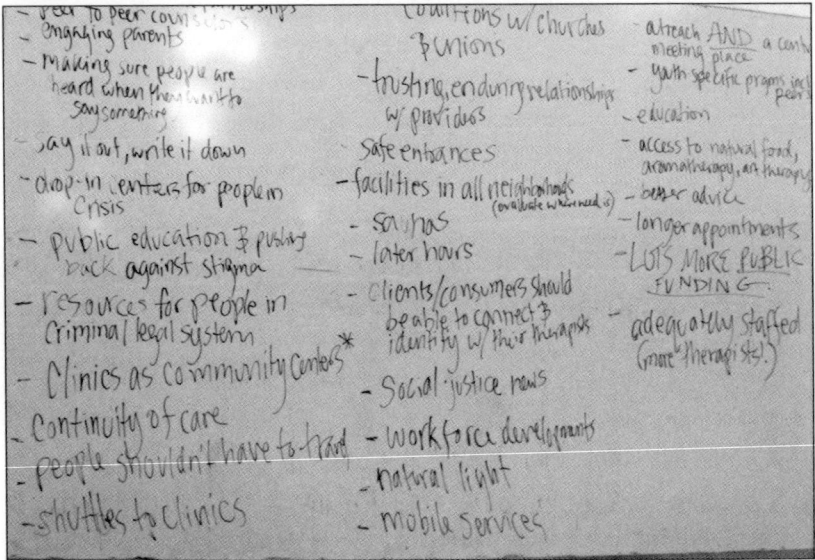

Figure C.1. List of ideal Chicago mental health center features generated at a Mental Health Coalition town hall meeting. Photograph by author.

and built coalitions with local churches and unions; a system that included a facility in *every* Chicago neighborhood, extended hours of operation, and free shuttle services between clinics and consumers' homes. "What about a sauna?" ventured one consumer with a smile. Delighted by this preposterous notion, others in the room joined in a whimsical aesthetic refashioning of Chicago's municipal facilities into luxurious spaces with upper-class amenities. Within ten minutes of discussion, a system of public mental health clinics complete with natural lighting, organic foods, art and aromatherapy—not to mention "better advice" dispensed by its therapists—had come into being on a large whiteboard in the church gathering room (figure C.1).

I conclude this book by dwelling on the above scene of collective fantasy-building and authority inversion because it serves as a reminder of the possibility—and value—of articulating alternatives to a system of power precisely at the moment in which that system feels most oppressive and inescapable. Moreover, it underscores the notion that these alternative ways of being are not necessarily or exclusively found in the social worlds that would seem most likely to potentiate and sustain them; they may emerge through ideological cracks and crevices—or out of paradoxical excesses of their opposite—and they may take the form of fleeting interruptions from the ordinary, or shadowy counterparts to the ongoing norm.

This book has examined how logics, policies, and practices of self-management—a term borrowed from the clinical paradigm that bears its name, but whose reach extends far beyond the treatment of psychiatric disorders to characterize many aspects of the contemporary neoliberal condition—insinuate themselves across various nodes of a mental healthcare apparatus so as to simultaneously reproduce and mystify structural inequalities. It has contended that the ideologies of entrepreneurship, self-responsibility, competition, and individualism contained within self-management migrate and reverberate across scales of governance, enabling state interests and anxieties to get decontextualized and transferred, through various mechanisms, onto the shoulders of structurally vulnerable actors. Furthermore, it has suggested that self-management—in both its more intentional and its most "unwilling" forms—determines and constrains the possibilities for agency and subjectivity available to disparate classes of citizens, while naturalizing these disparities.

Throughout this book, I have leveled various critiques of self-management as conceptually inaccurate, clinically ineffective, and politically conservative,[1] and have gestured toward the hope that there are, indeed, more livable, alternative models of selfhood and agency to be discovered—either from within the surprising heterotopic "otherwise" that self-management itself can occasionally produce, or inside the class contexts in which such alternatives are already socially sanctioned. And while I have tried to describe some of the more relational, distributive, or cybernetic qualities of these alternatives, I have yet to undertake the challenge, as the Mental Health Coalition did in its Town Hall meeting, of envisioning and articulating a paradigm outside of the one that I denounce. The absence of a clearly delineated alternative to self-management is certainly one of this ethnography's limitations—but it is a limitation that, I would argue, opens up a broader set of questions that linger in the margins of my analysis, and that warrant further consideration: What sorts of actors ought to bear the greatest responsibility for seeing and naming the structural problems plaguing the systems in which they are imbricated? Are these the same actors that are best positioned to imagine—and then to institute and enact—new social forms that might evade such problems? What modes of collective thought and praxis are required in order to effect a paradigm shift away from self-sovereignty? How, in other words, can the project of thinking about an outside to self-management be carried out in such a way that it does not become a self-managerial exercise in and of itself?

To put the matter in somewhat more narrow and concrete terms: Although I maintain that a mental healthcare system imbued with logics of self-management will only continue to reproduce and misrecognize its most pernicious forms of structural inequality, I find the question of the degree to which therapists should be asked to recognize and mitigate their own problematic, structurally compelled practices to be less straightforward. To be sure, there are many therapists who develop local structural critiques of some aspects of their workplace conditions, and who are able to put such critiques to use in the ethical provision of client care (Brodwin 2013). But to aspire to the full radicalization of low-status psychotherapists—wherein the therapists would not only have to survive, but also raise consciousness around and play a key role in unmaking their own structural constraints—is perhaps to posit an unfair division of political labor.

Rather than burdening therapists—or this author, or any individual actor—with the formidable task of escaping the dominant paradigm, I would suggest instead that we begin to think about collective ways of slowing down and interrupting those moments in which structural problems seamlessly flow into self-managerial narratives and practices. In the case of social work and psychotherapy, perhaps the notion of *structural competency* that has been rapidly gaining traction in clinical educational settings may provide a point of entry into this endeavor. Structural competency "directs clinical training and healthcare systems to intervene at the level of social structures, institutions, and policies that must be altered to improve population health and promote health equity" (Hansen and Metzl 2016, 180; cf. Jones 2025). Such initiatives raise the question: "How can clinical eyes be trained to see social structures?" (Hansen and Metzl 2016, 180). One answer to this question could be to introduce into clinical training processes a form of structural competency that aspires to the goals described above but that turns its gaze, reflexively, toward the problematic social structures, institutions, and policies impeding clinicians' practices in addition to those that more directly impact patients. Such an approach might equip therapists who are caught in the sorts of binds described in this ethnography with the critical tools to identify moments of structural impasse within their own professional activities, and to articulate—if not necessarily resolve—the ways in which their local institutional practices might be undermining the provision of structurally competent care. This, in turn, could provide therapists with options other than the individual self-management of structural constraints and the disavowal of market logics. As Biehl (2012, 249) asks, "the mixing of commodity and care *does* happen, and if we cannot explain the moral gravity of caregiving by merely defining good care as a pure, transcendent value and opposing it to the corrupting force of the market, how can we apprehend the ethics of care in today's consumer-capitalist society?" Training therapists to collectively see and acknowledge social structures in their own workplaces—to sit with their own inadequate sets of options rather than moving automatically to overcome or erase them—could, paradoxically, point the way to the beginning of an alleviation of deeply entrenched social inequalities.

ACKNOWLEDGMENTS

There is a certain irony in crediting oneself as the sole author of a book, when that book's central concern is with the violence done by an ideology that extracts the individual from her social and structural contexts. While the experience of writing *Therapeutic Inequalities*—first in the sleepless haze of new parenthood, and years later in the midst of a global pandemic—at times felt solitary, the project's existence is in fact owed to the many communities and institutions, both past and present, in which I am fortunate to be embedded. My words of acknowledgment here thus represent an effort, however inadequate, to pay tribute to the cybernetic distribution of self and agency that went into the production of this work; responsibility for the shortcomings of the book, on the other hand, falls on me alone.

First and foremost, I am deeply indebted to my interlocutors from the Chicago School for Psychoanalytic Psychotherapy, Wellness Behavioral Health, Community Recovery Center/RecoveryNet, and the Mental Health Coalition, all of whom welcomed me into their personal and professional communities, and generously shared their lived experiences. Over the course of my fieldwork, a number of these informants became trusted friends, colleagues, and political comrades; although I cannot thank them by name, I hope these folks will recognize in this book the wisdom that they have imparted to me. I am especially grateful to one therapist informant who disclosed that in agreeing to participate in my study, she had ventured far outside of her own comfort zone because she felt that the value of the research topic outweighed her anxiety and self-consciousness. I also wish to acknowledge an unnamed friend whose decision to withdraw from the study I respect, and whose influence on my thinking continues to be profound.

As a college student, I learned from Jeanne Marecek and Ken Gergen how to see psychology through the lens of culture, discourse and narrative. Subsequently, my graduate advisors served as invaluable sources of insight and encouragement as I worked toward writing this book. Jennifer Cole supported me with wit and friendship, believed in my work even at its most incoherent, and offered life advice on matters both pragmatic and existential. Judy Farquhar and Eugene Raikhel taught me, formally and by example, what psychological anthropology looks like at its best. Paul Brodwin felt like a kindred spirit since the first time we met, and has been an inspiration and guide as I've navigated the process of writing this book.

The list of friends and colleagues from my years in Chicago whose insights are reflected in the content of this book is too long to enumerate, but I am grateful to every one of you for steering my mind in directions that it would not otherwise have travelled. I am particularly thankful for ongoing or occasional interactions over the past several years with Elizabeth Fein, Nev Jones, Christine El Ouardani, Pinky Hota, Kim Walters, Adam Baim, Jen Karlin, Bambi Chapin, Eevie Smith, Kate Goldfarb, Colin Halverson, Duff Morton, Lainie Goldwert, Adam Sargent, Elise Berman, and Maddy Elfenbein.

I was fortunate to find a wonderful intellectual community in Cleveland, Ohio during the years that I spent as a postdoctoral trainee at Case Western Reserve University and University Hospitals. Bridget Haas, Allison Schlosser, Julia Knopes, and Kristi Westphaln were new colleagues who instantly felt like old friends. Sarah Ronis, Larry Kleinman, Louise Acheson, and Kurt Stange modeled transdisciplinarity and showed me how my clinical ethnographic work connects to conversations within primary care research, implementation science, epidemiology, and public health. Jill Korbin, Woody Gaines, Vanessa Hildebrand, Eileen Anderson, Sana Loue, and Jonathan Sadowsky were generous mentors and interlocutors. The teachers, staff, and other families at Fairmount Temple provided a loving home-away-from-home for my toddler (and often for me).

I could not have asked for a more intellectually creative, empathic, and delightfully quirky collection of colleagues than the people that I am privileged to work with in the psychology program at the University of West Georgia. Thank you to Marie-Cécile Bertau, Christine Simmonds-Moore, Richard LaFleur, Lisa Osbeck, Kathy Skott-Myhre, Jake Glazier, Nisha Gupta, Cassandra Bolar, John Roberts, Tobin Hart, Neill Korobov, Jeff Reber, Rossella Traversa, Chris Head, Jim Dillon and

Sheena Rowe—for creating a version of the field of psychology in which I belong.

Thank you to Jennifer Hammer, Brianna Jean, Alexia Traganas, and other NYU Press staff, for all of your editorial labor, responsiveness, patience, and encouragement. I am also grateful to the anonymous reviewers for their perceptive and generous feedback.

The ethnographic research that forms the backbone of this book was funded through fellowships from the National Institutes of Health, the Wenner-Gren Foundation, and the University of Chicago. A Ruth L. Kirschstein National Research Service Award in Primary Care Research and Bioethics afforded me the time and material support necessary to write a book proposal during my postdoctoral training at Case Western Reserve University.

For their unflagging love and support, I am incredibly grateful to my parents, Carol and Amram Weiner; my mother-in-law, Martha Fraenkel, and her husband Mike McGlynn; my siblings (by blood and marriage), Elan Weiner, Molly Thorkelson, and Saul Thorkelson; and my aunts, uncles, cousins, and late grandmother.

Above all, I want to thank my partner, Eli, and our kids, Claude and Faye, for working to create an otherwise in our family life.

NOTES

1 Like most of the organizations, institutions, fieldsites, and individuals that appear in this book, the Chicago School for Psychoanalytic Psychotherapy (CSPP) is a pseudonym; identifying details have been altered or removed to protect the confidentiality of those involved.

2 Of course, I am not the first to note such parallels: Calabrese writes that "[p]sychoanalysis can be seen as participant-observation in a single relationship: the same critical standards of length of analysis and development of trust apply in both ethnography and clinical psychoanalysis" (2013, 63). He traces this sentiment back to Geertz, who likened ethnography to "clinical inference" in medicine:

> To generalize within cases is usually called, at least in medicine and depth psychology, clinical inference . . . In the study of cultures the signifiers are not symptoms or clusters of symptoms but symbolic acts or clusters of symbolic acts, and the aim is not therapy but the analysis of social discourse. But the way in which theory is used—to ferret out the unapparent import of things—is the same. (Geertz 1973, 26; in Calabrese 2013, 64)

A helpful discussion of anthropologists' uses of psychoanalytic concepts can also be found in Hollan's "Psychoanalysis and Ethnography" (2016).

3 "Rule 132" (59 Ill. Adm. Code 132) was rolled out in 2007 as part of "comprehensive fee-for-service reforms" in the state of Illinois. It "establish[es] practice standards and billing rates for state-contracted community mental health services" (Spitzmueller 2016, 45).

4 In 2007, under "comprehensive fee-for-service reforms," Illinois eliminated most of its block grant funding for community mental health programs and adopted three funding streams: Medicaid Rehabilitation Option (MRO) fee-for-service; non-MRO fee-for-service; and capacity grants. Each of these streams placed caps on contracts and paid providers prospectively under an "advance and reconcile" model—a model that was later changed to a full reimbursement system for valid Medicaid services. The MRO stream "is the portion of an agency's contract that governs Medicaid fee-for-service money" (Spitzmueller 2014, 78). Under "Rule 132" (see above), the state defines the Medicaid services that it will purchase from providers, and sets billing rates in 15-minute increments for those services. Providers are paid only for validly billed case records (Spitzmueller 2014). Non-MRO advances, which were eliminated by Illinois in fiscal year 2010, were paid on the same fee-for-service model as MRO contracts, but they covered individuals who

were not eligible for Medicaid. Capacity grants existed on a limited basis to cover expenses that the state acknowledged could not be adequately captured in a fee-for-service billing schedule.

In 2010, Governor Quinn declared Illinois to be in a state of financial crisis, and signed into law the Emergency Budget Act and Budget Implementation Act, cutting the state's community mental health budget by $45 million.

> Budget reductions devolved to community mental health providers in three forms. DMH (Illinois Department of Human Services/Division of Mental Health) eliminated all non-MRO fee-for-service payments. This meant that individuals who were not yet Medicaid eligible but who had a serious mental illness would no longer qualify for public mental health services. DMH eliminated almost all remaining grants-in-aid . . . And DMH introduced a new utilization management program that narrowed Medicaid service definitions and tightened the link between medical necessity and social service provision. (Spitzmueller 2016, 46)

At the time of this research, agencies such as RecoveryNet were in the early phases of a transition from the MRO fee-for-service model to Medicaid Managed Care Entities and systems of "care coordination." The fee-for-service regime was still very much in effect, and practice standards and billing rates were still governed by the taxonomy laid out in Rule 132.

5 Throughout the book, I (loosely) follow the local terminological conventions of my informants and use the word "patient" when discussing CSPP, "client" when writing about agency settings (RecoveryNet/Community Recovery Center and Wellness Behavioral Health), and "consumer" in relation to the Chicago public mental health centers and the Mental Health Coalition.

6 At the time of this fieldwork, telemedicine did not occupy the prominent place in mental health service provision that it has since 2020. I would not be surprised if use of such technologies is now more widespread, and the technologies themselves more reliable and sophisticated, in agencies such as RecoveryNet. Nonetheless, we would undoubtedly find a similar division of therapeutic labor today, as was the case in the visit I attended, with lower-status clinicians such as social workers and counselors spending more time with clients in "the community" and psychiatrists engaging in briefer and less frequent interactions with clients at a greater remove.

7 Although my expansive interpretation and metaphorical usage of "self-management" is distinctive, the term itself is not my own. Rather, it refers in the first instance to a specific clinical treatment modality, described in detail later in the book.

INTRODUCTION

1 In a Keywords essay titled "Neoliberal Agency," Ilana Gershon notes that various anthropologists have argued "that the ethnographer's task should be to understand neoliberalism as situated, to analyze how neoliberal policies are transformed and

often reconfigured as they are transported and implemented in new locales" (2011, 537). Gershon goes on to contend that "insisting on the local is an important step but an insufficient one," calling on ethnographers to take up an "anthropological imagination" in order to discover an epistemological outside to neoliberal ways of being and forms of analysis (537). Following Gershon, in this book I aim to delineate the many forms that mood disorder self-management takes across the political economic landscape of Chicago precisely in order to discover how, in and through its situated enactments, self-management may invert itself and begin to suggest alternative modes of living.

2 Interestingly, a 2013 position statement published by the British Psychological Society's Division of Clinical Psychology (DCP) also renounced the *DSM* as lacking validity and utility, but for precisely the opposite reasons from the NIMH. According to the DCP, the *DSM* is *overly* oriented toward biological causes of mental illnesses, and "there is a need for a paradigm shift in relation to the experiences that [psychiatric] diagnoses refer to, towards a conceptual system which is no longer based on a 'disease' model" (Johnstone 2013).

3 This is an open question indeed, and the ethnographic record in fact suggests that the self-management of these prototypical physiological diseases is far from unproblematic. For examples of works that take up the difficulties experienced in diabetes self-management, see Borovoy and Hine (2008) and Mol (2008). For a discussion of the ways in which the outcomes of self-management policies and practices for coronary heart disease are impeded by a lack of consideration of "structural and psychosocial constraints," see Moore et al. (2015, 1254).

4 In outlining the historical and political shifts that enabled the interests of the psychiatric ex-patients movement and the disease self-management paradigm to converge, I am to some extent invoking a metanarrative that has been critiqued as underemphasizing the heterogeneity of the broader consumer/survivor/ex-patient (c/s/x) movement (e.g., Schrader et al. 2013). It is not my intent to imply that the radical message of the survivor/ex-patient movement was entirely "engulfed by neoliberal logics" (Coleman 2008, 343), or to suggest even that neoliberal logics can only be taken up and enacted in one single manner. Indeed, a chapter of this book concerns itself largely with the way in which differing positions vis-à-vis neoliberal logics of privatization between two racially distinct groups of disenfranchised mental health consumer activists in Chicago led to fracturing among would-be allies. It is important to recognize that the c/s/x movement today includes activists who "disavow neurological explanations of unusual states" (Schrader et al. 2013, 62) or who seek to normalize experiences such as voice-hearing (Luhrmann 2012a). Moreover, the willingness of psychiatric activists to "shift political messages and tactics within a tide of changing conditions" can be understood as a strategy that facilitated their "ability to survive as central protagonists in a critique of institutional psychiatry" rather than an abandonment of the movement's radical principles (Coleman 2008, 344).

5 Now the National Alliance on Mental Illness.

6 Originally named the National Alliance of Mental Patients (McLean 2000).

7 The term "managed care" is used to refer to a set of activities and policies that were implemented in the United States in the early 1980s with the intention of reducing the costs of health insurance and healthcare service delivery. Originally developed by health maintenance organizations (HMOs), managed care techniques have become nearly ubiquitous across both public and private health benefit programs in the United States today. Managed care's mechanisms of cost reduction include incentivizing physicians and patients to select less expensive forms of care, restricting or denying access to specific services, placing limitations on hospital inpatient admissions and lengths of stay, and increasing the proportion of healthcare costs paid by the patient (i.e., "beneficiary cost sharing"). A substantial body of clinical ethnographic research in the United States has examined the ways in which managed care—as a philosophy and as a collection of policies and procedures—has altered institutional cultures (Spitzmueller 2016), therapeutic practices (Kirschner and Lachicotte 2001), clinician-client interactions (Cohen et al. 2006), and negotiated formulations of selfhood and responsibility (Lester 2017).

8 "Obamacare" is the colloquial name for the Affordable Care Act (ACA), a momentous federal statute that was enacted by the 111th US Congress and signed into law by President Barack Obama in March 2010. The ACA marked the most significant expansion of healthcare coverage in the United States since the 1960s. As of the completion of this book in late 2024, in spite of dozens of Republican-led efforts to weaken or repeal Obamacare, most of the act's provisions are still in effect.

9 "Mixed episodes" include symptoms of both mania and depression.

10 Interestingly, a recent meta-analysis published in the journal *Molecular Psychiatry* concluded that "the serotonin theory of depression is not empirically substantiated" (Moncrieff et al. 2023, 3254). To date, however, serotonergic drugs are still the first-line medications prescribed to treat depression.

11 Jamison is a clinical psychologist and professor whose published work for lay audiences includes *Touched with Fire* (1993) and *An Unquiet Mind* (1995). In *Touched with Fire*, Jamison marshals historical evidence to assert that manic depression/bipolar disorder is associated with creativity and artistic ability, and that the diagnostic category can be retroactively applied to figures such as Virginia Woolf, Lord Byron, and Vincent van Gogh. Jamison subsequently revealed her own struggles with manic depressive illness in her memoir, *An Unquiet Mind*. As anthropologist Emily Martin notes, "it would be hard to exaggerate the impact of Jamison's work, which has been featured in major newspapers, magazines, and documentary films" (Martin 2007, 23).

12 These dynamics have shifted in the time that has passed between when I conducted my research and the writing of this book. I analyze these changes briefly in chapter 5.

CHAPTER 1. SITES AND SITUATIONS IN AN ETHNOGRAPHY OF HOME

1 My stance here is similar to that of other clinician-anthropologists who ethnographically study the clinical fields in which they have trained or practice (Baim
2022; Smith 2017; Schechter 2014; Lester 2021).

2 This is a bit of an over-simplification: While members of the Mental Health Coalition were accustomed to collaborating with clinician advocates and allies, some
were distrustful of those therapists who were affiliated with CDPH "community
partners" such as RecoveryNet and Wellness Behavioral Health. Such affiliations,
including my own employment at RecoveryNet's Community Recovery Center
(CRC), could reasonably be interpreted as tacit endorsements of the city's claim
that mental health services for the city's poor and uninsured were *improved*—
rather than jeopardized—by their privatization. In my own case, I had established
a relationship with the Mental Health Coalition for more than a year prior to
my involvement with RecoveryNet; MHC members understood and appreci-
ated some of the stakes of my research project, and could see how my gaining an
"insider's" perspective on RecoveryNet's treatment practices would provide an
important piece of the ethnographic story about the politics of mental healthcare
in contemporary Chicago. Other community partner clinicians, however, did
not always receive the "pass" I was given: At a large, open-to-the-public Mental
Health Coalition "Town Hall" event that I helped organize, one attendee identified herself as a therapist who worked for a RecoveryNet program. On hearing
this, the MHC leader who was facilitating the Town Hall insisted that the clinician leave the event at once. "You may not mean us any harm," the MHC leader
explained, "but we are here to talk about *our* vision of a public mental health care
system in Chicago—and you are the enemy."

3 A colleague rightly notes that these descriptions of first-instance Americanist anthropologists are less apt for characterizing those Americanists who are currently
residing in the United States but whose country of origin is elsewhere (Sargent,
personal correspondence).

4 These particular quotes are from current University of Chicago web pages (University of Chicago Community Impact n.d.; University of Chicago Civic Engagement n.d.), but the discourse is typical of decades of self-congratulation.

5 The University of Chicago's medical school and affiliated institutions have gone
by different names in different time periods. When I arrived in Chicago and as
it appears in this book, it was named the University of Chicago Medical Center
(UCMC). As of 2024, it is called University of Chicago Medicine (UCM).

6 The UCMC closed its adult trauma center in 1988, citing financial reasons. Soon
after, Michael Reese Hospital in Bronzeville followed suit, rendering the South
Side of Chicago a "trauma desert" with 50% longer ambulance transport times
to the nearest adult trauma center than for residents in other parts of the city
(Moore 2013). On August 15, 2010, 18-year-old community organizer Damian
Turner was critically injured in a drive-by shooting a few blocks away from the

UCMC. Because he was not a minor, he could not be admitted at the UCMC's pediatric trauma center, and instead had to be transported over 9 miles by ambulance to Northwestern Memorial Hospital, where he died. Turner's death ignited a grassroots direct action campaign, led by a Black youth community organization under the same umbrella organization as the Mental Health Coalition, for the University of Chicago to open an adult level 1 trauma center. After five years of protests that frequently brought community members and students into brutal contact with the University of Chicago Police Department, the UCMC announced a $270 million plan to open a trauma center on its own campus (Sailappan and Lalljee 2018). The trauma center opened in 2018.

7 Descriptions provided reflect the status of each site during the time period in which my ethnographic research was conducted. Where possible and appropriate, updates about changes that have occurred in the intervening years are noted.

8 Writing "process notes" after a session with a patient is a common practice among private psychotherapists. Unlike progress notes—which are basic records of dates and services provided that can be subpoenaed by a court—process notes are meant for the therapist's own use and are usually given special protection under the federal Health Insurance Portability and Accountability Act (HIPAA) (Clay 2007). Process notes are often used as a component of clinical supervision, so that the trainee may "recreate the therapeutic process for [the] supervisor" (Bender and Messner 2003, 97).

The form and content of a therapy process note are not unlike the ethnographer's fieldnote. As one practitioner explains in a published guide entitled *Becoming a Therapist: What Do I Say, and Why?*:

> To organize the notes, I divide a plain sheet of paper in half with a vertical line (or fold) down the center. On the left side of the paper, I write down as much as I can remember of the session's most meaningful moments (including names of important people in the patient's life, so I'll have them for future reference). Then, on the right side of the paper, I write any questions, ideas, or feelings I may have had during the hour. During supervision, I'll use my notes to formulate my questions and guide the discussion. (Bender and Messner 2003, 97)

9 Psychosocial Rehabilitation (PSR) programs were introduced in 1978 under President Jimmy Carter in a report—*Toward a National Plan for the Chronically Mentally Ill*—produced by the first Presidential Commission on Mental Health to address the early failures of the community mental health system. PSR centers are envisioned in the National Plan as social clubs "that facilitate rehabilitation by providing extended kinship and social support within a context of acceptance and positive expectation" (Spitzmueller 2014, 41). While the early PSR model was extremely flexible and provided only loose relational guidelines for day programs for clients, the shift to Medicaid financing in the 1980s and 1990s led to a redefinition of PSR as a set of services that "target specific skills deficits, are short-term in nature, and provide structured interventions that are curriculum-based" (88–89).

10 Many clinicians in private practice would also refrain from including certain types of personal artifacts, such as family photos, in the space where they conduct psychotherapy with patients, on the theory that an excessive display of the therapist's intimate memorabilia could interfere with the therapeutic process (Scharff 2004). However, in the case of these private practice settings—particularly, perhaps, those of psychoanalytically oriented therapists—the decision to include or omit a personal artifact is often part of a rather deliberate effort to curate a therapeutically conducive space for the therapist and patient. In addition to the iconic couch and the therapist's chair, many private practice clinicians appoint their therapy offices with certain *kinds* of personal objects that would be difficult to include in a shared room at an agency, such as diplomas, libraries, plants, wall art, evocative knick-knacks, or a pet. Some such therapists will even demarcate a portion of their own residence as the therapy space after carefully reflecting on ways to create an appropriate, but not excessive, degree of separation of the therapist's personal and professional lives—reflections that may incorporate and seek to represent salient psychoanalytic notions about qualities of intimacy of the therapeutic relationship (Frank 2014). A perusal of psychoanalyst/photographer Mark Gerald's fascinating photo series of his colleagues' offices conveys the care, intentionality, and distinctiveness with which private psychotherapy rooms are often designed (Gerald 2014), putting into perspective the aesthetic and symbolic stakes of the impossibility of such spaces in an agency setting. In different terms, psychological research has suggested that the clinician's control of the "orderliness," "personalization," and "softness" characteristics of a therapy office may influence clients' experiences of comfort and expectations about quality of care (Devlin and Nasar 2012).

11 As of the time of this research, Medicaid is a joint federal and state program that provides health coverage to more than 72.5 million Americans. It is the largest source of health coverage in the United States (Centers for Medicare and Medicaid Services 2017). Under the Affordable Care Act (ACA) of 2010, states were given the option to expand Medicaid, with an unlimited federal match, to cover nearly all low-income Americans under age 65 with an adjusted gross income of 133% or below the federal poverty level. As of early 2017, all but 19 states had expanded their Medicaid programs. In the state of Illinois, Medicaid expansion was authorized in July 2013 and went into effect on January 1, 2014. This expansion was fully financed by the federal government through 2016, with plans to gradually decrease federal support to 90% by 2020 (Norris 2017). Within the first six months of Medicaid expansion in Illinois, an overwhelming 350,000 new enrollees were approved (Frost 2014); by August 2016, that number had nearly doubled. In spite of the large number of people covered by Medicaid in the United States, there are very few mental health service providers (therapists, psychiatrists, psychologists, etc.) outside of agency settings who are contracted with a Medicaid health plan.

CountyCare is an Illinois Medicaid program for adult residents of Cook County. Expanded eligibility for CountyCare began in January 2013—a year ahead of Affordable Care Act (ACA) Medicaid expansion—due to the fact that Cook County applied for and received a federal waiver allowing the program to begin early. The waiver also enabled CountyCare to split costs between the Cook County Health and Hospital System and the federal government, bypassing the Illinois state Medicaid system for the year (Wallace 2012). Beginning on January 1, 2014, CountyCare transitioned from a Medicaid waiver program to become a Managed Care Community Network (MCCN) under the ACA. Individuals in Cook County applying for Medicaid subsequent to that date may choose coverage under CountyCare or through a commercial Medicaid managed care plan. During my research period, CountyCare (as well as IlliniCare Health Plan) subcontracted with a third-party administrator, Cenpatico, for the management of its covered behavioral health services.

12 During the time period in which I was conducting research, the state of Illinois passed a law requiring that at least 50% of its Medicaid recipients be assigned to a Managed Care Entity (MCE) and moved into "care coordination" by January 1, 2015. The law was part of a broader effort on the part of Illinois and other states to explore new ways of working with managed care organizations that contract with state Medicaid programs to coordinate and integrate care, and to move away from the fee-for-service model that preceded it. In 2017, the Illinois Healthcare and Family Services (HFS) website listed five types of Medicaid care coordination programs, into which it stated that more than 60% of its 3 million clients were enrolled. The five programs were designated as: Accountable Care Entities (ACEs) and Care Coordination Entities (CCEs); Medicare-Medicaid Alignment Initiative (MMAI); Integrated Care Program and Integrated Care Expansion (ICP); Managed Care Community Networks (MCCNs); and Health Homes. According to the Illinois care coordination statute (305 ILCS 5/5–30),

> [p]ayment for . . . coordinated care shall be based on arrangements where the State pays for performance related to health care outcomes, the use of evidence-based practices, the use of primary care delivered through comprehensive medical homes, the use of electronic medical records, and the appropriate exchange of health information electronically made either on a capitated basis in which a fixed monthly premium per recipient is paid and full financial risk is assumed for the delivery of services, or through other risk-based payment arrangements. (Illinois General Assembly n.d.)

The technical details of differences in payment arrangements between the five new care coordination programs—and between care coordination and the "fee-for-service" model—are beyond the scope of this book. I can say, however, that to the best of my knowledge, the introduction of care coordination programs in the greater Chicago region did not make an observable impact on the clinical interactions or institutional cultures of either WBH or RecoveryNet/CRC, both of which were still deeply entrenched in a fee-for-service managerial logic of efficiency and accountability (Spitzmueller 2016). For example, clinicians at both agencies were required to meet agency-set targets for billable productivity, a source of ongoing stress regularly glossed as a fee-for-service problem.

13 This Act was also known as the Community Mental Health Act of 1963.

14 The four clinics that were slated for closure in 2009 were Back of the Yards, Beverly/Morgan Park, Greater Grand/Mid-South, and Woodlawn.

15 Chicago's system of public mental health centers is intended for uninsured consumers, and therefore operates on funding streams that are distinct from the Medicaid fee-for-service structures utilized by private community mental health providers. Prior to July 2008, the state of Illinois issued mental health grants to fund the city clinics. Beginning in 2008, these grants were eliminated, and Illinois began requiring Chicago to bill the state for reimbursement for services rendered. According to Daley, the proposed clinic closures in 2009 had been necessitated by state-level budget cuts that were outside of the city's control. State officials countered Daley's explanation, blaming the city for failing to bill the state for mental health services under the new reimbursement system. Ultimately, the City of Chicago's health commissioner at the time, Dr. Terry Mason, acknowledged that a new computer system had caused billing delays on the city's end. Under pressure from the (soon-to-be-named) Mental Health Coalition, Daley agreed to find the money to keep the clinics open until the city's billing problems could be resolved (Spielman 2009).

16 Rogers Park, Logan Square, Woodlawn, Auburn-Gresham, Morgan Park, and Back of the Yards.

17 FQHCs "receive federal funding to serve an underserved area or population, and qualify for enhanced reimbursement from Medicaid and Medicare, among other benefits" (Health & Disability Advocates 2015, 8). The Health & Disability Advocates group ceased operations in December 2020. For more information about "The Role of Public Health in Chicago's Mental Health System," contact Barbara Otto, barbara@smartpolicyworks.com.

18 Not all MHC members agreed with this recommendation; some felt that even under the Affordable Care Act, there would always be some Americans who would not be able to afford health insurance and that, as such, it was important that the Chicago mental health centers remain dedicated to serving that population. However, many MHC members argued that by refusing to allow the city clinics to join insurance panels in the wake of the Affordable Care Act, the City of Chicago was choreographing its own obsolescence, which could then be used as a rationale for additional clinic closures.

19 A more detailed account of the creation of Chicago's first EMHSP—and of the controversy surrounding its establishment—is provided in chapter 5.

20 According to a report prepared by the Mental Health Coalition, prior to the closures, 61% of all city clinic consumers were African American and 17% were Hispanic. Additionally, 80% of the CDPH clinical therapists slated for layoffs due to the closures were African American (Mental Health Coalition 2012).

CHAPTER 2. ECONOMIES OF AGENCY AND THE (UN)MANAGED SELF

1   For a period of nine months, I attended nearly every weekly 90-minute support group meeting of the local chapter of a national, patient-directed organization for people living with depression and bipolar disorder. The support group later disaffiliated from the national organization but continued to meet. I often arrived early and socialized with my informants in a local coffee shop or in the meeting room, and usually stayed after the meetings, when people would hang out and smoke outside of the center. During the meetings, I participated in weekly introductions and closing "games" (each week, a different person was responsible for coming up with a question—which ranged from "What is your favorite food?" to "You have a bulldozer and can bulldoze one person or thing. What do you pick?"—for everyone to answer). I did not generally speak during the meetings, although on a few occasions I was asked personal questions and answered those honestly. Apart from attending support group meetings, I conducted semi-structured interviews with five members: Warren, James, Christine, Kevin, and Tricia.

   The individuals described in this chapter are those with a diagnosis of Bipolar Disorder 1 or 2 who regularly attended meetings and considered the support group to be an important component of their therapeutic regimen. I chose to focus on their narratives partly for pragmatic reasons—I had more of an opportunity to become well acquainted with regular support group attendees than with those who come only once or infrequently—but also theoretical ones: I wanted to study the cultivated subjectivities of people who not only accept and believe in their mood disorder diagnosis, but also make a constant, vigilant effort to self-manage.

2   Portions of this chapter appear in an article published in *Culture, Medicine, and Psychiatry* entitled "The (Un)managed Self: Paradoxical Forms of Agency in Self-Management of Bipolar Disorder" (Weiner 2011).

3   I use the phrase "bipolar person" (bipolar woman here) as opposed to "person with bipolar disorder" in order to avoid reinscribing the notions of the discreteness and separability of rational selfhood and disease that I seek to interrogate in this chapter. To further explore the ramifications of this choice, I take up debates about "I am" versus "I have" language ethnographically and within anthropological literature later in the chapter.

4   For the majority of my fieldwork at this site, the support group was peer-led by a man to whom I refer in this chapter as Warren. In the final weeks of my time there, a clinical leader (an intern who was in the process of completing their doctorate in clinical psychology) was added to the group.

5   I am grateful to Emily Martin for discussing this vignette with me at an early stage of my writing process and suggesting the term "distributed" for the style of agency that I was describing.

6   Because no single term for the diagnosed individual was dominant in the context of this support group, I use "patient" and "consumer" interchangeably in this chapter.

7 I employ the term "reification" following Taussig (1980). Drawing on his conversations with a terminally ill patient about the patient's search for meaning in her symptoms, Taussig illustrates that "medical practice is a singularly important way of maintaining the denial as to the social facticity of facts" (5). Here, I wish to emphasize that the delineation of rational self and bipolar symptom in the self-management literature similarly mystifies a set of social, political economic, intersubjective, and embodied relations.

8 Beryl Lawn, letter to the editor, *bp Magazine*, Spring 2007.

9 Richard K. Staggenborg, letter to the editor, *bp Magazine*, Fall 2007, 13.

10 Monica L. Gretter, letter to the editor, *bp Magazine*, Fall 2007, 13.

11 BobMinekheim, letter to the editor, *bp Magazine*, Fall 2007, 13.

12 Foucault writes that technologies of the self privilege self-knowledge over self-care, and "permit individuals to effect by their own means or with the help of others a certain number of operations on their own bodies and souls, thoughts, conduct, and way of being, so as to transform themselves in order to attain a certain state of happiness, purity, wisdom, perfection, or immortality" (Foucault et al. 1988, 18).

13 In the article "'Schizophrenic Person' or 'Person with Schizophrenia'?" Louis Sass offers a compelling argument that in bracketing out the schizophrenia "disease" and only listening to "what can be understood to emanate from [the patient's] supposed 'personhood'" (Sass 2007, 414), the biomedical model is, in unintended ways, inherently stigmatizing. Specifically, Sass shows, the "person with schizophrenia" formulation systematically obscures or dismisses important "schizophrenic modes of being"—including forms of intentionality, insight, and irony—by considering them to come from something wholly distinct from the self. Thus, the failure of biomedical models to listen to "the specifically schizophrenic qualities of the person" forecloses the possibility of encountering "points of view that can most deeply challenge as well as enrich our own" (Sass 2007, 415, emphasis in original).

14 Not every story or experience in the support group was one of self-management. A particularly striking and disturbing counterexample emerged one evening early in my fieldwork, when the wife of a bipolar man with whom several group members were acquainted showed up at the meeting on her own. Alternately tearing up and laughing in bitter disbelief, she described her husband's current manic state: He had stopped going to his real job in favor of staying up all night working on a "new business plan," was lying and using illegal drugs, had left their two-year-old daughter alone to play with an X-ACTO knife, and had drained the couple's savings by $20,000 at a casino. What upset her the most was the fact that her husband had seen the manic episode coming and was presently aware of his state, but was unbothered by it and felt no obligation to intervene and self-manage. "He knows he's manic but doesn't care," she had complained. "He's doing these things on purpose."

The discussion that ensued was a complex one for the group, but I believe that the direction it took is illustrative of the distinct and paradoxical form of self-managing bipolar subjectivity that many of the group members inhabit, and that this woman's husband was rejecting. Using their own personal histories as examples, group members found themselves in the uncomfortable position of explaining to the woman that it might not be worthwhile to try to reestablish trust with her bipolar husband. As James put it: "I imagine down the line he may feel remorse, but that may not matter. Lots of people feel remorse. Abusive people even feel remorse. But even if he is medicated, what happens the next time around? And there *will* be a next time around."

The group's consensus was that an awareness of one's mania implies a capacity and responsibility to distance oneself from and attempt to act upon it. Members explained: "Once you have any awareness you should be trying to take some responsibility."

15 Huxley and Baldessarini (2007), however, report that the "prognosis for BPD was once considered relatively favorable, but contemporary findings suggest that disability and poor outcomes are prevalent, despite major therapeutic advances" (183).

16 I borrow the phrase "culprit lesion" from Barry Saunders's fascinating ethnography of the historically genred reading, writing, and diagnosing practices that occur in a university hospital CT suite. Saunders demonstrates that even in the postmodern era of "non-invasive" diagnostic modalities, "CT technology . . . is haunted by nineteenth-century projects of comparing, interpreting, classifying morphological specimens and residues—including, ultimately, the residue of the cadaver" (Saunders 2008, 12). Furthermore, he asserts that even though the lesion, "once fixed, macroscopic, and retrieved from the cadaver," is now "microscopic, molecular, fluid," it nonetheless persists, particularly as the object of diagnostic aesthetics of detection and intrigue: "even if very small, the fixable, visible lesion remains important" (2–3).

In fact, contemporary psychiatry is often acutely aware that the success of its project will depend upon its ability to apply something analogous to the anatomo-clinical gaze to mental illnesses, describing its disease objects as, if not lesions per se, at least isolable neurochemical events that can (now or someday) be visualized (e.g., Insel and Quirion 2005, 2221).

17 Eugene Raikhel, personal communication.

CHAPTER 3. "I'VE PUT IN MY TIME"

1 Portions of this chapter first appeared in "The Recuperation of Moral Agency through Structural Erasure in Clinical Social Workers' Accounts of Career Path and Treatment Decisions" (Weiner 2020) and/or in "Billable Services and the 'Therapeutic Fee': On the Work of Disavowal of Political Economy and its Re-emergence in Clinical Practice" (Weiner 2019).

2 Because of the copious and ongoing paperwork that must be completed at WBH, clinicians often end up conducting therapy sessions with clients while sitting at their desks, with both parties facing the computer monitor. To streamline the

process, each computer is outfitted with an (often malfunctioning) electronic signature pad so that clients can sign documents on the spot. Furthermore, therapy interns are advised that to minimize their own backlog of paperwork, they should keep the agency's documentation software open and complete service notes together with clients during sessions, integrating the contents of the fields required by Medicaid into the therapeutic dialogue. Like most of my peers, however, I usually found that filling out the form was incompatible with maintaining rapport with my clients, and instead created, during sessions, empty "placeholder" service notes that needed to be completed later. The placeholder notes would accumulate rapidly, making the task of catching up a daunting and oft-dreaded one.

3 "Today Counts System News: Best Practices Yield Positive Results Across Wellness Health, Wellness Physician Performs First Two-level Artificial Disc Replacement in Illinois, New Models of Care Delivery Mean New Opportunity for Wellness Health, and More!"; "Poem for Feast of the Annunciation"; "It's Client Satisfaction Week!"

4 Parallel process is a concept that has its origins in psychoanalytic theories of transference and countertransference. In the context of clinical supervision, parallel process usually refers to the unconscious re-creation in a supervision session of the therapeutic difficulties that the supervisee has with a client. The recognition and examination of parallel process in supervision is theorized to facilitate growth and self-awareness in the supervisee (Searles 1955; Morrissey and Tribe 2001; Williams 1997).

5 In this chapter and throughout the book, I use the terms "psychotherapist" or "therapist" to refer to my clinician informants who provided direct mental health services either in an agency or in private practice. The majority of these informants held master's degrees in clinical social work, counseling, or a related field, and my analysis of the normative professional trajectory of psychotherapists focuses on this educational level. A very small number of my therapist informants had earned—or were working on—doctoral degrees, but this advanced training was typically undertaken later in the therapist's career, concurrently with full-time clinical work, and did not tend to significantly alter the therapist's professional trajectory. With regard to the particular master's credentials held by my informants, although counseling and social work have rather distinct historical lineages and potential career options—with a social work degree regarded as offering greater flexibility, particularly for those interested in policy work—these differences did not seem to exert themselves within the subset of clinicians pursuing careers in mental health treatment and psychotherapy that I studied: In the two community mental health agencies where I conducted research, and across similar sites, clinicians who had trained as either master's-level counselors or social workers were hired for identical positions and were compensated according to the same salary structure. In my observations of individual and group supervision, team meetings, or work with clients, I did not encounter any instance in which a distinction was made between these degree types. Likewise, those clinicians who

eventually move into full-time psychotherapy practice do not appear to differ in their clinical orientation or along other significant dimensions on the basis of their credentials. I therefore am comfortable grouping together counselors and social workers in my analysis.

6 As the youngest of the mental health professions, counseling has yet to undergo certain forms of national standardization that are found across its counterpart fields in the United States. For example, while the Council on Social Work Education, founded in 1952, serves as the sole accrediting agency for social work education programs recognized by the Council on Higher Education Accreditation, master's-level counseling programs may currently be accredited under either CACREP (the Council for the Accreditation of Counseling and Related Education Programs) or CORE (the Council on Rehabilitation Education), established in 1981 and 1972 respectively. One symptom of this lack of unified standards appears to be a discourse among clinicians about the need to define counseling's professional identity (Bobby and Urofsky 2011; Martin and Cannon 2010; Pistole 2001; Palmo 1999; Hanna and Bemak 1997) and—perhaps relatedly—a wildly varying assortment of titles awarded across different institutions for similar master's-level counseling degrees. As such, non-social worker therapists I encountered at my fieldsites held a variety of functionally equivalent credentials including Master of Arts or Master of Science in Counseling, Clinical Counseling, Clinical Mental Health Counseling, Family Counseling, and Marriage and Family Therapy.

7 Significantly, this shift from agency work to private practice entails not only a quantitative change in the therapist's remuneration (with private practice offering the potential for far higher earnings) but also a qualitative one: In the agency, the therapist receives a stable—if low—salary from their employer, paid irrespective of the amount of clinical service provided by the therapist during the given pay period. In private practice, the therapist's income is variable and comprises cash paid directly to the therapist by the patient (or the patient's insurance company, or both) in exchange for therapeutic services. Arguably, the distinction between these two models of remuneration has become less clear-cut in the wake of comprehensive fee-for-service Medicaid reforms, which have prompted agency clinicians to reorient their practices on the ground toward a new managerial logic (Spitzmueller 2016).

8 As is often the case in adjacent communities that are subject to similar types of structural subordination, I did occasionally witness moments characterized by a "narcissism of small differences" (Freud 1930), in which a psychotherapist would mobilize and accentuate the minor status differential between social work and counseling. In one such (perhaps overdetermined) case, a course instructor who was a licensed clinical social worker in private psychotherapy practice—and who frequently expressed frustration over never having completed the doctoral degree she began decades earlier—(half) joked to my counseling classmates and me on the first day of her "Professional Development" class: "We social workers were

glad when the profession of counseling was created; thanks to you folks, we're not the lowest on the totem pole anymore!"

9 Therapists who publish works chronicling their own personal and professional development (e.g., Dean 2000; Stricker 2001; Fodor 2001; Norcross and Farber 2005)—or who write about this topic in more general terms—describe the trajectory in many ways that suggest, but do not explicitly name (as either an aspiration or a source of ambivalence), the progressively upward shift in the social class of the therapist and their clientele that accompanies normative professional maturation. These narratives instead cite processes such as the acquisition of freedom in one's therapeutic work, the attainment of confidence in one's clinical intuitions, the outgrowing of one treatment paradigm and discovery of a more fulfilling theoretical orientation, or the taking on of clinical supervisory functions as driving the therapist's transition from early career work to private psychotherapy practice. Occasionally, a text will lament in passing the fact that the professional trajectory of psychotherapists supports a phenomenon in which inexperienced clinicians tend to treat the most "disturbed" and "challenging" patients, while better, more seasoned therapists keep the "YAVIS" (young, attractive, verbal, intelligent, successful) patients for themselves (Jennings 2010, 50), but even such accounts seldom acknowledge a correspondence between their categories and categories of social class. One notable, and controversial, exception is a book entitled *Unfaithful Angels: How Social Work Has Abandoned Its Mission* (Specht and Courtney 1994), which indicts the profession of social work for its movement "away from the poor" into private practice (106).

10 In the state of Illinois, in order to qualify to sit for the licensing examination, master's-level social workers must work for 3,000 hours under the supervision of an LCSW (Licensed Clinical Social Worker). Master's-level counselors must work for the equivalent of two years full-time under the supervision of a licensed clinical counselor, psychiatrist, clinical psychologist, or LCSW.

11 Klein et al. note that "for professional education in particular, including social work, adjuncts are apparently regarded as useful instructional resources" (1996, 255). They suggest that in addition to financial benefits, adjunct social work instructors contribute to universities their "expertise developed from their work-related experiences" (254), knowledge of current policy, and enthusiasm for teaching. Among the 43 adjunct social work instructors surveyed by the authors, the motivation to teach in addition to engaging in direct clinical practice was primarily not grounded in financial reward: While most of the respondents rated the supplemental income as "slightly important" and only 12% stated that the remuneration was "very important," 88% of respondents indicated that having a social and professional connection to an educational institution constituted a "very important" or "important" motivation to serve as adjunct faculty (259).

12 Understandably, agency clinicians would frequently invoke the theories of psychologist Abraham Maslow—in particular his concept of a "hierarchy of needs"—in considerations of the most appropriate order to address the many

problems with which their clients presented. In his 1943 paper "A Theory of Human Motivation," Maslow argues that human motivation for higher-order needs (e.g., self-esteem, love, self-actualization) is grounded in, and dependent upon, the fulfillment of a more basic set of physiological conditions. "In the human being who is missing everything in life in an extreme fashion," Maslow writes, "it is most likely that the major motivation would be the physiological needs rather than any others."

> If all the needs are unsatisfied, and the organism is then dominated by the physiological needs, all other needs may become simply non-existent or pushed into the background. It is then fair to characterize the whole organism by saying simply that it is hungry, for consciousness is almost completely preempted by hunger. All capacities are put into the service of hunger-satisfaction, and the organization of these capacities is almost entirely determined by the one purpose of satisfying hunger. The receptors and effectors, the intelligence, memory, habits, all may now be defined simply as hunger-gratifying tools. Capacities that are not useful for this purpose lie dormant, or are pushed into the background. The urge to write poetry, the desire to acquire an automobile, the interest in American history, the desire for a new pair of shoes are, in the extreme case, forgotten or become of secondary importance . . . For our chronically and extremely hungry man, Utopia can be defined very simply as a place where there is plenty of food . . . Freedom, love, community feeling, respect, philosophy, may all be waved aside as fripperies which are useless since they fail to fill the stomach. (Maslow 1943, 373–374)

> The iconic visual representation of Maslow's hierarchy of needs (though not in fact attributable to Maslow) as a pyramidal diagram was familiar to most clinicians at WBH and CRC, and could occasionally be found on display in a therapist's office. Coupled with the routinely cited metaphor of the therapist as firefighter—in other words, as needing to postpone the examination of non-urgent psychological issues in the interest of "putting out fires" or addressing the client's immediate crises—the image of Maslow's pyramid helped clinicians to see and articulate the mental health significance of activities that seemed outside of the scope of their training. At the same time, more often than not the pyramid seemed to offer a compelling rationale for working exclusively at its bottom rungs (as clients' physiological and safety needs were seldom fully satisfied) rather than serving as an order of operations that could be carried out in its entirety.

13 Typically during group supervision at WBH, one intern would be assigned each week to present on a clinical case with which they were struggling.

14 As Ehrenreich (1985) notes, social work salaries have historically "hover[ed] barely above the poverty level," in spite of the field's drive to professionalize (230). In 2015, the starting salary for a master's-level unlicensed therapist at the agencies where I conducted field research was just under $32,000 per year, with a nominal increase if the therapist obtained an initial or clinical license.

15 This therapist's preferred practice, I should note, was not particularly endorsed by his supervisor, who often encouraged the therapist to put less pressure on himself about billable productivity and enjoy his paid time off.

16 Relatedly, the emphases in the narratives on individual will, distinction, and sacrifice may work to deny the small amount of class privilege that even lower-status therapists do enjoy, and which has always already set them apart from their more disadvantaged clients (Judith Farquhar, personal communication).

CHAPTER 4. BILLABLE SERVICES AND THE "THERAPEUTIC FEE"

1 Emily's professional life course narrative is analyzed in chapter 3.

2 Portions of this chapter first appeared in an article in *Anthropological Quarterly* (Weiner 2019).

3 Psychotherapists have long been wary of the practice of accepting gifts from patients. The literature on this topic encompasses a spectrum of recommended approaches that the therapist might take when offered a gift, ranging from maintaining a policy of strict rejection, to accepting only gifts of nominal value, to making the decision on a case-by-case basis through an evaluation of the patient's motivation for offering the gift and the intersubjective significance of its acceptance or refusal (Knox 2008; Hahn 1998; Smolar 2003). In arguing here that private practice therapists' discourses about the "therapeutic fee" enable the fee to function similarly to a gift in the sociological sense, I do not mean to suggest that the fee represents a potentially problematic instance of the therapist accepting a gift qua gift of the type described in the clinical literature. Rather, I am drawing attention to the fact that the fee, as imagined in this discourse, indexes and entails an ongoing social relationship analogous to that accomplished through gift exchange, and that in both cases, the ability of the fee or gift to effect this social connection depends upon a mutual misrecognition of its mediating role as an object of economic exchange.

4 See Cole (2014) for a parallel case of actors' strategic and necessary misrecognitions (glossed by Cole as "working mis/understandings") producing the second-order effect of "naturaliz[ing] some of the structural inequalities already inherent" in the relationships in which the actors participate (547).

5 That therapists may take recourse to "moral talk" (Bennett 2014) as a way to performatively figure themselves as disinterested in money marks, I would argue, the popular uptake of the earlier definition of moral economy (i.e., as opposed to capitalist market logics). Indeed, the notion that morality and economy constitute disparate domains is pervasive in many contemporary discourses (Keane 2008).

6 In practice, this trust is something that therapists and patients may need to cultivate over time, as the consistency and endurance of the therapeutic relationship is established. While I do not have sufficient data to venture a generalization, my casual observations suggest that a private practice therapist may be more inclined to waive their required session fee for a last-minute cancellation if the patient is one whom the therapist regards as generally reliable, whereas the therapist might be

more likely to uphold their formal policy for a new or more erratic patient. These relational developments and case-by-case allowances exist, at times, in tension with a therapist's convictions regarding the need for firm and consistent payment procedures.

Furthermore, while private psychotherapists' common practice of deferring payment for sessions until the end of the month or some other agreed-upon time interval is indexical—and, to a certain extent, constitutive—of a relationship of trust, this is not to say that therapists are immune to incidents in which such trust may be ruptured. One therapist that I interviewed recounted her experiences with a former agency client who was simply unable to make the transition to a private practice billing arrangement:

> She got so furious and felt like I was abandoning her, betraying her, because she'd agreed to pay that $25, but she just wasn't paying, and we were doing 12 sessions and she wasn't paying the money and it just didn't work. She finally left, you know, and she still owes me money and I'm not going to go after her or anything like that, but yeah.

7 This discourse can be traced back to Freud, who famously cautioned in his notes on beginning psychoanalytic treatment that "the value of the treatment is not enhanced in the patient's eyes if a very low fee is asked" (1958, 131). Freud explained that a financial sacrifice made on the part of the clinician would not be counterbalanced by a benefit accrued to the patient; on the contrary, he insisted:

> Free treatment enormously increases some of a neurotic's resistances—in young women, for instance, the temptation which is inherent in their transference-relation, and in young men, their opposition to an obligation to feel grateful, an opposition which arises from their father-complex and which presents one of the most troublesome hindrances to the acceptance of medical help. The absence of the regulating effect offered by the payment of a fee to the doctor makes itself very painfully felt; the whole relationship is removed from the real world, and the patient is deprived of a strong motive for endeavouring to bring the treatment to an end. (1958, 132)

Interestingly, in the same essay Freud states that "[a]n analyst does not dispute that money is to be regarded *in the first instance as a medium for self-preservation and for obtaining power*" (1958, 131, emphasis added). He argues, furthermore, that the clinician should model for patients a treatment of "money matters with the same matter-of-course frankness with which he wishes to educate them in things relating to sexual life," adding that "it seems to me more respectable and ethically less objectionable to acknowledge one's actual claims and needs rather than, as is still the practice among physicians, to act the part of the disinterested philanthropist" (131).

Later, psychologist Anthony Davids drew on Festinger's (1957) theory of cognitive dissonance to provide a non-Freudian theoretical rationale for the therapeutic effectiveness of relatively high fees for middle-class private practice patients:

In accord with dissonance theory, these individuals should be motivated to reduce the dissonance engendered by payment of the fee which can be accomplished either by getting out of the situation that causes the dissonance or by coming to view the therapeutic situation as one worth the money and one deserving of the individual's investment of thought, judgment, energy, and effort. In this latter happy state of affairs, the therapist charges his high fee which the patient pays unbegrudgingly, and the payment of the fee helps to generate the inner motivation that eventuates in therapeutic success. (Davids 1964, 331)

Occasional studies have pointed to a lack of empirical evidence supporting the therapeutic purpose of the fee (Pope et al. 1975). In spite of these findings, the rhetorical force of the discourse does not appear to have been diminished.

8　In the Illinois Department of Human Services, Division of Mental Health's "Title 59: Mental Health, Chapter IV: Department of Human Services, Part 132, Medicaid Community Mental Health Services Program" (colloquially referred to as "Rule 132"), Therapy/Counseling is further defined as "a treatment modality that uses interventions based on psychotherapy theory and techniques to promote emotional, cognitive, behavioral or psychological changes" (59 Ill. Adm. Code 132).

9　The anthropological record demonstrates that agency workers adopt many heterogeneous practices—some deliberate and strategic, others embodied and unarticulated—in order to enact "everyday ethics" (Brodwin 2013) and preserve professional integrity in the face of managed care constraints (Kirschner and Lachicotte 2001; Lester 2009). While in some instances these practices are oriented toward actively subverting managed care policies that therapists find unethical (Cohen et al. 2006; Ware et al. 2000), my example illustrates a different phenomenon in which therapists' ethical standards and consequent therapeutic practices are structured by—but ideologically decoupled from—managed care's economic constraints.

10　At the time of this research, under Rule 132 both Community Support Individual (CSI) and Therapy/Counseling services were reimbursed at the following rates:

$16.65 per ¼ hour when administered on site by a Mental Health Professional (MHP);

$18.02 per ¼ hour when administered on site by a Qualified Mental Health Professional (QMHP);

$19.31 per ¼ hour when administered at the client's home or off site by an MHP;

$20.90 per ¼ hour when administered at the client's home or off site by a QMHP.

While Rule 132 lists a variety of ways in which an individual can meet the designation of MHP or QMHP, at WBH and CRC an MHP nearly always referred to a bachelor's-level clinician providing services under the supervision of a QMHP (e.g., a student intern in the process of completing a master's degree in social work or counseling). A QMHP usually referred to a clinician possessing a master's degree in social work or counseling.

The only notable difference in reimbursement policies for CSI and Therapy/
Counseling found in Rule 132 is that while the lowest practice level permitted for Therapy/Counseling is MHP, CSI services may also be provided by a
Rehabilitative Services Associate (RSA), defined as a person at least 21 years of
age with a high school diploma or GED certificate and "demonstrated skills in
the field of services to adults or children" (59 Ill. Admin. Code 132 [§132.25 Defi-
nitions]). Neither WBH nor CRC employed RSAs to provide direct services to
clients. However, this difference can be seen as indicative of the lower thresh-
olds of education and training viewed by the state as appropriate to the needs
of agency clients.

11 Lest we imagine that patients at private practices are socialized into a utopian
paradigm that replaces the notion of the isolated, autonomous individual with a
model of community and interdependence, Tolleson (2009) warns us that
"[d]oing psychotherapy, with its contemporary democratizing thrust (i.e., empathy, mutuality, anti-authoritarianism) provides possibilities for clinicians to
fashion a social utopia in the privacies of their work . . . in lieu of social action on
the streets . . . Like a mother who comforts her child after he has endured a beat-
ing by his father, we help our patients feel better but stop short of confrontation
with the system" (192).

CHAPTER 5. "IF YOU CLOSE MY CLINIC, I WILL DIE"

1 The four were Auburn/Greshem, Back of the Yards, Woodlawn, and Morgan Park.

2 My characterization of the key actors in this chapter as "disenfranchised individuals who are forced to self-manage in quite a literal sense" is both analytically
useful and overly homogenizing. As the ethnographic material presented in the
forthcoming pages will reveal, the practices and lived experiences of my mental
health consumer activist informants are better apprehended through an appreciation of the fractures within and across this population than by any unified
descriptions.

3 See chapter 1 for further details.

4 In conversations and in speeches at public events, MHC members recounted
various versions of the legend of their victory against Mayor Daley in 2009. One
consumer leader maintained that

The Mental Health Coalition was smart enough to sit in in [Daley's] office.
And he didn't know we were there, so when a reporter said to him "what
are you gonna do about the closing mental health clinics?" he said "Oh! I'm
gonna keep them open! I'll take care of it!" He didn't tell his staff! So mean-
while *we* were in his office and the staff said, "there is nothing we can do."
And then it was announced that Daley had said the clinics will stay open!

Other narratives held that the mayor knew about the MHC sit-in and had
granted the reprieve for public relations reasons, as the sit-in had been timed
to coincide with a meeting between the mayor and a representative from the

International Olympic Committee who was in town to review Daley's proposal for hosting the 2016 games.

5 The MHC's action was undoubted influenced by the zeitgeist of the Occupy Wall Street (OWS) protest movement that began in New York City's financial district in September 2011 and quickly expanded to become a wide-reaching critique of the income and wealth inequality characteristic of late capitalism in the United States. Indeed, the OWS slogan highlighting the disparity between the wealthiest 1% of the country and the rest of the population—"We are the 99%"—inspired a nickname for Chicago's Mayor Rahm Emanuel: "Mayor 1%" (Lydersen 2013).

6 Members of the Mental Health Coalition did not typically advance arguments linking mental illness to violent behavior, and in fact often worked to dispel this form of stigma and misinformation. As recently as June 2022, in the wake of a cluster of shootings across the United States, several MHC members circulated articles via email entitled "The Dangers of Linking Gun Violence and Mental Illness" (Ranney and Gold 2019) and "Mental illness and reduction of gun violence and suicide: bringing epidemiologic research to policy" (Swanson et al. 2015). We might read Jones's comments to the police officer, therefore, as further demonstrating the degree to which Mental Health Coalition members felt compelled to rehearse stereotypes about the social categories to which they belonged in order to receive public recognition.

7 These are all pseudonyms.

8 As the next section will demonstrate, emotion rules and race-based stereotypes about affective comportment also seemed to play a significant role in shaping the MHC's relationship with peer consumer activists of only marginally higher social status.

9 Fioretti's statement of regret, as well as those of other public servants made at the time of the City Hall hearing, did not lead to real policy change and instead may have been made as political maneuvers that had little to do with the Mental Health Coalition's concerns. In fact, after attempting unsuccessfully to unseat his longtime rival Rahm Emanuel in the 2015 mayoral election, Bob Fioretti stunned Chicago's mental health consumers by endorsing Emanuel in the runoff election that year between Emanuel and the more progressive Jesus "Chuy" Garcia. Fioretti's backing of Emanuel inspired the Mental Health Coalition to stage an action to "Buy Back Bob," in which consumers crashed a private lunch between the two former enemies to deliver "Funds for Fioretti's Friendship" to their supposed ally. Referencing Fioretti's apology at the press conference before the City Hall hearing, a video of the "Buy Back Bob" action shared on YouTube explains that consumers felt betrayed by Fioretti given that he had been one of the few aldermen to express regret about voting for Mayor Emanuel's budget that closed half of Chicago's mental health clinics. Shaking a jar of loose change, Mental Health Coalition members carrying signs reading "NEED $ TO BUY BACK BOB" entered the restaurant where Fioretti and Emanuel were dining, and addressed the other diners: "Fioretti

needs money! He is with Rahm Emanuel now. His vote is *clearly for sale!*" They were soon forced to leave the restaurant.

Although Fioretti and others did not deliver on the repentant vows they issued at the time of the hearing—and even though the hearing itself was marked by disappointment and frustration for public mental health clinic consumers—it would be a mistake to underestimate the positive outcomes that resulted from these events from the perspective of the MHC's visibility and public opinion about the group. These positive outcomes both helped to sustain the Mental Health Coalition's momentum in the short term and served as stepping stones toward the partial victories that the MHC would eventually win in the years that followed (e.g., Mayor Lightfoot's sevenfold increase in funding for mental health services from $12 million in 2019 to $89 million in 2022 [City of Chicago Office of the Mayor]). At the time of the completion of this book, although a good number of Chicago city clinic consumer activists had shifted their political goals away from the reopening of the original public clinics and toward the growth of community-funded expanded mental health services programs, some MHC members were celebrating a plan announced by Chicago Mayor Brandon Johnson to reopen and expand several shuttered public mental health clinics by the end of 2024 (City of Chicago Office of the Mayor 2024).

10 Sociologist Patricia Hill Collins (2010) rightly notes that "the construct of community is versatile, malleable, and easy to use" yet simultaneously "unexamined, taken-for-granted, and difficult to define," holding "varied and often contradictory meanings that reflect diverse and conflicting social practices" (11). These attributes of the construct, Collins argues, make it "a promising candidate for examining the changing-same nature of social inequalities, and the intersecting power relations that animate them, especially within the United States" (10).

11 Drawing on the rationale that free market competition ensured a better quality of services, the CDPH insisted, from the early 2000s onward and especially beginning in 2011, that private agencies were better equipped to fund mental health services than the city was, and that the city could not afford to entice clinicians—particularly psychiatrists, of which there was a national shortage—with market-rate salaries.

12 Much has changed in the intervening years between the time when this research was conducted and the time of the book's completion. In November 2016, more than 86% of voters in Chicago's West Side community (including the neighborhoods of North Lawndale, East and West Garfield Park, and the Near West Side) approved a property tax increase to fund their own Expanded Mental Health Services Program (EMHSP), the Encompassing Center, which opened in October 2019. Residents of Logan Square and surrounding communities in Northwest Chicago followed suit in 2018, followed by Bronzeville in 2020 and West Town Humboldt Park and mid-South Side Chicago in 2022. Of the over 25,000 votes on ballots within Chicago's 4th, 5th, 6th, 7th, 8th, and 20th wards—encompassing the neighborhoods of Kenwood, Hyde Park, Woodlawn, and South Shore—93.54% were in support of establishing an EMHSP and 88.14% supported a property tax increase

of 0.025% to fund the new center (Pharo 2022; Coalition to Save Our Mental Health Centers n.d.). Inasmuch as I can discern, the umbrella organization under which the MHC still exists continues to fight for (among other causes) the reopening of the original mental health centers, to be operated by the Chicago Department of Public Health. At the same time, today the division between those whose sights are set on reopening Chicago's original public clinics and those who favor community-based, privately funded expanded mental health services programs does not fall neatly along racial, geographic, or socioeconomic lines anymore.

13 In their discussion of the ways in which ideologies construct difference, linguistic anthropologists Gal and Irvine describe a process of *recursiveness* that "involves the projection of an opposition, salient at some level of relationship, onto some other level . . . Reminiscent of fractals in geometry . . . , the myriad oppositions that can create identity may be reproduced repeatedly, either within each side of a dichotomy or outside it" (1995, 974). In the case of the MHC and North Side clinic consumers, the race- and class-based dichotomy dividing "Chicago public mental health clinic consumers" from other groups of psychiatric service users is reproduced internally so as to create two opposing groups of city clinic consumers.

14 I am indebted to Pinky Hota for pointing me to Muehlmann's analysis.

CHAPTER 6. USE OF THE SELF

1 While sovereignty, autonomy, and self-determination are, throughout this book, subject to critique as ideological formations that obscure political economy and are at times ascribed to marginalized individuals as a means to rationalize their social exclusion, I recognize that there are communities for whom these constructs hold different, deeply significant and positive meanings. For example, in the field of anthropology, recent scholarship has raised concerns that collaborative or community-oriented archeological research with Indigenous groups, "despite its good intentions, has the potential to do harm to Indigenous rights and self-determination" (Supernant and Warrick 2014, 563). Such work has sparked important dialogue across the discipline about knowledge production and "data sovereignty" (Gupta et al. 2023; Kukutai and Taylor 2016), leading to calls for "co-production scholars [to] move away from seeking to better 'integrate' Indigenous knowledges into western science and make way for Indigenous research leadership" (Latulippe and Klenk 2020, 7). Indeed, Supernant and Warrick (2014) even go as far as to advise their colleagues: "For archaeologists who are intent on de-colonizing archaeology in solidarity with Indigenous peoples, there may be situations where archaeologists should refrain from doing archaeology" (563). I take seriously these critical interventions and their potential implications for ethnographic research such as my own that tends to valorize distributed, co-produced, or "cybernetic" modes of being and knowing. Methodologically, I have endeavored to ensure that my informants are comfortable with and supportive of the manner in which the research in this book was carried out. Where possible and appropriate, I have also tried to refrain from including data or knowledge that an

informant would consider to be, in the above sense, "sovereign" and not my place
to share. Thematically, I have aimed to represent the full range of existential and
structural binds, social inequities, *and* positive affordances of self-management
(which I take as intimately linked to notions of sovereignty, self-determination,
etc.) experienced and described by my informants, including the eventual embrace by some MHC consumers of "self-determination" in the form of private,
neighborhood-funded Expanded Mental Health Services Programs.

2 Of course, it was noted in our class, there could be rare exceptions. As psychoanalyst Nancy McWilliams (2004) writes in a chapter on boundaries and the frame
that we were assigned to read at the time:

> Once the frame is clear to both parties, the security of the therapeutic couple
> depends on observing a mutually understood set of boundaries consistently.
> But, somewhat paradoxically, it is also true that the most moving and healing
> moments in treatment are often the times when the therapist does some-
> thing exceptional, stepping out of the frame and responding to the patient
> with a spontaneous gesture . . . When patients and ex-patients are asked
> about the most pivotal incidents in their treatments, they tend to talk about
> moments when their therapist surprised them, often by deviating from the
> frame. (103)

McWilliams goes on to emphasize that "[f]or such moments to have any power,
they must be genuinely spontaneous, and they must be the exceptions to an
established pattern" (104).

3 I am reminded of existential psychiatrist Irvin Yalom's reflections on the possibility that many of the "off the record" "throw-ins" (as he terms them) that therapists
perform without theorization may in fact constitute crucial components of the
therapeutic process. Writing on Freud's account of his successful treatment of
Fraulein Elisabeth von R, Yalom observes:

> Freud explained his therapeutic success solely by his technique of abreaction,
> of de-repressing certain noxious wishes and thoughts. However, in studying
> Freud's notes, one is struck by the vast number of his other therapeutic activ-
> ities. For example, he sent Elisabeth to visit her sister's grave and to pay a call
> upon a young man whom she found attractive. He demonstrated a "friendly
> interest in her present circumstances" by interacting with the family in the
> patient's behalf . . . He helped untangle the family financial tangle. . . . Finally,
> after the termination of therapy, Freud, hearing that Elisabeth was going to
> a private dance, procured an invitation so he could watch her "whirl past in
> a lively dance." One cannot help but wonder what really helped Fraulein von
> R. Freud's extras, I have no doubt, constituted powerful interventions; to
> exclude them from theory is to court error. (1980, 4)

CONCLUSION

1 I am indebted to Paul Brodwin for this succinct summary of my critiques of
self-management.

REFERENCES

59 Illinois Administrative Code 132. 2007. Illinois Department of Human Services.

Agamben, Giorgio. 1998. *Homo Sacer: Sovereign Power and Bare Life*. Stanford University Press.

Agha, Asif. 2007. *Language and Social Relations: Studies in the Social and Cultural Foundations of Language no. 24*. Cambridge University Press.

Ahearn, Laura M. 2001. "Language and Agency." *Annual Review of Anthropology* 30:109–137.

Altman, Neil. 2013. "Psychoanalysis In and Out of the Office." *Psychoanalysis, Culture, & Society* 18 (2):128–139.

Altman, Neil. 2020. *White Privilege: Psychoanalytic Perspectives*. Routledge.

American Psychiatric Association: DSM-5 Task Force. 2013. *Diagnostic and Statistical Manual of Mental Disorders: DSM-5*. 5th ed. American Psychiatric Association.

Angell, M. 1993. "The Doctor as Double Agent." *Kennedy Institute of Ethics Journal* 3 (3):279–286.

Ansell, David A. 2011. *County: Life, Death, and Politics at Chicago's Public Hospital*. Academy Chicago Publishers.

Appadurai, Arjun. 1988. *The Social Life of Things: Commodities in Cultural Perspective*. 1st ed. Cambridge University Press.

Aron, Lewis. 2003. "The Paradoxical Place of Enactment in Psychoanalysis." *Psychoanalytic Dialogues* 13 (5):623–631.

Auestad, Lene, ed. 2012. *Psychoanalysis and Politics: Exclusion and the Politics of Representation*. Routledge.

Augustine, and Albert Cook Outler. 1955. *Confessions and Enchiridion, The Library of Christian Classics*. Westminster Press.

Baim, Adam. 2022. "Eyes in Sight: Embodiment, Affect, and Learning to See in Ophthalmology." *Medicine Anthropology Theory* 9 (1):1–25.

Bakhtin, M. M. 1981. *The Dialogic Imagination: Four Essays*. University of Texas Press.

Baldwin, M., ed. 2013. *The Use of Self in Therapy*. 3rd ed. Routledge.

Bandura, A. 1989. "Human Agency in Social Cognitive Theory." *American Psychologist* 44 (9):1175–1184.

Basco, Monica Ramirez. 2006. *The Bipolar Workbook: Tools for Controlling Your Mood Swings*. Guilford Press.

Bateson, Gregory. 1972. *Steps to an Ecology of Mind: Collected Essays in Anthropology, Psychiatry, Evolution, and Epistemology*. Jason Aronson Inc.

Belluck, Pam, and Benedict Carey. 2013. "Psychiatry's Guide Is Out of Touch with Science, Experts Say." *New York Times Online*, (May 6. Accessed March 1, 2017. www .nytimes.com.

Benabarre, A., E. Vieta, F. Colom, A. Martínez-Arán, M. Reinares, and C. Gastó. 2001. "Bipolar Disorder, Schizoaffective Disorder and Schizophrenia: Epidemiologic, Clinical and Prognostic Differences." *European Psychiatry* 16 (3):167–172.

Bender, Suzanne, and Edward Messner. 2003. *Becoming a Therapist: What Do I Say, and Why?* Guilford Press.

Bennett, Joe. 2014. "Avoiding Emotivism: A Sociolinguistic Approach to Moral Talk." *Language & Communication* 39:73–82.

Benveniste, Emile. 1971. *Problems in General Linguistics*. University of Miami Press.

Berzoff, Joan, ed. 2012. *Falling Through the Cracks: Psychodynamic Practice with Vulnerable and Oppressed Populations*. Columbia University Press.

Bettelheim, Eric C. 2022. "Acting Out and Enactment: An Effort at Clarity." *Neuropsychoanalysis* 24 (1):71–85.

Biehl, João Guilherme. 2005. *Vita: Life in a Zone of Social Abandonment*. University of California Press.

Biehl, João Guilherme. 2012. "Care and Disregard." In *A Companion to Moral Anthropology*, edited by D. Fassin, 242–263. Wiley.

Binkley, Sam. 2014. *Happiness as Enterprise: An Essay on Neoliberal Life*. State University of New York Press.

Bion, W. R. 2013 [1959]. "Attacks on Linking." *Psychoanalytic Quarterly* 82 (2):285–300.

Blacksher, Erika. 2002. "On Being Poor and Feeling Poor: Low Socioeconomic Status and the Moral Self." *Theoretical Medicine and Bioethics* 23 (6):455–470.

Bleger, Jose. 1967. "Psycho-analysis of the Psycho-analytic Frame." *International Journal of Psychoanalysis* 48 (4):511–519.

Bobby, Carol, and Robert Urofsky. 2011. "Counseling Students Deserve a Strong Professional Identity." *Counseling Today* 53 (11):52.

Bodenheimer, T., K. Lorig, H. Holman, and K. Grumbach. 2002. "Patient Self-Management of Chronic Disease in Primary Care." *JAMA* 288 (19):2469–2475.

Bogira, S. 2009. "Starvation Diet: Coping with Shrinking Budgets in Publicly Funded Mental Health Services." *Health Affairs* 28 (3):667–675.

Bohleber, W., P. Fonagy, J. P. Jiménez, D. Scarfone, S. Varvin, and S. Zysman. 2013. "Towards a Better Use of Psychoanalytic Concepts: A Model Illustrated Using the Concept of Enactment." *International Journal of Psychoanalysis* 94 (3):501–530.

Bondi, Liz. 2005. "Working the Spaces of Neoliberal Subjectivity: Psychotherapeutic Technologies, Professionalisation and Counselling." *Antipode* 37 (3):497–514.

Borenzweig, Herman. 1981. "Agency vs. Private Practice: Similarities and Differences." *Social Work* 26 (3):239–244.

Borovoy, Amy, and Janet Hine. 2008. "Managing the Unmanageable: Elderly Russian Jewish Émigrés and the Biomedical Culture of Diabetes Care." *Medical Anthropology Quarterly* 22 (1):1–26.

Bourdieu, Pierre. 1977. *Outline of a Theory of Practice*. Cambridge University Press.

Bourdieu, Pierre. 1984. *Distinction: A Social Critique of the Judgment of Taste*. Routledge & Kegan Paul.

Bourdieu, Pierre. 1989. "Social Space and Symbolic Power." *Sociological Theory* 7 (1):14–25.

Bowlby, John. 1979. *The Making and Breaking of Affectional Bonds*. Routledge.

Bowlby, John. 1988. *A Secure Base: Parent-Child Attachment and Healthy Human Development*. Basic Books.

Bradley, James. 2021. "The University of Chicago, Urban Renewal, and the Black Community." *Black Perspectives*, April 12. Accessed June 20, 2024. www.aaihs.org.

Brennan, Teresa. 2004. *The Transmission of Affect*. Cornell University Press.

Brenner, Neil, Jamie Peck, and N.I.K. Theodore. 2010. "Variegated Neoliberalization: Geographies, Modalities, Pathways." *Global Networks* 10 (2):182–222.

Brickman, Celia. 2018. *Race in Psychoanalysis: Aboriginal Populations in the Mind*. Routledge.

Briggs, Jean L. 2008. "Daughter and Pawn: One Ethnographer's Routes to Understanding Children." *Ethos* 36 (4):449–456.

Brijnath, Bianca, and Josefine Antoniades. 2016. "'I'm Running My Depression': Self-Management of Depression in Neoliberal Australia." *Social Science & Medicine* 152:1–8.

Britt, Sonya L., Brad Klontz, Racquel Tibbetts, and Linda Leitz. 2015. "The Financial Health of Mental Health Professionals." *Journal of Financial Therapy* 6 (1):17–32.

Brodwin, Paul. 2008. "The Coproduction of Moral Discourse in U.S. Community Psychiatry." *Medical Anthropology Quarterly* 22 (2):127–147.

Brodwin, Paul. 2010. "The Assemblage of Compliance in Psychiatric Case Management." *Anthropology & Medicine* 17 (2):129–143.

Brodwin, Paul. 2011. "Futility in the Practice of Community Psychiatry." *Medical Anthropology Quarterly* 25 (2):189–208.

Brodwin, Paul. 2013. *Everyday Ethics: Voices from the Front Line of Community Psychiatry*. University of California Press.

Buch, Elana D. 2013. "Senses of Care: Embodying Inequality and Sustaining Personhood in the Home Care of Older Adults in Chicago." *American Ethnologist* 40 (4):637–650.

Buchman, D. Z., E. L. Borgelt, L. Whiteley, and J. Illes. 2013. "Neurobiological Narratives: Experiences of Mood Disorder through the Lens of Neuroimaging." *Sociology of Health and Illness* 35 (1):66–81.

Butler, Judith. 2001. "Giving an Account of Oneself." *Diacritics* 31 (4):22.

Butler, Judith. 2005. *Giving an Account of Oneself*. 1st ed. Fordham University Press.

Byrne, John. 2023. "An Important Early Test for Mayor Brandon Johnson: Reopening the City's Mental Health Clinics." *Chicago Tribune*, June 7. www.chicagotribune.com.

Byrnes, Dave. 2023. "Seventh Circuit Upholds Chicago's 75-Year Parking Privatization Deal." *Courthouse News Service*, April 7. Accessed June 24, 2024. www.courthousenews.com.

Cain, Carole. 1991. "Personal Stories: Identity Acquisition and Self-Understanding in Alcoholics Anonymous." *Ethos* 19 (2):210–253.

Calabrese, Joseph D. 2013. *A Different Medicine: Postcolonial Healing in the Native American Church.* Oxford University Press.

Callard, Felicity, Diana Rose, Emma-Louise Hanif, Jody Quigley, Kathryn Greenwood, and Til Wykes. 2012. "Holding Blame at Bay? 'Gene Talk' in Family Members' Accounts of Schizophrenia Aetiology." *BioSocieties* 7 (3):273–293.

Carpenter-Song, E. 2009. "Caught in the Psychiatric Net: Meanings and Experiences of ADHD, Pediatric Bipolar Disorder and Mental Health Treatment among a Diverse Group of Families in the United States." *Culture, Medicine, and Psychiatry* 33 (1):61–85.

Carr, Danielle. 2021. "Scientology's Lonely Turf War: How the Left Learned to Love Psychiatry." *Pioneer Works*, April 20. Accessed January 11, 2024. https://pioneerworks.org.

Carr, E. Summerson. 2010. "Enactments of Expertise." *Annual Review of Anthropology* 39:17–32.

Carr, E. Summerson. 2011. *Scripting Addiction: The Politics of Therapeutic Talk and American Sobriety.* Princeton University Press.

Carr, E. Summerson. 2013. "Signs of Sobriety: Rescripting American Addiction Counseling." In *Addiction Trajectories*, edited by E. Raikhel and W. Garriott, 160–187. Duke University Press.

Carr, E. Summerson. 2015. "Occupation Bedbugs: Or, the Urgency and Agency of Professional Pragmatism." *Cultural Anthropology* 30 (2):257–285.

Carr, E. Summerson, and Michael Lempert. 2016. *Scale: Discourse and Dimensions of Social Life.* University of California Press.

Casement, Patrick J. 1991. *Learning from the Patient.* Guilford Press.

Cattelino, Jessica R. 2010. "Anthropologies of the United States." *Annual Review of Anthropology* 39 (1):275–292.

Centers for Medicare and Medicaid Services. 2017. "Medicaid.gov: Eligibility." Accessed February 3, 2017. www.medicaid.gov.

Chamberlin, J. 1984. "Speaking for Ourselves: An Overview of the Ex-Psychiatric Inmates' Movement." *Psychosocial Rehabilitation Journal* 8 (2):56–63.

Chapman, R., and H. Carel. 2022. "Neurodiversity, Epistemic Injustice, and the Good Human Life." *Journal of Social Philosophy* 53:614–631.

Chicago Department of Public Health. 2014. "Ensuring Access to Mental Health Services for All Chicagoans," August 19. Accessed July 29, 2024. www.chicago.gov. PowerPoint slides.

Choudhury, Suparna, Saskia Kathi Nagel, and Jan Slaby. 2009. "Critical Neuroscience: Linking Neuroscience and Society through Critical Practice." *BioSocieties* 4 (1):61–77.

City of Chicago. 2012. "Chicago Department of Public Health Mental Health Reforms Continue to Expand Access to Care Funding Awarded to Increase Psychiatry Services for Over 1,000 People Across Chicago." Accessed May 1, 2017. www.cityofchicago.org.

City of Chicago Office of the Mayor. 2022. "Mayor Lightfoot and the Chicago Department of Public Health Announce Expansion of Citywide Mental Health Network," June 13. Accessed February 10, 2024. www.chicago.gov.

City of Chicago Office of the Mayor. 2024. "Mayor Johnson Announces Plans to Reopen Shuttered Roseland Mental Health Clinic on Far South Side, Expand Mental Health Services Across the City," , May 30. Accessed June 24, 2024. www.chicago.gov.

Clarke, John. 2005. "New Labour's Citizens: Activated, Empowered, Responsibilized, Abandoned?" *Critical Social Policy* 25 (4):447–463.

Clarke, J., J. Newman, and L. Westmarland. 2007. "Creating Citizen-Consumers? Public Service Reform and (Un)willing Selves." In *On Willing Selves: Neoliberal Politics vis-à-vis the Neuroscientific Challenge*, edited by Sabine Maasen and Barbara Sutter, 125–145. Palgrave Macmillan.

Clarke, Laura Hurd, and Erica V. Bennett. 2013. "Constructing the Moral Body: Self-Care Among Older Adults with Multiple Chronic Conditions." *Health* 17 (3):211–228.

Clay, Rebecca A. 2007. "Keeping Track: New Professionals Need to Know How to Keep, Safeguard and Destroy Records." Accessed March 1, 2017. www.apa.org.

Coalition to Save Our Mental Health Centers. 2017a. "About the Coalition." Accessed May 1, 2017. http://saveourmentalhealth.org.

Coalition to Save Our Mental Health Centers. 2017b. "Expanded Mental Health Services Programs." Accessed May 1, 2017. http://saveourmentalhealth.org.

Coalition to Save Our Mental Health Centers. n.d. "Current Expanded Mental Health Services Programs (EMHSPs)." Accessed June 21, 2024. www.saveourmentalhealth.org.

Cohen, Julie, Jeanne Marecek, and Jane Gillham. 2006. "Is Three a Crowd? Clients, Clinicians, and Managed Care." *American Journal of Orthopsychiatry* 76 (2):251–259.

Cole, Jennifer. 2014. "Working Mis/understandings: The Tangled Relationship between Kinship, Franco-Malagasy Binational Marriages, and the French State." *Cultural Anthropology* 29 (3):527–551.

Coleman, G. 2008. "The Politics of Rationality: Psychiatric Survivor's Challenge to Psychiatry." In *Tactical Biopolitics*, edited by K. Phillip and B. de Costa, 341–363. MIT Press.

Collins, Patricia Hill. 2010. "The New Politics of Community." *American Sociological Review* 75 (1):7–30.

Collins, Patricia Hill. 1998. "The Tie That Binds: Race, Gender, and US Violence." *Ethnic and Racial Studies* 21 (5):917–938.

"Community Psychiatry and Social Work Introduction Statement." 1966. *Social Service Review* 40 (3):245–245.

Congress.gov. 2017. "H.R.1275—World's Greatest Healthcare Plan of 2017." Accessed May 1, 2017. www.congress.gov.

Cook, Joanna. 2016. "Mindful in Westminster: The Politics of Meditation and the Limits of Neoliberal Critique." *HAU: Journal of Ethnographic Theory* 6 (1):141–161.

Cooper, Amy. 2015. "Time Seizures and the Self: Institutional Temporalities and Self Preservation among Homeless Women." *Culture, Medicine, and Psychiatry* 39 (1):162–185.

Crawshaw, P. 2012. "Governing at a Distance: Social Marketing and the (Bio)politics of Responsibility." *Social Science and Medicine* 75 (1):200–207.

Creer, Thomas L., and Walter P. Christian. 1976. *Chronically Ill and Handicapped Children, Their Management and Rehabilitation*. Research Press.

Dardick, Hal. 2014. "Council to Hold Hearing on Closing of City Mental Health Clinics." *Chicago Tribune*, August 19. Accessed May 1, 2017. www.chicagotribune.com.

Davids, A. 1964. "The Relation of Cognitive-Dissonance Theory to an Aspect of Psychotherapeutic Practice." *American Psychologist* 19 (5):329–332.

Davis, Elizabeth Ann. 2012. *Bad Souls: Madness and Responsibility in Modern Greece*. Duke University Press.

DBSA. 2017a. "Depression." Accessed April 10, 2017. www.dbsalliance.org.

DBSA. 2017b. "Bipolar Disorder." Accessed April 2, 2017. www.dbsalliance.org.

DBSA. 2017c. "Bipolar Disorder Statistics." Accessed January 3, 2017. www.dbsalliance.org.

Dean, M. 1999. "Risk, Calculable and Incalculable." In *Risk and Sociocultural Theory: New Directions and Perspectives*, edited by D. Lupton, 131–159. Cambridge University Press.

Dean, Ruth G. 2000. "Making the Personal Professional and the Professional Personal." In *Odysseys in Psychotherapy*, edited by J. Shay Joseph and Joan Wheelis, 67–95. Ardent Media Inc.

Depp, Colin, John Stricker, David Zagorsky, Lisa Goodale, Lisa Eyler, Thomas Patterson, Barry Lebowitz, and Dilip Jeste. 2009. "Disability and Self-Management Practices of People with Bipolar Disorder: A Web-Based Survey." *Community Mental Health Journal* 45 (3):179–187.

Derrida, Jacques. 1992. *Given Time. I. Counterfeit Money*. Translated by Peggy Kamuf. University of Chicago Press.

Desjarlais, Robert. 1994. "Struggling Along: The Possibilities for Experience Among the Homeless Mentally Ill." *American Anthropologist* 96 (4):886–901.

Desjarlais, Robert. 1997. *Shelter Blues: Sanity and Selfhood Among the Homeless*. University of Pennsylvania Press.

Devlin, Ann Sloan, and Jack L. Nasar. 2012. "Impressions of Psychotherapists' Offices: Do Therapists and Clients Agree?" *Professional Psychology: Research and Practice* 43 (2):118–122.

Dewane, Claudia J. 2006. "Use of Self: A Primer Revisited." *Clinical Social Work Journal* 34 (4):543–558.

Donald, A. 2001. "The Wal-Marting of American Psychiatry: An Ethnography of Psychiatric Practice in the Late 20th Century." *Culture, Medicine, and Psychiatry* 25 (4):427–439.

Drake, St. Clair, and Horace R. Cayton, Jr. 1945. *Black Metropolis: A Study of Negro Life in a Northern City*. Harcourt, Brace and Company.

Dumit, Joseph. 2003. "Is It Me or My Brain? Depression and Neuroscientific Facts." *Journal of Medical Humanities* 24 (1):35–47.

Duncombe, Stephen. 2016. "Affect and Effect: Artful Protest and Political Impact." In *The Democratic Public Sphere: Current Challenges and Prospects*, edited by Christina Fiig, Jørn Loftager, Henrik Kaare Nielsen, Thomas Olesen, Jan Løhmann Stephensen, and Mads P. Sørensen, 433–452. Arhaus University Press.

Eberstadt, Nick. 2012. *A Nation of Takers: America's Entitlement Epidemic*. West Templeton Press.

Edwards, Jana K., and Jennifer M. Bess. 1998. "Developing Effectiveness in the Therapeutic Use of Self." *Clinical Social Work Journal* 26 (1):89–105.

Ehrenreich, John H. 1985. *The Altruistic Imagination: A History of Social Work and Social Policy in the United States*. Cornell University Press.

Ehrenreich, Barbara. 2009. *Bright-Sided: How the Relentless Promotion of Positive Thinking Has Undermined America*. Henry Holt and Company.

Epstein, Steven. 1996. *Impure Science: AIDS, Activism, and the Politics of Knowledge*. University of California Press.

Estroff, Sue E. 1989. "Self, Identity, and Subjective Experiences of Schizophrenia: In Search of the Subject." *Schizophrenia Bulletin* 15 (2):189–196.

Evans, Louwanda, and Wendy Leo Moore. 2015. "Impossible Burdens: White Institutions, Emotional Labor, and Micro-Resistance." *Social Problems* 62:439–454.

Ewing, Katherine P. 1990. "The Illusion of Wholeness: Culture, Self, and the Experience of Inconsistency." *Ethos* 18 (3):251–278.

Fassin, Didier. 2005. "Compassion and Repression: The Moral Economy of Immigration Policies in France." *Cultural Anthropology* 20 (3):362–387.

Fassin, Didier. 2009. "Les Économies Morales Revisitées." *Annales. Histoire, Sciences Sociales* 64 (6):1237–1266.

Festinger, Leon. 1957. *A Theory of Cognitive Dissonance*. Stanford University Press.

Fodor, Iris E. 2001. "Making Meaning of Therapy: A Personal Narrative of Change Over 4 Decades." In *How Therapists Change: Personal and Professional Reflections*, edited by Marvin R. Goldfried, 123–146. American Psychological Association.

Foley, Henry A. 1975. *Community Mental Health Legislation: The Formative Process*. Lexington Books.

Fortino, Ellyn. 2014. "Chicago Activists, Progressive Aldermen Call for the Reopening of Mental Health Clinics." Accessed May 1, 2017. http://progressillinois.com.

Foucault, Michel. 1967. *Madness and Civilization: A History of Insanity in the Age of Reason*. Tavistock Publications.

Foucault, Michel. 1973. *The Birth of the Clinic: An Archaeology of Medical Perception*. 1st American ed., *World of Man*. Pantheon Books.

Foucault, Michel. 1977. *Discipline and Punish: The Birth of the Prison*. 1st American ed. Pantheon Books.

Foucault, Michel. 1978. *The History of Sexuality*. 1st American ed. Pantheon Books.

Foucault, Michel. 1984 [1967]. "Of Other Spaces: Utopias and Heterotopias." *Architecture/Mouvement/Continuité* October.

Foucault, Michel, Luther H. Martin, Huck Gutman, and Patrick H. Hutton. 1988. *Technologies of the Self: A Seminar with Michel Foucault*. University of Massachusetts Press.

Frank, Kenneth A. 2014. "Out from Hiding." In *Clinical Implications of the Psychoanalyst's Life Experience: When the Personal Becomes Professional*, edited by Steven Kuchuck, 65–80. Routledge.

Freedberg, Sharon. 2007. "Re-examining Empathy: A Relational-Feminist Point of View." *Social Work* 52 (3):251–259.

Freire, P. 1970. *Pedagogy of the Oppressed*. Seabury Press.

Freud, Sigmund. 1927. *The Ego and the Id, International Psycho-analytical Library No. 12*. L. & Virginia Woolf at the Hogarth Press, and the Institute of Psycho-analysis.

Freud, Sigmund. 1930. *Civilization and Its Discontents*. J. Cape & H. Smith.

Freud, Sigmund. 1958. "On Beginning the Treatment (Further Recommendations on the Technique of Psycho-analysis I)." In *The Standard Edition of the Complete Psychological Works of Sigmund Freud*, 123–144. The Hogarth Press and the Institute of Psycho-Analysis.

Fricker, Miranda. 2007. *Epistemic Injustice: Power and the Ethics of Knowing*. Oxford University Press.

Frost, Peter. 2014. "Medicaid Applications Keep Piling Up in Illinois." *Chicago Tribune*, June 15. Accessed March 1, 2017. http://articles.chicagotribune.com.

Fryers, T., T. Brugha, Z. Morgan, J. Smith, T. Hill, M. Carta, V. Lehtinen, and V. Kovess. 2004. "Prevalence of Psychiatric Disorder in Europe: The Potential and Reality of Meta Analysis." *Social Psychiatry and Psychiatric Epidemiology* 39 (11):899–905.

Fullagar, S. 2009. "Negotiating the Neurochemical Self: Anti-Depressant Consumption in Women's Recovery from Depression." *Health (London)* 13 (4):389–406.

Funahashi, D. 2021. *Untimely Sacrifices: Death and Work in Finland*. Cornell University Press.

Gal, Susan. 2016. "Sociolinguistic Differentiation." In *Sociolinguistics: Theoretical Debates*, edited by N. Coupland, 113–136. Cambridge University Press.

Gal, Susan, and Judith T. Irvine. 1995. "The Boundaries of Languages and Disciplines: How Ideologies Construct Difference." *Social Research* 62 (4):967–1001.

Geertz, Clifford. 1973. *The Interpretation of Cultures: Selected Essays*. Basic Books.

Gelso, C. J. 2011. *The Real Relationship in Psychotherapy: The Hidden Foundation of Change*. American Psychological Association.

Gelso, C. J., D. M. Kivlighan, Jr., J. Busa-Knepp, E. B. Spiegel, S. Ain, A. M. Hummel, Y. E. Ma, and R. D. Markin. 2012. "The Unfolding of the Real Relationship and the Outcome of Brief Psychotherapy." *Journal of Counseling Psychology* 59 (4):495–506.

Gerald, Mark. 2014. "In the Shadow of Freud's Couch." Accessed April 2, 2017. www.markgeraldphoto.com.

Gergen, Kenneth J. 2009. *Relational Being: Beyond Self and Community*. Oxford University Press.

Gergen, Kenneth J. 2010. "The Acculturated Brain." *Theory & Psychology* 20 (6):795–816.

Gershon, Ilana. 2011. "Neoliberal Agency." *Current Anthropology* 52 (4):537–555.

Ginsburg, Faye. 2006. "Ethnography and American Studies." *Cultural Anthropology* 21 (3):487–495.

Goffman, Erving. 1961. *Asylums: Essays on the Social Situation of Mental Patients and Other Inmates*. Anchor Books.

Good, Byron J. 2012. "Theorizing the 'Subject' of Medical and Psychiatric Anthropology." *Journal of the Royal Anthropological Institute* 18 (3):515–535.

Good, B. J., H. Herrera, M. J. Good, and J. Cooper. 1982. "Reflexivity and Countertransference in a Psychiatric Cultural Consultation Clinic." *Culture, Medicine, and Psychiatry* 6 (3):281–303.

Gostin, Lawrence O. 2000. "Managed Care, Conflicts of Interest, and Quality." *Hastings Center Report* 30 (5):27–28.

Grand, S. 2014. "Skin Memories: On Race, Love and Loss." *Psychoanalysis, Culture & Society* 19 (3):232–249.

Greco, Monica. 1993. "Psychosomatic Subjects and the 'Duty to Be Well': Personal Agency Within Medical Rationality." *Economy and Society* 22 (3):357–372.

Greenberg, P. E., R. C. Kessler, H. G. Birnbaum, S. A. Leong, S. W. Lowe, P. A. Berglund, and P. K. Corey-Lisle. 2003. "The Economic Burden of Depression in the United States: How Did It Change between 1990 and 2000?" *Journal of Clinical Psychiatry* 64 (12):1465–1475.

Greenwood, Davydd J., William Foote Whyte, and Ira Harkavy. 1993. "Participatory Action Research as a Process and as a Goal." *Human Relations* 46 (2):175–192.

Gregory, Steven. 1998. *Black Corona: Race and the Politics of Place in an Urban Community*. Princeton University Press.

Gupta, Neha, Andrew Martindale, Kisha Supernant, and Michael Elvidge. 2023. "The CARE Principles and the Reuse, Sharing, and Curation of Indigenous Data in Canadian Archaeology." *Advances in Archaeological Practice* 11 (1):76–89.

Hackey, Robert B. 1998. *Rethinking Health Care Policy: The New Politics of State Regulation, American Governance and Public Policy*. Georgetown University Press.

Hahn, William K. 1998. "Gifts in Psychotherapy: An Intersubjective Approach to Patient Gifts." *Psychotherapy: Theory, Research, Practice, Training* 35 (1):78–86.

Hanna, Fred J., and Fred Bemak. 1997. "The Quest for Identity in the Counseling Profession." *Counselor Education and Supervision* 36 (3):194–206.

Hansen, H., and J. Metzl. 2016. "Structural Competency in the U.S. Healthcare Crisis: Putting Social and Policy Interventions Into Clinical Practice." *Bioethical Inquiry* 13:179–183.

Haraway, Donna Jeanne. 2008. *When Species Meet*. University of Minnesota Press.

Harlow, Roxanna. 2003. "'Race Doesn't Matter, But . . .': The Effect of Race on Professors' Experiences of Emotion Management in the Undergraduate College Classroom." *Social Psychology Quarterly* 66 (4):348–363.

Health & Disability Advocates. 2015. "The Role of Public Health in Chicago's Mental Health System." Accessed January 2, 2017. http://resources.hdadvocates.org (site discontinued).

Healy, D. 2006. "The New Medical Oikumene." In *Global Pharmaceuticals: Ethics, Markets, Practices*, edited by Adriana Petryna et al., 61–84. Duke University Press.

Henneberger, Melinda. 1994. "Managed Care Changing Practice of Psychotherapy." *New York Times*, October 9. Accessed March 1, 2017. www.nytimes.com.

Herron, William G., and Sheila R. Welt. 1992. *Money Matters: The Fee in Psychotherapy and Psychoanalysis*. Guilford Press.

Hilgers, Mathieu. 2010. "The Three Anthropological Approaches to Neoliberalism." *International Social Science Journal* 61 (202):351–364.

Hill, Laurence D., and James L. Madara. 2005. "Role of the Urban Academic Medical Center in US Health Care." *JAMA* 294 (17):2219–2220.

Hirsch, Arnold R. 1983. *Making the Second Ghetto: Race and Housing in Chicago, 1940–1960*. University of Chicago Press.

Hochschild, Arlie Russell. 1979. "Emotion Work, Feeling Rules, and Social Structure." *American Journal of Sociology* 85 (3):551–575.

Hollan, Douglas. 2008. "Being There: On the Imaginative Aspects of Understanding Others and Being Understood." *Ethos* 36 (4):475–489.

Hollan, Douglas. 2016. "Psychoanalysis and Ethnography." *Ethos* 44 (4):507–521.

Hopper, Kim. 2001. "Commentary: On the Transformation of the Moral Economy of Care." *Culture, Medicine, and Psychiatry* 25 (4):473–484.

Hopper, Kim. 2006. "Redistribution and its Discontents: On the Prospects of Committed Work in Public Mental Health and Like Settings." *Human Organization* 65 (2):218–226.

Howard, Matthew O., Curtis K. McMillen, and David E. Pollio. 2003. "Teaching Evidence-Based Practice: Toward a New Paradigm for Social Work Education." *Research on Social Work Practice* 13 (2):234–259.

Huxley, Nancy, and Ross J. Baldessarini. 2007. "Disability and Its Treatment in Bipolar Disorder Patients." *Bipolar Disorders* 9 (1–2):183–196.

Illinois Department of Human Services. 2017. "Consumer Eligibility, Enrollment and Benefit Status." Accessed March 1, 2017. www.dhs.state.il.us.

Illinois General Assembly. n.d. "Illinois Compiled Statutes." Accessed June 20, 2024. www.ilga.gov.

Insel, Thomas. 2013. "Post by Former NIMH Director Thomas Insel: Transforming Diagnosis." Accessed June 1, 2015. www.nimh.nih.gov.

Insel, Thomas R., and Remi Quirion. 2005. "Psychiatry as a Clinical Neuroscience Discipline." *JAMA* 294 (17):2221–2224.

Ispa-Landa, Simone, and Sara Thomas. 2019. "Race, Gender, and Emotion Work Among School Principals." *Gender & Society* 33 (3):387–409.

Jackson, Brandon A. (2018). "Beyond the Cool Pose: Black Men and Emotion Management Strategies." *Sociology Compass* 12 (4):e12569. https://doi.org.

Jacobs, T. J. 1986. "On Countertransference Enactments. *Journal of the American Psychoanalytic Association* 34 (2):289–307.

Jakobson, Roman. 1971. *Word and Language, Selected Writings / Roman Jakobson*. The Hague; Mouton.

Jamison, Kay R. 1993. *Touched with Fire: Manic-Depressive Illness and the Artistic Temperament.* Free Press; Maxwell Macmillan Canada; Maxwell Macmillan International.

Jamison, Kay R. 1995. *An Unquiet Mind: A Memoir of Moods and Madness.* 1st ed. Knopf.

Jasper, James M. 1998. "The Emotions of Protest: Affective and Reactive Emotions in and around Social Movements." *Sociological Forum* 13 (3):397–424.

Jasper, James M. 2011. "Emotions and Social Movements: Twenty Years of Theory and Research." *Annual Review of Sociology* (37):285–303.

Jenkins, Janis H. 2011. *Pharmaceutical Self: The Global Shaping of Experience in an Age of Psychopharmacology.* School for Advanced Research Press.

Jennings, Len. 2010. "Practicum Pain, Professional Gain." In *Voices from the Field: Defining Moments in Counselor and Therapist Development,* edited by Michelle Trotter-Mathison, 50–52. Routledge.

Johnstone, Lucy. 2013. "UK Clinical Psychologists Call for the Abandonment of Psychiatric Diagnosis and the 'Disease' Model." Accessed March 1, 2017. www.madinamerica.com.

Jolly, David, and Matthew Saltmarsh. 2009. "Suicides in France Put Focus on Workplace." *New York Times,* September 29. www.nytimes.com.

Jones, Nev. 2025. " 'Structural Competency' Meets Mad Studies: Reckoning with Madness and Mental Diversity Beyond the Social and Structural Determinants of Mental Health." In *Mad Studies Reader: Interdisciplinary Innovations in Mental Health,* edited by Bradley Lewis, Alisha Ali, and Jazmine Russell, 244–257. Routledge.

Jones, S., M. Deville, D. Mayes, and F. Lobban. 2011. "Self-Management in Bipolar Disorder: The Story So Far." *Journal of Mental Health* 20 (6):583–592.

Karlin, Jennifer. 2013. "Loss and Gain in Translation: Financial Epidemiology on the South Side of Chicago." *Public Culture* 25 (3):523–550.

Keane, Webb. 2008. "Market, Materiality and Moral Metalanguage." *Anthropological Theory* 8 (1):27–42.

Kellam, Sheppard G., and Sheldon K. Schiff. 1966. "The Woodlawn Mental Health Center: A Community Mental Health Center Model." *Social Service Review* 40 (3):255–263.

Kirmayer, L., and I. Gold. 2012. "Re-socializing Psychiatry: Critical Neuroscience and the Limits of Reductionism." In *Critical Neuroscience: A Handbook of the Social and Cultural Contexts of Neuroscience,* edited by S. Choudhury and J. Slaby, 307–330. Wiley-Blackwell.

Kirmayer, L. J. 2007. "Psychotherapy and the Cultural Concept of the Person." *Transcultural Psychiatry* 44 (2):232–257.

Kirmayer, L. J. 2008. "Empathy and Alterity in Cultural Psychiatry." *Ethos* 36 (4):457–474.

Kirmayer, L. J. 2015. "Mindfulness in Cultural Context." *Transcultural Psychiatry* 52 (4):447–469.

Kirschner, S. 2015. "Subjectivity as Socioculturally Constituted Experience." In *The Wiley Handbook of Theoretical and Philosophical Psychology: Methods, Approaches and New Directions for Social Science*, 1st ed., edited by Jack Martin, Jeff Sugarman, and Kate Slaney, 293–307. Wiley.

Kirschner, Suzanne, and William Lachicotte. 2001. "Managing Managed Care: Habitus, Hysteresis and the End(s) of Psychotherapy." *Culture, Medicine, and Psychiatry* 25 (4):441–456.

Kitanaka, Junko. 2012. *Depression in Japan: Psychiatric Cures for a Society in Distress*. Princeton University Press.

Klein, Waldo C., Dan Weisman, and Thomas Edward Smith. 1996. "The Use of Adjunct Faculty: An Exploratory Study of Eight Social Work Programs." *Journal of Social Work Education* 32 (2):253–263.

Knox, Sarah. 2008. "Gifts in Psychotherapy: Practice Review and Recommendations." *Psychotherapy: Theory, Research, Practice, Training* 45 (1):103–110.

Kohli, Martin. 1987. "Retirement and the Moral Economy: An Historical Interpretation of the German Case." *Journal of Aging Studies* 1 (2):125–144.

Kukutai, T., and J. Taylor, eds. 2016. *Indigenous Data Sovereignty: Toward an Agenda* (Vol. 38). ANU Press.

Lakoff, Andrew. 2005. *Pharmaceutical Reason: Knowledge and Value in Global Psychiatry*. Cambridge University Press.

Lammers, J. C., and P. Geist. 1997. "The Transformation of Caring in the Light and Shadow of 'Managed Care.'" *Health Communication* 9 (1):45–60.

Lane, Charles. 2017. "The GOP's Health-Care Plan Goes in the Exact Wrong Direction." *Washington Post*, March 22. Accessed May 10, 2017. www.washingtonpost.com.

Lapping, Claudia. 2011. *Psychoanalysis in Social Research: Shifting Theories and Reframing Concepts*. Routledge.

Latour, Bruno. 1987. *Science in Action: How to Follow Scientists and Engineers Through Society*. Harvard University Press.

Latulippe, Nicole, and Nicole Klenk. 2020. "Making Room and Moving Over: Knowledge Co-production, Indigenous Knowledge Sovereignty and the Politics of Global Environmental Change Decision-making." *Current Opinion in Environmental Sustainability* 42:7–14.

Layton, L., N. C. Hollander, and S. Gutwill, eds. 2006. *Psychoanalysis, Class and Politics: Encounters in the Clinical Setting*. Routledge.

Lemke, Thomas. 2001. "'The Birth of Bio-politics': Michel Foucault's Lecture at the Collège de France on Neo-liberal Governmentality." *Economy and Society* 30 (2):190–207.

Lester, Rebecca. 2009. "Brokering Authenticity: Borderline Personality Disorder and the Ethics of Care in an American Eating Disorder Clinic." *Current Anthropology* 50 (3):281–302.

Lester, Rebecca. 2017. "Self-governance, Psychotherapy, and the Subject of Managed Care: Internal Family Systems Therapy and the Multiple Self in a US Eating-Disorders Treatment Center." *American Ethnologist* 44 (1):23–35.

Lester, Rebecca. 2021. *Famished: Eating Disorders and Failed Care in America*. University of California Press.

Leys, Ruth. 2011. "The Turn to Affect: A Critique." *Critical Inquiry* 37 (3):434–472.

Lorig, Kate, and Halsted Holman. 2003. "Self-Management Education: History, Definition, Outcomes, and Mechanisms." *Annals of Behavioral Medicine* 26 (1):1–7.

Luhrmann, Tanya. 2000. *Of Two Minds: The Growing Disorder in American Psychiatry*. 1st ed. Knopf.

Luhrmann, Tanya. 2012a. "Living With Voices." *The American Scholar* (Summer). Accessed April 2, 2017. https://theamericanscholar.org.

Luhrmann, Tanya. 2012b. "Beyond the Brain." *The Wilson Quarterly* (Spring):28–34. Accessed October 10, 2012. http://archive.wilsonquarterly.com.

Lydersen, Kari. 2013. *Mayor 1%: Rahm Emanuel and the Rise of Chicago's 99%*. Haymarket Books.

Maasen, Sabine, and Barbara Sutter. 2007. *On Willing Selves: Neoliberal Politics vis-à-vis the Neuroscientific Challenge*. Palgrave Macmillan.

MacAskill, E. 2012. "Mitt Romney Under Fire After Comments Caught on Video." *The Guardian*. Accessed May 10, 2017. www.theguardian.com.

Mahmood, Saba. 2001. "Feminist Theory, Embodiment, and the Docile Agent: Some Reflections on the Egyptian Islamic Revival." *Cultural Anthropology* 16 (2):202–236.

Mahmood, Saba. 2005. *Politics of Piety: The Islamic Revival and the Feminist Subject*. Princeton University Press.

Malabou, Catherine. 2008. *What Should We Do With Our Brain?* Fordham University Press.

Marcus, George A. 1995. "Ethnography in/of the World System: The Emergence of Multi-Sited Ethnography." *Annual Review of Anthropology* 24:95–117.

Markus, Hazel R., and Shinobu Kitayama. 1991. "Culture and the Self: Implications for Cognition, Emotion, and Motivation." *Psychological Review* 98 (2):224–253.

Martin, Emily. 1994. *Flexible Bodies: Tracking Immunity in American Culture from the Days of Polio to the Age of AIDS*. Beacon Press.

Martin, Emily. 2007. *Bipolar Expeditions: Mania and Depression in American Culture*. Princeton University Press.

Martin, Francis A., and W. Cris Cannon. 2010. "A Profession in Peril." *Counseling Today* 52 (11):50.

Maslow, A. H. 1943. "A Theory of Human Motivation." *Psychological Review* 50 (4):370–396.

Mattingly, C. 1994. "The Concept of Therapeutic 'Emplotment.'" *Social Science and Medicine* 38 (6):811–822.

Mauss, Marcel. 1990. *The Gift: The Form and Reason for Exchange in Archaic Societies*. Translated by William D. Halls. Routledge.

Mazzarella, William. 2006. "Internet X-Ray: E-Governance, Transparency, and the Politics of Immediation in India." *Public Culture* 18 (3):473–505.

McDonnell, Celena. 2017. "President Trump, Stop Implying that Americans on Welfare Aren't Working." *Washington Post*, February 1. Accessed April 1, 2017. www.washingtonpost.com.

McLean, Athena. 2000. "From Ex-Patient Alternatives to Consumer Options: Consequences of Consumerism for Psychiatric Consumers and the Ex-Patient Movement." *International Journal of Health Services* 30 (4):821–847.

McWilliams, Nancy. 2004. *Psychoanalytic Psychotherapy: A Practitioner's Guide.* Guilford Press.

Mental Health Coalition [pseud.]. 2012. "Dumping Responsibility: The Case Against Closing CDPH Mental Health Clinics." Accessed March 1, 2017. www.stopchicago.org.

Metzl, Jonathan. 2010. "The Protest Psychosis: How Schizophrenia Became a Black Disease." Beacon Press.

Miklowitz, David Jay. 2002. *The Bipolar Disorder Survival Guide: What You and Your Family Need to Know.* Guilford Press.

Miller, Jean Baker, Judith V. Jordan, Irene P. Stiver, Maureen Walker, Janet L. Surrey, and Natalie S. Eldridge. 1999. "Therapists' Authenticity." *Work in Progress* 82:1–14.

Miller, Peter. 2001. "Governing by Numbers: Why Calculative Practices Matter." *Social Research* 68 (2):379–396.

Minkler, Meredith, and Thomas R. Cole. 1992. "The Political and Moral Economy of Aging: Not Such Strange Bedfellows." *International Journal of Health Services* 22 (1):113–124.

Mol, Annemarie. 2002. *The Body Multiple: Ontology in Medical Practice.* Duke University Press.

Mol, Annemarie. 2008. *The Logic of Care: Health and the Problem of Patient Choice.* Routledge.

Molé, Noelle J. 2008. "Living It on the Skin: Italian States, Working Illness." *American Ethnologist* 35 (2):189–210.

Molé, Noelle J. 2012. *Labor Disorders in Neoliberal Italy: Mobbing, Well-being, and the Workplace.* Indiana University Press.

Moncrieff, J., R. E. Cooper, T. Stockmann, et al. 2023. "The Serotonin Theory of Depression: A Systematic Umbrella Review of the Evidence." *Molecular Psychiatry* 28:3243–3256.

Monger, Jane. 1998. "The Gap between Theory and Practice: A Consideration of the Fee." *Psychodynamic Counselling* 4 (1):93–106.

MoodSurfing. 2017. "Mood Tracking." Accessed April 2, 2017. http://moodsurfing.com.

Moore, L., J. Frost, and N. Britten. 2015. "Context and Complexity: The Meaning of Self-Management for Older Adults with Heart Disease." *Sociology of Health and Illness* 37 (8):1254–1269.

Moore, Natalie. 2013. "Report Links Chicagoans' Distance from Trauma Centers to Higher Mortality Rates." *WBEZ Chicago*, April 18. Accessed April 16, 2024. www.wbez.org.

Moore, Natalie Y. 2016. *The South Side: A Portrait of Chicago and American Segregation.* Picador.

Morrissey, Jean, and Rachel Tribe. 2001. "Parallel Process in Supervision." *Counselling Psychology Quarterly* 14 (2):103–110.

Muehlmann, Shaylih. 2009. "How Do Real Indians Fish? Neoliberal Multiculturalism and Contested Indigeneities in the Colorado Delta." *American Anthropologist* 111 (4):468–479.

Mulvey, T. A. 2011. "Debt, Salaries, and Careers in Psychology: What You Need to Know." Accessed July 10, 2016. www.apa.org.

Myerhoff, Barbara G. 1980. *Number Our Days.* Simon & Schuster.

Myers, Neely Laurenzo. 2010. "Culture, Stress and Recovery from Schizophrenia: Lessons from the Field for Global Mental Health." *Culture, Medicine, and Psychiatry* 34 (3):500–528.

Myers, Neely Laurenzo. 2015. *Recovery's Edge: An Ethnography of Mental Health Care and Moral Agency.* Vanderbilt University Press.

National Institutes of Health. 2017. "The BRAIN Initiative: About." Accessed March 15, 2017. www.braininitiative.nih.gov.

Norcross, John C., and Barry A. Farber. 2005. "Choosing Psychotherapy as a Career: Beyond 'I Want to Help People.'" *Journal of Clinical Psychology* 61 (8):939–943.

Norris, Louise. 2017. "Illinois and the ACA's Medicaid Expansion: Medicaid Expansion Enrollment Far Above Projections." Accessed April 3. 2017. www.healthinsurance.org.

Novak, Tim, and Chris Fusco. 2008. "U. of C. Shunning Poor Patients? Obama's Wife, Aides Tied to Plan to Free Space." *Chicago Sun Times,* August 23. Accessed June 2, 2024. https://chicago.suntimes.com.

Novas, Carlos, and Nikolas Rose. 2000. "Genetic Risk and the Birth of the Somatic Individual." *Economy and Society* 29 (4):485–513.

OccupyWallStreet. 2012. "Chicago: #SaveOurClinics Occupies Mental Health Clinic Slated for Closure." Accessed May 1, 2017. http://occupywallst.org.

Ortega, Francisco. 2009. "The Cerebral Subject and the Challenge of Neurodiversity." *BioSocieties* 4 (4):425–445.

Ortner, Sherry. 2006. *Anthropology and Social Theory: Culture, Power, and the Acting Subject.* Duke University Press.

Pacyga, Dominic A. 2009. *Chicago: A Biography.* University of Chicago Press.

Palmo, Artis J. 1999. "The MHC Child Reaches Maturity: Does the Child Seem Short for Its Age?" *Journal of Mental Health Counseling* 21 (3):215.

Papoulias, Constantina, and Felicity Callard. 2010. "Biology's Gift: Interrogating the Turn to Affect." *Body & Society* 16 (1):29–56.

Peck, Jamie. 2001. *Workfare States.* Guilford Press.

Perlstein, Rick. 2015a. "There Goes the Neighborhood: The Obama Library Lands on Chicago." *The Baffler* 28:100–112.

Perlstein, Rick. 2015b. "How to Sell Off a City." *In These Times,* January 21. Accessed April 10, 2017. http://inthesetimes.com.

Petryna, Adriana. 2004. "Biological Citizenship: The Science and Politics of Chernobyl-Exposed Populations." *Osiris* 19:250–265.

Pharo, Zoe. 2022. "Mid-South Siders Vote to Establish and Fund a Community Mental Health Center." *Hyde Park Herald*, November 11. Accessed June 1, 2024. www.hpherald.com.

Pickering, Andrew. 2010. *The Cybernetic Brain: Sketches of Another Future*. University of Chicago Press.

Pickersgill, Martyn, Sarah Cunningham-Burley, and Paul Martin. 2011. "Constituting Neurologic Subjects: Neuroscience, Subjectivity and the Mundane Significance of the Brain." *Subjectivity* 4 (3):346–365.

Pistole, M. Carole. 2001. *Mental Health Counseling: Identity and Distinctiveness. ERIC/ CASS Digest*.

Pitts-Taylor, V. 2010. "The Plastic Brain: Neoliberalism and the Neuronal Self." *Health (London)* 14 (6):635–652.

Poovey, Mary. 1998. *A History of the Modern Fact: Problems of Knowledge in the Sciences of Wealth and Society*. University of Chicago Press.

Pope, K. S., J. D. Geller, and L. Wilkinson. 1975. "Fee Assessment and Outpatient Psychotherapy." *Journal of Consulting and Clinical Psychology* 43 (6):835–841.

Povinelli, Elizabeth A. 2011. *Economies of Abandonment: Social Belonging and Endurance in Late Liberalism*. Duke University Press.

Prioleau, Brian. 2013. "Reflecting on JFK's Legacy of Community-Based Care." Accessed April 1, 2017. www.samhsa.gov.

Purser, Ron, and David Loy. 2013. "Beyond McMindfulness." *Huffington Post*. Accessed June 21, 2023. www.huffingtonpost.com.

Ramon, Shulamit. 2007. "Inequality in Mental Health: The Relevance of Current Research and Understanding to Potentially Effective Social Work Responses." *Radical Psychology* 6 (1). Accessed February 1, 2013. www.radpsynet.org.

Ranney, Megan L., and Jessica Gold. 2019. "The Dangers of Linking Gun Violence and Mental Illness." *Time*, August 7. https://time.com.

Reveley, James. 2015. "Foucauldian Critique of Positive Education and Related Self Technologies: Some Problems and New Directions." *Open Review of Educational Research* 2 (1):78–93.

Ridgeway, Cecilia L., and Tamar Kricheli-Katz. 2013. "Intersecting Cultural Beliefs in Social Relations: Gender, Race, and Class Binds and Freedoms." *Gender & Society* 27 (3):294–318.

Rivkin-Fish, Michele. 2011. "Learning the Moral Economy of Commodified Health Care: 'Community Education,' Failed Consumers, and the Shaping of Ethical Clinician-Citizens." *Culture, Medicine, and Psychiatry* 35 (2):183–208.

Roberts, M. 2010. "Where Are They Now?" *bp Magazine* (Winter):40.

Rose, Nikolas. 1996. *Inventing Our Selves: Psychology, Power, and Personhood*. Cambridge University Press.

Rose, Nikolas. 1999. "The Psychiatric Gaze." Working paper, Department of Sociology, Goldsmiths College University of London.

Rose, Nikolas. 2003. "Neurochemical Selves." *Society* 41 (1):46–59.

Rose, Nikolas. 2007. *The Politics of Life Itself: Biomedicine, Power, and Subjectivity in the Twenty-First Century*. Princeton University Press.

Rose, Nikolas, and Carlos Novas. 2008. "Biological Citizenship." In *Global Assemblages*, edited by A. Ong and S. J. Collier, 439–463. Blackwell Publishing.

Sahlins, Marshall David. 1981. *Historical Metaphors and Mythical Realities: Structure in the Early History of the Sandwich Islands Kingdom*. University of Michigan Press.

Sahlins, Marshall David. 1985. *Islands of History*. University of Chicago Press.

Sailappan, Deepti, and Jason Lalljee. 2018. "Rallies, Sit-ins, and Padlocks: The History of Trauma Center Activism." *The Chicago Maroon*, April 26. Accessed June 20, 2024. https://chicagomaroon.com.

Sampson, Edward E. 1988. "The Debate on Individualism: Indigenous Psychologies of the Individual and Their Role in Personal and Societal Functioning." *American Psychologist* 43 (1):15–22.

Sass, Louis Arnorsson. 1994. *The Paradoxes of Delusion: Wittgenstein, Schreber, and the Schizophrenic Mind*. Cornell University Press.

Sass, Louis Arnorsson. 2007. "'Schizophrenic Person' or 'Person with Schizophrenia'? An Essay on Illness and the Self." *Theory Psychology* 17 (3):395–420.

Satir, Virginia. 2013. "The Therapist Story." In *The Use of Self in Therapy*. 3rd ed., edited by Michèle Baldwin, 19–27. Routledge.

Saunders, Barry F. 2008. *CT Suite: The Work of Diagnosis in the Age of Noninvasive Cutting*. Duke University Press.

Scharff, K. 2004. *Therapy Demystified: An Insider's Guide to Getting the Right Help—Without Going Broke*. Marlowe.

Schechter, Kate. 2014. *Illusions of a Future: Psychoanalysis and the Biopolitics of Desire*. Duke University Press.

Scheff, Thomas J. 1966. *Being Mentally Ill: A Sociological Theory*. Aldine.

Schrader, S., N. Jones, and M. Shattell. 2013. "Mad Pride: Reflections on Sociopolitical Identity and Mental Diversity in the Context of Culturally Competent Psychiatric Care." *Issues in Mental Health Nursing* 34 (1):62–64.

Schüll, Natasha. 2006. "Machines, Medication, Modulation: Circuits of Dependency and Self-Care in Las Vegas." *Culture, Medicine, and Psychiatry* 30 (2):223–247.

Scott, James C. 1976. *The Moral Economy of the Peasant Rebellion and Subsistence in Southeast Asia*. Edited by James C. Scott. Yale University Press.

Scull, Andrew. 1989. *Social Order/Mental Disorder: Anglo-American Psychiatry in Historical Perspective*. University of California Press.

Searles, H. F. 1955. "The Informational Value of the Supervisor's Emotional Experiences." *Psychiatry* 18 (2):135–146.

Sedgwick, P. 1982. *Psychopolitics*. Pluto Press.

Segal, C. 2012. "'We're Cool, You and Me' A Relational Approach to Clinical Social Work in the City: Psychodynamic Psychotherapy Within a Homeless Shelter for Formerly Incarcerated Women and Their Children." In *Falling Through the Cracks: Psychodynamic Practice with Vulnerable and Oppressed Populations*, edited by Joan Berzoff, 75–106. Columbia University Press.

Seligman, Amanda I. 2005. *Block by Block: Neighborhoods and Public Policy on Chicago's West Side*. University of Chicago Press.

Shields, John D. 1996. "Hostage of the Fee: Meanings of Money, Countertransference, and the Beginning Therapist." *Psychoanalytic Psychotherapy* 10 (3):233–250.

Shweder, Richard. 1991. *Thinking Through Cultures: Expeditions in Cultural Psychology*. Harvard University Press.

Silverstein, Michael. 2003. "Indexical Order and the Dialectics of Sociolinguistic Life." *Language & Communication* 23 (3–4):193–229.

Silverstein, Michael. 2004. "'Cultural' Concepts and the Language-Culture Nexus." *Current Anthropology* 45 (5):621–652.

Simmel, Georg. 1950. *The Sociology of Georg Simmel*. Edited by Kurt H. Wolff. Free Press.

Sinclair, Upton. 1906. *The Jungle*. Doubleday, Jabber, and Co.

Slochower, Joyce Anne. 1996. *Holding and Psychoanalysis: A Relational Perspective*. Analytic Press.

Smith, Yvonne. 2017. "'Sense' and Sensitivity: Informal Apprenticeship among Youth Care Workers in a Residential Treatment Center for Children." *Child and Family Social Work* 22:1330–1337.

Smolar, Andrew I. 2003. "When We Give More: Reflections of Intangible Gifts from Therapist to Patient." *American Journal of Psychotherapy* 57 (3):300–323.

Specht, Harry, and Mark E. Courtney. 1994. *Unfaithful Angels: How Social Work Has Abandoned Its Mission*. Edited by Mark E. Courtney. Free Press; Maxwell Macmillan Canada; Maxwell Macmillan International.

Spiegel, Alix. 2005. "The Dictionary of Disorder: How One Man Revolutionized Psychiatry." *The New Yorker* January 3:56–63.

Spielman, Fran. 2009. "Daley Halts Closure of Mental Health Clinics." *Chicago Sun-Times*. Accessed March 2, 2017. www.illinoispsychiatricsociety.org.

Spitzmueller, Matthew C. 2014. "The Making of Community Mental Health Policy in Everyday Street-Level Practice: An Organizational Ethnography." ProQuest Dissertations Publishing.

Spitzmueller, Matthew C. 2016. "Negotiating Competing Institutional Logics at the Street Level: An Ethnography of a Community Mental Health Organization." *Social Service Review* 90 (1):35–82.

Stanford Medicine. 2017a. "Stanford Small-Group Self-Management Programs in English." Page now available at: https://archive.is/dh9D2.

Stanford Medicine. 2017b. "Meet Our Staff." Page now available at: https://archive.is/dh9D2.

Star, Susan Leigh, and James R. Griesemer. 1989. "Institutional Ecology, 'Translations' and Boundary Objects: Amateurs and Professionals in Berkeley's Museum of Vertebrate Zoology, 1907–39." *Social Studies of Science* 19 (3):387–420.

Strathern, Marilyn. 2000. *Audit Cultures: Anthropological Studies in Accountability, Ethics, and the Academy*. Routledge.

Strauss, John S. 1989. "Subjective Experiences of Schizophrenia: Toward a New Dynamic Psychiatry—II." *Schizophrenia Bulletin* 15 (2):179–187.

Stricker, George. 2001. "How I Learned to Abandon Certainty and Embrace Change." In *How Therapists Change: Personal and Professional Reflections*, edited by Marvin R. Goldfried, 67–81. American Psychological Association.

Sunder Rajan, Kaushik. 2005. "Subjects of Speculation: Emergent Life Sciences and Market Logics in the United States and India." *American Anthropologist* 107 (1):19–30.

Supernant, Kisha, and Gary Warrick. 2014. "Challenges to Critical Community-based Archaeological Practice in Canada." *Canadian Journal of Archaeology* 38 (2):563–591.

Swanson, J. W., E. E. McGinty, S. Fazel, and V. M. Mays. 2015. "Mental Illness and Reduction of Gun Violence and Suicide: Bringing Epidemiologic Research to Policy." *Annals of Epidemiology* 25 (5):366–376.

Szasz, Thomas Stephen. 1974. *The Myth of Mental Illness: Foundations of a Theory of Personal Conduct*. Harper & Row.

Taussig, M. T. 1980. "Reification and the Consciousness of the Patient." *Social Science & Medicine* 14b (1):3–13.

Teghtsoonian, Katherine. 2009. "Depression and Mental Health in Neoliberal Times: A Critical Analysis of Policy and Discourse." *Social Science & Medicine* 69 (1):28–35.

Terry, Don. 2011. "A Sit-In Fails to Save Clinics, but the Fight Continues." *New York Times*, November 19. Accessed May 1, 2017. www.nytimes.com.

Thompson, E. P. 1963. *The Making of the English Working Class*. Gollancz.

Thompson, E. P. 1971. "The Moral Economy of the English Crowd in the Eighteenth Century." *Past & Present* (50):76–136.

Thompson, E. P. 1991. *Customs in Common*. New Press, distributed by W.W. Norton.

Tolleson, Jennifer. 2009. "Saving the World One Patient at a Time: Psychoanalysis and Social Critique." *Psychotherapy and Politics International* 7 (3):190–205.

Trachtman, Richard. 1999. "The Money Taboo: Its Effects in Everyday Life and in the Practice of Psychotherapy." *Clinical Social Work Journal* 27 (3):275–288.

UChicagoMedicine. n.d. "Urban Health Initiative (UHI)." Accessed June 12, 2024. www.uchicagomedicine.org.

Ungar, Michael. 2019. "Put Down the Self-Help Books. Resilience Is Not a DIY Endeavour." *The Globe and Mail*, May 25. Accessed June 1, 2024. www.theglobeandmail.com.

Ungar, Michael, and Lou Costanzo. 2007. "Supervision Challenges When Supervisors Are Outside Supervisees' Agencies." *Journal of Systemic Therapies* 26 (2):68–83.

University of Chicago Civic Engagement. n.d. "Economic Opportunity and Entrepreneurship." Accessed February 25, 2024. https://civicengagement.uchicago.edu.

University of Chicago Community Impact. n.d. "Committed to Our Community." Accessed February 25, 2024. www.uchicago.edu.

Valverde, Mariana. 1998. *Diseases of the Will: Alcohol and the Dilemmas of Freedom*. Cambridge University Press.

Vaughans, K. C., and L. Harris. 2016. "The Police, Black and Hispanic Boys: A Dangerous Inability to Mentalize." *Journal of Infant, Child, and Adolescent Psychotherapy* 15 (3):171–178.

Wallace, Lewis. 2012. "Cook County Begins Enrolling 250,000 New Medicaid Recipients." WBEZ News. Accessed March 1, 2017. www.wbez.org.

Walley, Christine J. 2012. *Exit Zero: Family and Class in Postindustrial Chicago.* University of Chicago Press.

Ware, N. C., W. S. Lachicotte, S. R. Kirschner, D. E. Cortes, and B. J. Good. 2000. "Clinician Experiences of Managed Mental Health Care: A Rereading of the Threat." *Medical Anthropology Quarterly* 14 (1):3–27.

Weber, Max. 1978. *Economy and Society: An Outline of Interpretive Sociology.* University of California Press.

Weick, Ann. 2015. "Guilty Knowledge." *Families in Society: The Journal of Contemporary Social Services* 96 (1):35–39.

Weiner, Talia. 2011. "The (Un)managed Self: Paradoxical Forms of Agency in Self-Management of Bipolar Disorder." *Culture, Medicine, and Psychiatry* 35 (4):448–483.

Weiner, Talia. 2019. "Billable Services and the 'Therapeutic Fee': On the Work of Disavowal of Political Economy and Its Re-emergence in Clinical Practice." *Anthropological Quarterly* 92 (3):697–728.

Weiner, Talia. 2020. "The Recuperation of Moral Agency through Structural Erasure in Clinical Social Workers' Accounts of Career Path and Treatment Decisions." *Smith College Studies in Social Work* 90 (1):115–138.

Weiner, Talia. 2025. "Relationality, Contextual Embeddedness, and the Inextricable Self of the Researcher in Ethnographic Interviewing." *Qualitative Psychology* 12 (1):69–84.

Whitaker, T. 2008. "In the Red: Social Workers and Educational Debt." National Association of Social Workers. Accessed July 10, 2016. www.socialworkers.org.

Wilkins, Amy. 2012. "'Not Out to Start a Revolution': Race, Gender, and Emotional Restraint among Black University Men." *Journal of Contemporary Ethnography* 41 (1):34–65.

Wilkinson, R. Tyler, and Suhyun Suh. 2012. "Professional Counselors' Experiences Pursuing State Licensure." *Alabama Counseling Association Journal* 38 (1):20–30.

Williams, Abi B. 1997. "On Parallel Process in Social Work Supervision." *Clinical Social Work Journal* 25 (4):425–435.

Wingfield, Adia Harvey. 2007. "The Modern Mammy and the Angry Black Man: African American Professionals' Experiences with Gendered Racism in the Workplace." *Race, Gender, & Class* 14 (1/2):196–212.

Wingfield, Adia Harvey. 2010. "Are Some Emotions Marked 'Whites Only'? Racialized Feeling Rules in Professional Workplaces." *Social Problems* 57 (2):251–268.

Winnicott, D. W. 1953. "Transitional Objects and Transitional Phenomena: A Study of the First Not-Me Possession." *International Journal of Psychoanalysis* 34 (2):89–97.

Winnicott, D. W. 1960. "The Theory of the Parent-Infant Relationship." *International Journal of Psychoanalysis* 41:585–595.

Winnicott, D. W. 1971. *Playing and Reality.* Tavistock/Routledge.

Wolfson, Elizabeth R. 1999. "The Fee in Social Work: Ethical Dilemmas for Practitioners." *Social Work* 44 (3):269–273.

World Health Organization. 2008. "The Global Burden of Disease: 2004 Update, Table A2: Burden of Disease in DALYs by Cause, Sex and Income Group in WHO Regions, Estimates for 2004." Geneva, Switzerland.

Wortham, Stanton. 2001. *Narratives in Action: A Strategy for Research and Analysis.* Teachers College Press.

Wortham, Stanton. 2006. Learning Identity: The Joint Emergence of Social Identification and Academic Learning. Cambridge University Press.

Yalom, Irvin D. 1980. *Existential Psychotherapy.* Basic Books.

Yankellevich, Ariel, and Yehuda C. Goodman. 2017. "'You Can't Choose These Emotions . . . They Simply Jump Up': Ambiguities in Resilience-Building Interventions in Israel." *Culture, Medicine, and Psychiatry* 41:56–74.

Yoon, Intae. 2012. "Debt Burdens Among MSW Graduates: A National Cross-Sectional Study." *Journal of Social Work Education* 48 (1):105–125.

Young, Allan. 1993. "A Description of How Ideology Shapes Knowledge of a Mental Disorder (Posttraumatic Stress Disorder)." In *Knowledge, Power, and Practice: The Anthropology of Medicine and Everyday Life*, edited by Shirley Lindenbaum and Margaret Lock, 108–128. University of California Press.

Young, Allan. 1995. *The Harmony of Illusions: Inventing Post-Traumatic Stress Disorder.* Princeton University Press.

Zimmerman, F. J., and W. Katon. 2005. "Socioeconomic Status, Depression Disparities, and Financial Strain: What Lies Behind the Income-Depression Relationship?" *Health Economics* 14 (12):1197–215.

Žižek, Slavoj. 2001. "From Western Marxism to Western Buddhism." *Cabinet*, 2. Accessed June 21, 2023. www.cabinetmagazine.org.

INDEX

Page numbers in italics indicate Figures

ABOUT THE AUTHOR

TALIA ROSE WEINER is Assistant Professor of Psychology in the School of Social Sciences at the University of West Georgia.